Reframing health and health policy in Ireland

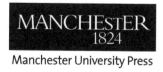
MANCHESTER
1824

Manchester University Press

Reframing health and health policy in Ireland

A governmental analysis

Edited by
Claire Edwards and Eluska Fernández

Manchester University Press

Published by Manchester University Press
Altrincham Street, Manchester M1 7JA

www.manchesteruniversitypress.co.uk

British Library Cataloguing-in-Publication Data
A catalogue record for this book is available from the British Library

ISBN   978 0 7190 9587 0   hardback

First published 2017

Typeset
by Toppan Best-set Premedia Limited
Printed in Great Britain
by CPI Group (UK) Ltd, Croydon, CR0 4YY

For
Ihintza
Cillian, Charlotte and Alice

Contents

List of figures and tables   *page* ix
Notes on contributors   x
Acknowledgements   xiv
List of abbreviations   xv

1 Analysing health and health policy: introducing the
   governmentality turn   *Claire Edwards and*
   Eluska Fernández   1

Part I   Constructing health problems and (un)healthy subjects
2 Governing the future: children's health and biosocial
   power   *Kevin Ryan*   25
3 Doing the 'right thing'? Children, families and fatness
   in Ireland   *Michelle Share and Perry Share*   46
4 32 and 37 inches – the healthy body and the politics of
   waist circumference: a governmental analysis of the *Stop*
   the Spread campaign   *Fiona Dukelow*   72
5 The contemporary self in tobacco control: exploring
   the introduction of the smoking ban in Ireland
   Eluska Fernández   96
6 When health means illness: analysing mental health
   discourses and practices in Ireland   *Derek Chambers*   117
7 Governing organ donation: the dead body, the
   individual and the limits of medicine
   Órla O'Donovan   137

Part II   Governing neoliberal healthcare agendas: politics,
         strategies and practices
8 Neoliberal governmentality and public health policy
   in Ireland   *Joanne Wilson and Lindsay Prior*   161
9 Governing healthcare: the case of Universal Health
   Insurance – by competition   *Cliona Loughnane*   182

10 Assessment of Need as a technology of government
    in Ireland's Disability Act 2005   *Claire Edwards*   203
11 Long-term care policy for older people in Ireland:
    a governmental analysis   *Ciara O'Dwyer*   226

12 Conclusion: governmentality, health policy and the
    place of critical politics   *Eluska Fernández and
    Claire Edwards*   247

Index   258

Figures and tables

Figures

2.1 Childhood as networked governance   *page* 39

Tables

3.1 Overweight and obesity amongst Irish children and
     young people   54
3.2 Obesity: *GUI* and prior studies compared   57
3.3 Conflation of overweight and obese in *GUI* reports   61

Notes on contributors

Derek Chambers is a doctoral student at the School of Applied Social Studies in University College Cork (UCC) and Director of Programmes and Policy at ReachOut Ireland. He has co-authored a number of peer-reviewed publications and book chapters, including Understanding Irish Suicide(s) (with Kieran Keohane, in *Collision Culture: Transformations in Everyday Life in Ireland*, by Keohane and Kuhling, 2004). Derek previously worked in the public sector with the Irish Health Service Executive and he was project manager and lead author of Ireland's National Strategy for Action on Suicide Prevention, 2005–2014. During his time with the HSE, Derek also project managed Ireland's first state-funded public mental health awareness campaign, *Your Mental Health*. Derek left the state sector in 2009 to oversee the delivery of *ReachOut.com*, an online mental health resource for young people aimed at promoting a broad-based model of mental health literacy at a population level, informed by the approaches outlined within the discipline of critical psychiatry.

Fiona Dukelow is a lecturer in social policy at the School of Applied Social Studies, UCC. Her recent research has focused on welfare state change, the impact of economic crisis and the evolution of neoliberalism. She is co-author, with Mairéad Considine, of *Irish Social Policy: A Critical Introduction* (Gill and Macmillan, 2009), and has recently co-edited *Defining Events: Power, Resistance and Identity in Twenty-First-Century Ireland* (Manchester University Press, 2015) with Rosie Meade, and *The Irish Welfare State in the Twenty First Century: Challenges and Change* (Palgrave, 2016) with Mary P. Murphy.

Claire Edwards is a lecturer in the School of Applied Social Studies, UCC. Her teaching and research interests are in the areas of disability rights, urban regeneration and the relationship between research and policy. She has published widely in a range of journals, including *BioSocieties*, *Health & Place*, *Disability and Society*, *Sociology*, *Critical Social Policy* and *Urban Studies*. Her most recent research has explored disabled people's encounters with the criminal justice system as victims of crime, and the dynamics and barriers of access to justice.

Eluska Fernández is a lecturer in the School of Applied Social Studies, UCC. Her teaching and research interests include contemporary discourses of health, the politics of public health and tobacco control. She has published on the topics of smoking, the smoking ban in Ireland and more recently, on vaping, in journals such as *Social Theory and Health* and the *Irish Journal of Sociology*. Currently, she is undertaking an ethnographic study of vaping in Cork city.

Cliona Loughnane is a doctoral candidate at the School of Applied Social Studies, UCC and Policy and Research Manager at the Irish Heart Foundation. Her doctoral work focuses on the increasing role which corporate interests play in the development of public health policy, particularly the influence of the food industry on anti-obesity policy. She has worked for over a decade in public affairs and policy roles in health and disability not-for-profit organisations. She holds a BA in English and History, HDip in Social Policy and MEconSc in European Economics and Public Affairs.

Órla O'Donovan is based in the School of Applied Social Studies, UCC. She has a long-standing interest in questions about the tensions between democracy and expertise, and how the production and use of science and technology for public purposes can be promoted. In recent years, her concern with the search for radically alternative ways of living, beyond the alienations of patriarchy and consumer capitalism, has led her to explore the promises of the commons as a route to what Ivan Illich referred to as a 'convivial society'. Together with Mary McDermott and Tom O'Connell, in 2014 she co-edited a Special Supplement to the *Community Development Journal* called 'Commons Sense – New thinking about an old idea'.

Ciara O'Dwyer is the Co-ordinator of a European Project on *The Human Rights of Older Persons and Long-term Care*, being carried out by the European Network of National Human Rights Institutions (ENNHRI) and funded by the European Commission. Her primary research interests are on care policies for older people and the social inclusion of older people in society. She completed her PhD (Trinity College Dublin) in 2012 on the use of regulations to monitor the quality of residential care settings for older people in Ireland and its impact on older people themselves. Before joining ENNHRI, she was a Post-Doctoral Research Fellow in the Collegio Carlo Alberto, Turin, Italy. She also worked as a Research Fellow at the Social Policy and Ageing Research Centre (SPARC), Trinity College Dublin, where she led and assisted with projects in the area of home care, community-based services, the quality of life of older people in residential care and the contribution of older people to society.

Lindsay Prior is a Professor Emeritus in the Centre of Excellence for Public Health at Queen's University, Belfast, UK. Recent publications have included journal papers on physical activity and health (*Social Science & Medicine*), architecture and health, and end-of-life care (*Sociology of Health & Illness*). He also contributes regularly to edited collections, dictionaries and encyclopaedias on social research methods and he is author and editor of the four-volume collection, *Using Documents and Records in Social Research* (Sage, 2011), and *Using Documents in Social Research* (Sage, 2003). He is currently writing a book on exploratory methods in social research. His most recent publication is entitled 'In praise of small N, and of N =1 in particular', *Critical Public Health*, 2016.

Kevin Ryan is a lecturer at the School of Political Science and Sociology, National University of Ireland, Galway. His research focuses on degrees of freedom, that is, arenas of practice which are formed by historically constituted conditions of possibility and relations of power. Kevin is the author of *Social Exclusion and the Politics of Order* (Manchester University Press, 2007) and co-editor (with Mark Haugaard) of *Political Power: The Development of the Field* (Barbara Budrich, 2012). His articles have been published in *Childhood*, *Critical Horizons*, *Critical Sociology*, the *International Journal of Sport Policy and Politics* and *The Journal of Political Power*.

Michelle Share is a Senior Research Fellow at the School of Education, Trinity College Dublin. Her doctoral thesis 'Risk, responsibility and choice: food and eating in Irish second level schools' examined food provision and education issues amongst students, teachers, parents and caterers in different school types in Northern Ireland/Republic of Ireland using a Foucauldian governmentality perspective. Michelle has also designed and conducted large-scale programme evaluations in child and youth settings in relation to nutrition, smoking, mental health and school health education. She has researched and published on dietary and food issues amongst women dieters, asylum seekers, older people in community settings, and children and young people. She is currently leading a research project on grandparental childcare, with a focus on transnational care practices in the Polish community in Ireland.

Perry Share is Head of School of Business and Social Sciences, Institute of Technology, Sligo. He is a sociologist with diverse research interests, most of which can ultimately be traced to a concern for the operation of language and discourse: these include the relationship between evidence, policy and practice; professionalisation and the social professions; the sociology of food and eating; and intertextuality in academic writing. He is the co-author of *A Sociology of Ireland*, and co-editor of *Applied Social Care*, both bestselling Irish social science texts, as well as numerous papers, chapters, articles and posters among three decades of academic work in Ireland and Australia.

Joanne Wilson is the Managing Editor of the Cochrane Developmental, Psychosocial and Learning Problems Group, currently based at the School of Sociology, Social Policy and Social Work at the Queen's University Belfast.

Acknowledgements

We would like to thank the individual authors for their willingness to contribute to the volume and for their patience and responsiveness in terms of our various requests. Many thanks also to our colleagues in the School of Applied Social Studies, UCC, for providing support at different times throughout the process, particularly Fiona Dukelow who provided a sounding board and encouragement when the idea for the book was still in its infancy, and Gill Harold who provided fantastic support through her careful proofreading and editing. We would also like to acknowledge Tony Mason and Alun Richards at Manchester University Press for their guidance and advice in the preparation and delivery of the book.

Finally, we would like to thank our families and friends for their constant encouragement, and particularly those who have lived with us day to day through this long-running project: James, Cillian, Charlotte, Alice and Ihintza.

Abbreviations

AO	Assessment Officer
AoN	Assessment of Need
AVFC	*A Vision for Change: Report of the Expert Group on Mental Health Policy*
BMI	Body Mass Index
DCYA	Department of Children and Youth Affairs
DoH	Department of Health
DoHC	Department of Health and Children
GP	General Practitioner
GUI	*Growing Up in Ireland*
HCP	Home Care Package
HIQA	Health Information and Quality Authority
HSE	Health Service Executive
NDA	National Disability Authority
NHSS	Nursing Home Support Scheme
NPAS	National Positive Ageing Strategy
OECD	Organisation for Economic Co-operation and Development
PHI	Private Health Insurance
STS	*Stop the Spread*
TD	Teachta Dála (Irish Member of Parliament)
UHI	Universal Health Insurance
UHI-C	Universal Health Insurance-by Competition
VHI	Voluntary Health Insurance
WHO	World Health Organization

1 Claire Edwards and Eluska Fernández

Analysing health and health policy: introducing the governmentality turn

Introduction

Recent years have witnessed a burgeoning international literature which seeks to analyse the construction of health and health policy through an analytical lens drawn from post-Foucauldian ideas of *governmentality* (Petersen and Lupton, 1996; Lupton, 1995, 2003; Joyce, 2001; Petersen and Bunton, 1997; Lovell, Kearns and Prince, 2014; Ferlie, McGivern and FitzGerald, 2012). From analyses of constructions of welfare citizens and patients deemed to be 'at risk' from particular health conditions to strategies of governance in healthcare systems, a trawl through sociological health-based journals reveals an enduring interest in deploying analytical tools drawn from governmentality studies. Following Dean's (1999) book of the same name, governmentality implies a repositioning of the state and state power in advanced neoliberal societies: a move away from a centralised state wielding power, to government as a series of agencies, institutions and actors through which power becomes manifest, and in which the state does not act *on* individual citizens, but *through* them, shaping their sensibilities and behaviours. Governmentality as the 'conduct of conduct' (Foucault, 1982), then, is concerned with the *how* of governing and with the specific techniques and strategies through which citizen subjectivities come to be constructed in the management of populations.

Analysis of health issues and policy in Ireland has, however, been relatively untouched by such an analysis, with a few notable exceptions (see for example Share and Strain, 2008; McDonnell and O'Donovan, 2009; Fernández, 2016, and for a critique see Porter, 1996). We believe this to be a significant absence for a number of reasons. First, like many developed countries in the Western world, Ireland is witnessing the emergence of a number of health and healthcare dilemmas: the (disputed) emergence of obesity as a public health issue, the increasing visibility of dementia, and concerns regarding the mental health of the population, to name but a few. In such a context, there is a need to critically analyse how, or why, certain health issues emerge into public view as significant health conditions which require governmental intervention; how governmental strategies and techniques have sought to manage these health issues; and how the citizens 'at risk' in these contexts are constructed through such strategies. Ireland has arguably witnessed a number of contentious legislative and policy developments in the health arena which have sought to construct and manage the health identities of individual citizens over the past fifteen years: the introduction of the smoking ban in 2004, for example, turned on multiple discourses in which smokers were simultaneously constructed as uncivilised, irrational and irresponsible (Fernández, 2016). In other cases, strategies of governance have sought to bring into being a particular category of citizen as a means of managing health issues and scarce resources. For example, under Ireland's Disability Act 2005, access to assessment and resources is predicated on the adoption of a particular definition of disability, whilst the legislation has introduced a whole series of processes and techniques through which knowledge about the disabled population might be generated.

Second, a governmental perspective allows us to reflect on health policy as an expression of the actions of advanced neoliberal government (see for example, Lovell, Kearns and Prince, 2014; Ferlie, McGivern and FitzGerald, 2012). Ireland's healthcare system is in many ways an example par excellence of advanced neoliberal society, whereby the free market, through privatisation, has created a two-tier healthcare system (Considine and Dukelow, 2009; Mercille and Murphy, 2015) in which patients are expected to exercise freedom as consumers whilst regulatory bodies seek to manage health risks and regulate healthcare professionals 'at a distance'. As in many jurisdictions, health policy in Ireland has often been contentious, and Ireland's health system has constantly found itself in a perilous position, subject to severe budgetary constraints, and accused of inefficiencies and inequitable service provision (Mercille and Murphy, 2015; Tussing and Wren, 2006). How, then, do the rationalities associated with advanced liberal societies and welfare regimes shape the governance of health and health policy in Ireland?

This edited collection builds on these themes by providing empirical examples of the application of ideas drawn from governmentality studies to health and health policy in Ireland. Drawing on contributions from writers based in the disciplines of social policy, sociology, public health and political science, the book seeks to answer three related questions: (1) How have certain health issues become constructed as 'problematic' and in need of intervention in Ireland? (2) Through what strategies, discourses and technologies have health policies and initiatives sought to manage specific groups of citizens in the state? (3) How have spaces of resistance to such strategies been mobilised, if at all? Governmentality studies have in the past been criticised for failing to provide clear empirical applications of key ideas and concepts and for focusing on the 'how' of government at the expense of the 'so what?' (O'Malley, Weir and Shearing, 1997; Larner, 2000; McKee, 2009). Discussing the latter, for example, O'Malley, Weir and Shearing (1997) and Larner (2000) have argued that despite the clear potential for linking the governmentality approach to critical politics, by and large this potential has not been realised. As Larner argues (2000: 14), 'the governmentality literature has not paid a great deal of attention to the politics surrounding specific programmes and policies'. We seek to address these criticisms by providing empirical analyses of governance strategies deployed, whilst recognising that these strategies always have a political effect or outcome, and cannot be divorced from social relations and political struggle.

This introductory chapter establishes some of the conceptual cornerstones associated with governmentality thinking and considers their implications for an analysis of health and health policy in Ireland. One of these implications is that studying health policy means moving beyond formal government prescriptions set down in policy documents or statements issued by government ministers, and excavating the multifarious actors and actions that lead to particular issues becoming problematised as health issues in the first place. This requires an exploration of how bodies and disease categories are constructed, spoken about and understood through particular discourses and interventions, which in turn brings into focus the role that expert knowledge systems play in rendering particular bodies and subjectivities visible. One of the key contributions of Foucault's work has been to show how knowledge is intimately tied up with the everyday exercise of power in the management of individual bodies and the social problems of populations – a form of power he termed *biopower*, or 'the set of mechanisms through which the basic biological features of the human species became the object of a political strategy' (Foucault, 2007: 1). Taking up these ideas, for example, philosopher Ian Hacking (2006) has shown how the disciplines of medicine, psychiatry and sociology have all been implicated in creating new (statistical) social categories of being or *human kinds*, categories which in turn beget the creation of new identities, behaviours and knowledges by those who are members of these groupings. For Foucault, the disciplining gaze and regulatory practices of medicine cannot be underestimated, and his legacy has prompted a range of studies which question the normalising status of, and power inherent in (medical) explanations of disease and disease interventions (Lupton, 1995; Howson, 1999). Allied to this, governmentality approaches have placed an emphasis on investigating the practices and technologies through which governing health and healthcare takes place, particularly in the context of neoliberal welfare reform. These include the specific processes, strategies and calculative regimes which have sought to gently or not so gently encourage citizens to become healthy subjects or 'civilised selves' in the context of health-promoting agendas, and which also have implications for the subjectivities and practices of those working within the health policy or healthcare arena (see for example, Brownlie and Howson, 2006; Kurunmäki and Miller, 2008). We begin the chapter, then, by laying out Foucault and others' understandings of governmentality, and follow this by exploring how governmentality literature has been deployed within studies of health and health policy analysis.

We then move on to situate the volume by introducing the Irish health policy arena and system. Our concern here is not to reposition the formal state or government apparatus as centre stage in our analysis, but rather to provide a context to some of the specificities and contingencies of Irish health policy debates. Chief amongst these are the principles of subsidiarity which have characterised the approach to welfare more generally since the inception of the Irish Republic in 1922, but also more recently, the increasingly neoliberal principles shaping current health policy and healthcare reforms. Situated in a context where Ireland has often been described in welfare terms as 'between Boston and Berlin' (Finn, 2011), successive administrations have put an ever-increasing emphasis on the for-profit sector in addressing health service shortfalls; meanwhile, a public–private split in care has entrenched inequity between those who can pay for access and those who cannot, reflecting what some commentators have referred to as a form of 'apartheid' in Irish healthcare (Burke, 2009). Moreover, recent economic and political contingencies – including most significantly, the politics of austerity – have created a climate in which commentators have argued that the burden of health and healthcare is being transferred to a range of actors beyond the remit of the formal state, including the individual, family and community (Mercille and Murphy, 2015; McDonnell and O'Donovan, 2009). We conclude by providing an overview of the volume and its chapters.

Governmentality: some conceptual starting points

That Foucault's work has had such an influence on sociological studies of health and illness, medicine and health policy perhaps reflects the fact that so much of his work focused explicitly on the discipline of medicine and the growth of health institutions in seeking to understand the practice(s) of government, and also as a basis for developing and elaborating his ideas about power/knowledge. In pulling together this collection, however, our concern is not just with Foucault's own work, but with the vast literature which has sought to interpret and deploy his ideas in various different guises. From the 1980s, a growing body of literature within sociology, political science and cognate disciplines has developed (both empirically and conceptually) strands of Foucault's work: in this respect, Mitchell Dean's work and that of Peter Miller and Nikolas Rose stand out particularly as articulating and making practicable Foucault's exposition of governmentality. Similarly, in applying these ideas to the sociology of health, illness and medicine, the work of Deborah Lupton, Alan Petersen and Sarah Nettleton, amongst others, has had a significant role to play in developing our conceptual and empirical understandings of disease categories, health subjectivities and mapping using Foucauldian-inspired literature; increasingly, they have been joined by contributions from those within health-based disciplines, social policy and geography, to name but a few.

In this section, we set out a brief exposition of Foucault's ideas about governmentality, and explore how others have interpreted and developed these ideas. From the outset, it is important to note that Foucault did not have one coherent 'grand theory' of governmentality (Huxley, 2008: 1636), and nor can there be said to be a single governmentality perspective. Rather governmentality is reflective of a set of evolving ideas developed over a period of time, but always a reflection of Foucault's preoccupation with 'revealing the historical and sociocultural contingencies of conceptions of the human – however necessary, essential and written in stone they might seem to be to those who have embraced them' (Faubion, 2014: 1).

A key part of Foucault's understanding of governmentality emerged from his genealogical work excavating the historical changes in the practices of modern power in Europe. From the eighteenth century, Foucault observed a shift in the mode of governing which he described as a move from a regime based on sovereign power, in which allegiance to the monarch and defence of territory took prominence, to one in which management of the health and welfare of the population, and of social and economic stability became much more important (Huxley, 2008; Legg, 2005). The consequence of this shift, as Legg (2005) summarises, was twofold. In the first instance, a disciplining imperative could be witnessed in the growth of specific spaces and institutions – the asylum, prison, school or workhouse – for those perceived to be a threat to the body politic, and requiring reform at the level of the individual body. In the second instance, there emerged a growing concern with the regulation of the population, a regulation that was made possible by the growth of human and economic sciences, demography and statistics. These sciences made the problems of populations calculable and knowable, whether in terms of their biosocial characteristics (expressed in terms of morbidity, mortality or fertility, for example) or their economic and/or social stability and security. In this context, the aim of governmental practices was less on exerting influence through the disciplining of individual bodies, but rather through the creation of a 'self-regulating subject who would vote conscientiously, invest responsibly and work diligently, while moving about and maintaining the modern city with suitable civic pride' (Legg, 2005: 139–140). To that list, we could also add, 'live healthily'.

Biopower, then, reflects the emergence of a form of power focused on techniques of knowing and acting which move between the individual, body and the social body, or body politic. In terms of health and medicine,

Lupton (2005) articulates these two dimensions as the difference between
the disciplining gaze of the individual medical encounter, and regulatory
tendencies inherent in programmes, such as public health initiatives, on
the overall health of the population. As Foucault himself noted, and as
empirical analyses such as Evans and Colls's (2009) analysis of the Body
Mass Index (BMI) in relation to obesity have demonstrated, however, these
two imperatives (the disciplinary and the regulatory) need not be mutually
exclusive, but rather may co-exist together in governmental practices and
techniques.

The notion of biopower is simultaneously connected to Foucault's ideas
about governmentality in the context of the continued historical metamor-
phosis of modern practices of governing, and specifically, the emergence
of advanced liberal government in the twentieth century (Huxley, 2008).
Foucault's exposition of governmentality, which he set out in a lecture at the
Collège de France in 1978, and has been further developed by authors such
as Rose (1996, 2007) and Dean (1999), has to be understood against the
backdrop of the long-term recession of the ideal of a welfare state and the
revitalisation of claims of a form of economic liberalism (or neoliberalism).
In social and political theory, neoliberalism has often been analysed as a
policy framework, or as an ideology driven by the philosophy of the New
Right, and has focused on exposing the 'retreat of the state' or the 'domination of the market'. While the study of governmentality continues with
such a theoretical framework, in that the exercise of power and authority
remains at the centre of analysis, it differs significantly from many of the
key assumptions of many theories of the state.

Key to this difference, and central to the notion of governmentality, is
Foucault's understanding of power, insofar as the meaning of government
is not seen as necessarily tied to the nation state (and nor is power seen
as inhering within the state), but rather is understood as the 'conduct of
conduct' (Foucault, 1982). Gordon (1991: 2) explains Foucault's definition
of 'the conduct of conduct' as 'a form of activity aiming to shape, guide or
affect the conduct of some person or persons'. There are two key related
elements that arise from this definition of government: the first of these
is that power functions in terms of the relations between different fields,
institutions, bureaucracies and other groups (such as the private media and
other businesses) within the state. These relations of power are understood
as mobile and contingent; thus, power can flow very quickly from one
point or area to another, moving through different groups, institutions
and individuals, depending on changing alliances and circumstances. This
extends the scope of political analysis beyond the domain of the state and
institutional politics, that is, the analysis of political power beyond the state
(Rose and Miller, 1992).

Second, Foucault (1991) used the term 'rationality of government' interchangeably with 'art of government'. He was interested in government as

a *strategic* activity or practice, and in areas of government as a way of knowing what that activity consisted of, and how it might be carried out. According to Gordon (1991: 3),

> A 'rationality of government' will thus mean a way or system of thinking about the nature of the practice of government (who can govern; what governing is; what or who is governed), capable of making some form of activity thinkable and practicable both to its practitioners and to those upon whom it was practiced.

This is what Dean (1999: 33) also refers to as the 'utopian element of government', because, within this understanding, to govern 'is to believe that government is not only necessary but possible ... [this] implies that it is possible to re-form human beings, to form or shape them or their attributes in some way'. Within the conceptualisation of power adopted by a governmentality approach, the political vocabulary structured by oppositions between state and civil society, public and private, government and market, coercion and consent, sovereignty and autonomy and the like, does not adequately characterise the diverse ways in which rule is exercised today (Rose and Miller, 1992; Lupton, 1995; Dean, 1999).

Governmentality then is often described as having two elements: the rationalities or mentalities of rule, which describe the aspirational visions of governmental projects and programmes; and the actual practices, techniques or technologies through which processes of governing are rendered actionable and operable (Rose and Miller, 1992). In the context of advanced liberal governmentality, moreover, *technologies of the self* have a key role to play in the creation of the autonomous and self-determining liberal subject. Defined as techniques that allow individuals to effect change in the forms in which they govern their body, thought and conduct 'so as to transform themselves in order to attain a certain state of happiness, purity, wisdom, perfection, or immortality' (Foucault, 1988: 18), technologies of the self seek to enhance 'our possibilities of agency' (Dean, 1999: 167) and foster the development of particular subjectivities. Thus, a central element within a governmentality approach is attention to the formation of governmental subjects and identities as a basis for governing.

Perhaps somewhat ironically given Foucault's ideas about the dispersed nature of power and his exposing of all truths as socially and historically contingent, there is a danger that governmentality can appear as a somewhat linear (top-down) framework explaining modern modes of governing, with governmental aspirations giving rise to specific programmatic actions, and the (successful) creation of individual and collective citizen identities as a means of exacting programme aims. Some commentators have criticised the way in which 'post-Foucauldian governmentality' (McKee, 2009) has been applied empirically in social policy analysis, highlighting that there has been an overemphasis on the aims or

rationalities of government and the seemingly contained discursive subjectivities they engender, with rather less attention paid to the messy contingencies of how these aims get put into practice (including by those who
are charged with implementing or working with particular governmental
programmes), or how individuals respond to, and sometimes resist, particular identities in numerous, and often small-scale, actions (Barnett *et
al.*, 2008; for an excellent review, see McKee, 2009). It is important to
note, however, that Foucault recognised government as an action which
was often doomed to failure. Thus, as he and others have acknowledged,
there is often a mis-match between project rationalities and practices: governmental aspirations may often conflict with one another, and individuals
do not embody 'ideal type' subjectivities presupposed by governmental
objectives (Huxley, 2008; Rose and Miller, 1992). This being so, it would
seem to us that understanding the dynamics of governmentality requires
even more careful attention directed towards the specific contexts of governing and the 'realpolitiks' they engender (McKee, 2009: 474; Lippert and
Stenson, 2010).

Deploying governmentality in health and health policy

Since the 1980s and 1990s, poststructuralist and postmodernist theoretical approaches, influenced by Foucault's ideas, have stimulated a significant body of research in the field of the sociology of health and illness
(Armstrong, 1995, 1997; Petersen and Bunton, 1997), and critiques of
public health and health promotion strategies and policies (Nettleton, 1991;
Lupton, 1995; Petersen and Lupton, 1996; Bunton, Nettleton and Burrows,
1995; Petersen and Bunton, 2002; O'Malley and Valverde, 2004). The
appeal of Foucault's work – so much of which dealt directly with the role
of the medical profession, medical expertise and biosocial strategies aimed
at the health of the population (what we might refer to as public health, or
health promotion) – lies particularly in its challenging of accepted assumptions about (biomedical) truth(s) and knowledge(s). Structural critics have
generally accepted the knowledge claims of medicine and public health,
questioning the uses to which they are put rather than seeking to explore the
assumptions that underlie them (Lupton, 1995). Poststructural critiques, on
the other hand, drawing on Foucault's concept of power/knowledge, have
highlighted the social construction of knowledge and the social processes
involved in the production of medical knowledge. Through texts such as
The Birth of the Clinic (1973) and *Madness and Civilisation* (1967), Foucault was concerned to show how biomedicine as an expert system had a
strongly normalising imperative, and was intimately tied up in the creation
of medical categories separating the 'sick' from the 'well', or 'normal' from
'deviant', categories which in and of themselves were often taken as givens

and provided the justification for particular medical interventions and processes (Philo, 2000).

In the context of governmentality, analyses have explored how these normalising discourses are made actionable in particular strategies and practices which seek to discipline the individual body, regulate the social body and engender self-responsible health-seeking behaviours in individual citizens. For some, for example, advanced neoliberal societies can increasingly be associated with 'surveillance medicine', particularly in the context of public health, health promotion and health education (Armstrong, 1995; Howson, 1999; Lupton, 1995). Thus as Lupton (1995: 10) describes it, 'The institution of public health has served as a network of expert advice, embodied in professionals such as doctors and health promoters, who have dispensed wisdom directed at improving individual's health through self-regulation.'

At the level of the social body, health promotion strategies and public health often turn on the creation of particular (healthy/unhealthy) subjectivities and it is perhaps unsurprising that much governmentality-inspired analysis has explored the creation of these subjectivities and identities. Barcelos's (2014: 477) analysis of the 'problem' of teenage pregnancy and related prevention programmes, for example, notes that

> a variety of biopolitical techniques have emerged [in managing teen pregnancy], ranging from abstinence to 'comprehensive' sexual health education; the pathologisation of pregnant teen bodies; an admonishment to engage in contraceptive use; the promotion of the two-parent, heterosexual, middle-class family; restrictions on welfare assistance; and the creation of multi-sector coalitions to reduce teen childbearing.

As she recognises, these strategies are underpinned by particular ideas and constructions – informed by relevant experts – about appropriate norms in relation to sexual behaviour, the childbearing body and motherhood, and seek to responsibilise women in making 'right' sexual and childbearing choices. In unpicking these constructions, a governmental analysis facilitates a broader questioning of the problematisation of teen pregnancy in the first place: that is, as Barcelos (2014: 486) asks, when, or at what point, did the 'teenage mother' become 'a particular, universal, and essential subject?' (*ibid.*).

From the study of pregnancy (Weir, 2006), through to obesity (Evans and Colls, 2009; Lupton, 2013), mental health (Fullagar, 2008; Teghtsoonian, 2009) and specific medical procedures, including medical screening (Armstrong and Eborall, 2012), a vast range of studies have sought to explore how medicine, public health strategies and health promotion are implicated in promoting self-responsible, healthy, citizens. At the heart of many of these studies is an awareness of discourses and governmental strategies of *risk* in how health programmes seek to construct health truths and engender

health-seeking behaviours. Armstrong's (2005) study of a cervical screening programme in the UK, for example, describes how the programme
encourages women to 'self-position' as at risk from cervical cancer, with
official discourse promoting the idea that *all* women need to see themselves
as at risk. As her analysis shows, however, women frequently resist these
official constructions, drawing on more localised, lay discourses in interpreting and self-identifying individual risks in relation to cervical cancer.
Armstrong's (2005) study provides a useful example of work that seeks to
challenge any notion of governmentality as a 'univocal' (O'Malley, 2008:
69) approach to understanding and interpreting mentalities and processes of
government.

While many health-based studies drawing on governmentality echo these
themes about the building of subjectivities through particular health technologies and practices, another arena of work has explored more specifically the implications of advanced liberal governing for the focus and
management of healthcare and health systems. Thus studies have explored
the implications of health policy and health-service reconfigurations, which
increasingly place the onus on individuals, or communities, to take responsibility for their care through a network of agencies and institutions: Junne
and Huber's (2014) study of the reconfiguration of services for people with
disabilities in Germany around the goal of 'personalisation' – made practicable in the provision of direct payments to individuals to purchase their
own support and assistance – provides one such example of how neoliberal
approaches to health and social welfare seek to govern citizens at a distance,
and, in the context of direct payments, have arguably transferred certain
risks from the state to individuals.

Other studies take their lead from the use of Foucauldian ideas in understanding organisational change, whether this be in the context of health and
social care, local government reform, or the specific task of organisational
management (see for example, McKinlay and Starkey, 1998; Kurunmäki
and Miller, 2008, 2011), and place a specific focus on the implications of
organisational change for those working within health-based organisations.
Thus, Ferlie, McGivern and FitzGerald's (2012) work on the emergence of
Managed Cancer Services in the UK, for example, explores the emergence of
'clinical managerial hybrids', that is, medical and health-based professionals
who are increasingly drawn into clinical governance and managerial roles.
In the neoliberal reconfiguration of healthcare, tools such as audit, financial
management and performance indicators increasingly provide a way of both
managing disparate institutional actors and entities, whilst also creating
healthcare workers as 'calculating selves' (Miller, 2001).

In total, these studies – whether focusing on the creation of subjectivities,
institutional configurations or specific technologies and techniques – have
undoubtedly opened up new and exciting understandings and analyses of
health issues and healthcare policies and systems. However, as in other

disciplinary arenas, so too have there been criticisms of the limits of governmentality within the sociology of health and illness and the health policy arena. Reiterating McKee's (2009) critique, for example, Armstrong (2005), in the context of her aforementioned study on cervical cancer, argues that a governmentality perspective on risk is in danger of focusing too much attention on the discourses and strategies employed to discipline individuals, at the expense of exploring how individuals themselves respond to these discourses (see also Lovell, Kearns and Prince, 2014, in the context of health promotion professionals). Osborne's (1997) exposition of the relevance of Foucault's ideas to health policy also repays a careful reading. As he notes, Foucault's work provides no easy answers about how, or to what end, health policy should be constructed. Indeed, the one thing that can be said about health as a governmental project is its indeterminacy, such that health is an indirect by-product of governmental intervention. While, as he notes, Foucault's work offers no 'positive conceptions as to how health might be regulated', he suggests that Foucault's ideas provide the potential to rethink how we understand health policy as less about a reactive response to 'objective health needs' (Osborne, 1997: 173) and rather more about the construction of a series of creative problematisations.

Contextualising Irish health policy

This volume takes a specific focus on Ireland and Irish health policy as a basis for its analysis. As in so many countries, health, health policy and, indeed, healthcare issues in Ireland are often high-profile, politically charged and form the basis for considerable public debate, with Considine and Dukelow (2009: 235) arguing that 'Health is the most contested and debated area of social policy in contemporary Irish society.' Like many other Western nations, stories about disease epidemics – whether in terms of obesity, Alzheimer's or mental illness – frequently feature in media debates and are constructed in different ways, and ascribed different meanings (not least in terms of 'who' or 'what' is to blame, and how it should be tackled). Battles over health – not least in terms of access to services, or medical treatments – are increasingly fought between different parties and allegiances, as Ireland has witnessed the growth of patients' organisations and advocacy groups seeking to articulate the concerns of those with particular conditions. In this regard, Ireland and the Irish context is perhaps no different to other Western nations. Yet insofar as governmentality draws attention to the historically contingent nature of modes of governing and governmental strategies in relation to health, it is also important to set out some of the specificities of the Irish context, which emerge from the broader governance and politics of the Irish state.

As outlined earlier, governmentality develops an understanding of governing in the context of the advanced neoliberal states, and the historical dismantling of state welfare structures, or state retrenchment. In Ireland, it cannot be said that state welfare structures – at least in the form of a Keynesian welfare state – ever existed in the same way. Rather, following the creation of the Irish state in 1922, charitable religious organisations played a key role in the provision of healthcare and social services, influenced by the Catholic principle of subsidiarity, which stressed that the state 'should not take on the responsibility for providing social services where needs could be met by smaller entities such as individuals themselves, their families or voluntary organisations' (Considine and Dukelow, 2009: 30). Indeed, the Catholic Church saw itself as equal in power to the state, and its moral teachings and authority were intimately tied up in approaches and medical practices towards specific health issues (most notably, women's reproductive health) (McDonnell and Allison, 2006). This involvement has waned today, with the Department of Health (DoH) and Health Service Executive (HSE) taking overall responsibility for the direction of health policy, and semi-state bodies, such as the Health Information and Quality Authority (HIQA), being established to regulate health institutions, but religious organisations still run many hospitals and social services within Ireland's mixed economy of healthcare. Meanwhile remnants of Catholic attitudes still remain in terms of certain medical procedures and debates, most notably abortion, which remains illegal in most circumstances and is highly contested (McDonnell and Allison, 2006).

Ireland's healthcare system today involves a complex number of actors, but can be seen as exhibiting many of the features of advanced neoliberal societies. It is a system that is frequently criticised for being underfunded, but also one which is seen as hugely inequitable due to a significant public–private split in the way in which care is provided. Primary care, through General Practitioners (GPs), for example, is only available free to Medical Card holders (and since 2015, to all children under 6). The Irish hospital system contains a mix of public and private hospitals, but somewhat unusually, private care can be provided in public hospitals, which 'has produced many inequities and inefficiencies' (Considine and Dukelow, 2009: 244). During the 1980s, in a context of welfare cutbacks, the provision of private health services grew and the public/private mix in the system became more entrenched, as the extra revenue hospitals could raise by providing private accommodation acted as an incentive to increase the number of private beds. The growth in private medicine has been paralleled by the growth in private health insurance. Private health coverage grew from 26.1% of the population in 1979 to 34.4% by 1990 (Considine and Dukelow, 2009). Despite the fact that free hospital care was extended to the entire population in 1991, the percentage of the population who purchased private health insurance continued to grow: in 2008 it stood at

52% (McDonnell and O'Donovan, 2009). While numbers have fallen since, due in large part to Ireland's recession, it still remains comparatively high, recorded as 45.8% of the population in December 2015 (Health Insurance Authority, 2016).

The main reasons for the growing levels of private healthcare purchase, and the fact that it still continues to be very high, are linked to the existing inequalities between public patients and private patients in accessing timely healthcare (Nolan and Wiley, 2001; Watson and Williams, 2001). As Wren (2003: 14) explains, 'This is a system in which patients are treated according to income rather than need. Private patient care is delivered promptly and, generally, by consultants in person. Public patient care comes tardily and is frequently delivered by doctors in training.' In Ireland, the two-tier system refers to the two tiers in both access and care in the public hospital system. From a governmentality perspective, these political changes (the shift towards privatisation) can be understood not as a decline of state sovereignty but as a promotion of forms of government that foster and enforce individual responsibility (Rose and Miller, 1992), privatised risk-management (Rose, 1996) and the play of market forces and entrepreneurial models in a variety of social domains (Dean, 1999). In the context of Irish health policy, the purchase of private health insurance has been promoted by various governments through a number of strategies and mechanisms. For example, the private component of the public health system in Ireland has been heavily subsidised by the state: public hospitals have not charged the full costs of providing private care and there is tax relief on insurance premiums.

More recently, there has also been significant analysis of the impacts of austerity on the Irish health system. Marking the end of Ireland's economic 'boom' years, when the country became known as the Celtic Tiger, the economic crash and recession, accompanied by the EU-IMF bailout in 2010 and subsequent austerity politics, have further entrenched neoliberal agendas, with deleterious effects for the health system. Thus, it is argued that the effects of austerity on the health system have been to reinforce existing inequalities and increasingly shift the costs of healthcare on to individual citizens (Mercille and Murphy, 2015; see also Thomas, Burke and Barry, 2014). As Thomas, Burke and Barry (2014: 1545) note, 'From 2009 to 2013 financing of the HSE fell by 22%, which amounted to almost €3·3 billion less in public funding.' Meanwhile, individuals are paying more for existing services, such as for charges for prescriptions, or visits to emergency departments. The impacts of the economic realm require acknowledgement in understanding processes of governmentality within Ireland's health arena, not least in terms of recognising the way in which the economic domain intrudes into and intersects with other governmental projects and programmes designed to preserve and manage the biosocial stability of both the social, and individual, body (Legg, 2005).

Overview of the volume

Our aim in this volume is to put governmentality to use in exploring the specific contexts and contingencies that have given rise to particular problematisations of health within Ireland, and have led to specific, delimited, sets of techniques and strategies enacted in the name of health policy. Following Osborne (1997: 173), the chapters in the book therefore seek to move away from many analyses of health policy which may be described as 'reactive': 'that is, on the one hand, policy is viewed as a reaction to objective problems and health needs and provision, and on the other, the state of health is viewed as the product of the relative effectiveness of policy'. Rather, by examining health issues and policies ranging from obesity, to mental health, smoking, older age, disability and even the dead body, the contributions elucidate the *relativity* of health as a construct and ideal in the way in which it is understood and addressed by various governmental practices and assemblages.

While not seeking to stress a dichotomy between the subjectivities produced through governmental programmes, and the specific technologies and practices of the (neoliberal) governance of health and healthcare, the chapters in the volume are divided into two key parts based on their analytical focus. Part I, 'Constructing health problems and (un)healthy subjects', focuses on the way in which different health issues, through sources including policy documents, television health promotion campaigns, letters in broadsheet newspapers, documents from professional bodies and parliamentary debates, have sought to 'bring into being' particular health problems and construct particular health behaviours as problematic. The chapters in this section explore how the subjects of health policy and public health initiatives more generally have become constituted in the process of governing, as well as how these identities have been subject to contestation and resistance.

Reflecting the contingencies, and often moral panics, which lead to particular dimensions of health becoming visible at particular times in history, three of the chapters in this section deal with the issues of obesity and childhood, albeit in very different ways. In Chapter 2, Kevin Ryan begins the section by developing a historical analysis of the figure of the child as a locus of biosocial and moral concerns about the health of the (Irish) population. Moving from the eighteenth century to the present day, Ryan draws on the work of Rousseau and Foucault to excavate 'the story of how childhood has come to articulate a moralised conception of health which is also a medicalised pedagogy' (p. 26). Insofar as children have long been constructed as representing the future population, so concerns about their discipline, health and morality have been continuing targets of governmental strategies within the Irish state, whether in the form of the nineteenth-century reformatory schools or more recently, public health strategies which accord a central role to childhood in stabilising and securing the future of the nation. Through a process of detailed empirical investigation, Ryan traces the way in which historical discourses continually inform our understanding of the present, and project forward into our constructions of the future.

The theme of childhood is continued in Chapter 3, albeit this time in relation to concerns about childhood obesity in contemporary Irish society. Like many other Western nations, concerns about a childhood obesity epidemic since the 2000s have featured prominently in Irish media and government discourses. In a critical reading of these discourses, Michelle Share and Perry Share seek to unpick the ways in which particular truths are created about childhood obesity by a complex range of institutional actors, and become the basis for interventions and actions targeted at particular groups. Specifically, they explore how data from the National Longitudinal Study of Children, *Growing Up in Ireland* (*GUI*), has been used to construct a particular reality of the 'problem' of childhood obesity, grounded in an uncritical acceptance of medical norms and instruments (such as the BMI). Their analysis points to the sheer complexity of both the institutional actors (medical and social scientists, policymakers and the media) and types of knowledges invoked in the problematisation of obesity, and also points to the limits of interventions that place responsibility for tackling the risk of obesity at the feet of children, parents (primarily mothers) and schools through individualised interventions to act on the behaviours and bodies of children (witnessed through the visual metaphor of the measuring tape, for example). Recognising that *GUI* is in itself a technology of government, their analysis demonstrates how a governmentality approach can be used to build into, and develop, a critical politics of obesity.

The measuring tape as a visual image and metaphor also lies at the heart of Fiona Dukelow's chapter. While Share and Share's chapter provides a wider overview of the different institutional actors engaged in generating intersecting, and sometimes conflicting, discourses about childhood obesity, Dukelow focuses on a specific instance of health promotion, in the form of the 2011 *Stop the Spread* campaign, part of which involved the distribution of measuring tapes to the population via pharmacies to encourage people to measure their waists. Drawing on an analysis of campaign materials, the chapter explores the significance of *Stop the Spread* as a governmental technology in which medical discourse was utilised in an effort to not only reprogramme ideas of what a normal healthy body should measure and look like, but also to more directly attempt to change behaviour by gifting people the technology to measure themselves, and to ultimately inscribe those numbers on their bodies. Dukelow's analysis provides insights into how neoliberal governmentality is evolving in relation to public health policy, not least in the context of soft paternalism, which is more directive in its use of techniques and strategies to steer norms and behaviour, but which remains highly individualised in terms of its understanding of health and its determinants.

In Chapter 5, our attention turns to the rather different public health issue of smoking. Ireland was the first country in the world to introduce an outright ban on smoking in the workplace in 2004, an initiative that was widely regarded by Irish politicians, public health and anti-smoking advocates as a story of success, despite 'common sense' commentaries at the time which suggested that the ban would be too radical a proposal. Drawing on commentaries from broadsheet newspapers and political speeches from the time, Eluska Fernández analyses the introduction of the smoking ban in Ireland as a successful exercise in 'the conduct of conduct' (Foucault, 1982) by exploring the types of conduct that were embraced and promoted in the context of the debates over the ban. Informed by the centrality of notions of rational, responsible and civilised selfhood in contemporary public health and health promotion discourses, the chapter reveals how notions of what came to be promoted as rational, responsible and civilised behaviours, and their flip side, irrational, irresponsible and uncivilised ones, were central to the exercise of power in the context of the ban.

The identities and subjectivities produced through governmental programmes also form the basis of Derek Chambers's chapter, which focuses on the area of mental health policy. As an arena in which expert systems, in the form of biomedical discourses and psychiatry, have played a central role in constituting mental health subjects, Chambers seeks to analyse the discourses emerging from recent mental health policy documents, including Ireland's main mental health strategy, *A Vision for Change*. Drawing on Dean's (2010) ideas about fields of visibility and valued knowledge, Chambers suggests that despite a broadening of understanding of mental health beyond medicalised discourses, seen most recently in health promotion campaigns and suicide prevention strategies, in practice, the focus remains on the mental health service user, and the provision of services for those who are mentally 'ill'. Attempts to reconfigure mental health as something which affects 'all of us', and moves beyond mental 'illness' – which, Chambers argues, may have the potential to open up less stigmatising modes of understanding about mental health – are hampered by the continuing dominance of the biomedical frameworks of understanding.

The final chapter in this section (Chapter 7) focuses on governmental dilemmas and practices around the dead body as they have been played out in recent political debates about organ donation. Drawing on a public consultation process initiated by the Joint Committee on Health and Children in 2013 on proposals to change the organ donation system in Ireland from one based on 'opting in' to one based on 'presumed consent' (where it is assumed a person will donate their organs unless they express an opinion to the contrary during their lifetime), Órla O'Donovan explores the political rationalities and modes of thinking that underpinned the construction of organ donation as a problem, and the ways in which the Irish state has sought 'to act *through* its citizens to transform the prevailing cultural attitude to organ donation whereby … (almost) everybody's cadaveric organs become available for transplantation' (p. 156). As she argues, the governmental shaping of people's subjectivities and dispositions in relation to organ donation was necessarily complex and messy, reflected in the different rationalities articulated in public hearings which invoked ideas about the dead body (how we think about death), the rights of the individual and the family, and the limits to medicine. The chapter draws attention to the significance of counter-conducts or forms of resistance in defining and articulating policy problems: thus, despite the overriding construction of the organ donation problem by the government as one of a scarcity of organs and a low donation rate in Ireland, counter-discourses articulated that the problem could be traced to an ineffective and poorly resourced health system.

Part II of the book, 'Governing neoliberal healthcare agendas: politics, strategies and practices', focuses on how the rationalities underpinning the governance of healthcare get played out within the different sites and spaces of Ireland's health landscape. Whilst these cannot be separated from the creation of subjectivities, the chapters in this section place a greater focus on the *mechanics* of governing – that is, the practices, strategies and techniques – through which neoliberal healthcare agendas are brought into being and implemented. The chapters also recognise the role of institutional relationships (for example, between the NGO sector and the state or between private and public sector bodies) and the politics of expertise that give shape to, and influence, the processes of governing health in Ireland.

In the first of these chapters (Chapter 8), Joanne Wilson and Lindsay Prior provide an analysis of some of Ireland's key public health-policy documents since 1994 in the context of advanced liberal government. As they note, public health strategies increasingly target the individual in terms of responsibilising behaviours, inculcating them to make healthy lifestyle choices and mitigate against health risks. Scrutinising the claims and arguments set out in three health documents – *Shaping a Healthier Future* (DoH, 1994), *Quality and Fairness – A Health Service for You* (DoHC, 2001), and *Healthy Ireland* (DoH, 2013) – they note the increasing shift to a market-based model of healthcare, and of the role of the state as one amongst many actors in the health policy arena. Health policymaking in Ireland, as they argue, has become an increasingly technocratic process, and their analysis raises significant questions about the implications of neoliberal modes of government in the context of the three documents' acknowledgement of persistent health inequalities in the state.

Chapter 9 echoes many of these themes in the context of a specific episode of Irish health policymaking in 2011, in which the government sought to initiate proposals regarding the introduction of Universal Health

Insurance (UHI). As outlined earlier, Ireland's health system is unusual in the context of its entanglement between public and private provision, and the fact that a substantial proportion of the population have private health insurance (albeit subsidised by tax breaks). Cliona Loughnane demonstrates how proposals to implement a system in which every member of the population would be expected to take out health insurance – and mooted by politicians as a way to end Ireland's two-tier health system – exhibited particular characteristics of advanced liberal modes of governing. Specifically, she takes Rose and Miller's (1992) conceptualisation of the aspirations of advanced liberal government – governing at a distance, the management of risk, engendering individuals to take responsibility through choice, and the fragmentation of the social state into multiple communities – as a basis for analysing the proposals. As this conceptualisation allows her to demonstrate, while political rhetoric may have stressed the significance of UHI as a basis for promoting 'solidarity' and 'fairness', it is hard to avoid the conclusion that the policy would have 'contradictorily tied healthcare delivery more strongly to market processes and controls' (p. 199) had it been implemented.

Claire Edwards's chapter is concerned with exploring a specific governmental technology – the Assessment of Need process in the Disability Act 2005 – which has initiated a new system of categorising children with disabilities in the Irish state. Subject to significant controversy, the AoN exposes not just the way in which governmental rationalities and strategies seek to bring new categories of individuals into being, but also how these projects are often incomplete and fraught with tension, insofar as they are played out within and across institutional and professional boundaries. In particular, Edwards's concern is to document how those charged with working within the health system interpret, make sense of and sometimes subvert the categorisations and obligations which the AoN process places upon them, thereby pointing to the messy realities of governing which are sometimes absent from governmentality-inspired analyses of policy programmes.

These realities, and the process of government as a 'congenitally failing operation' (Rose and Miller, 1992), also become apparent in Ciara O'Dwyer's analysis of long-term care policy for older people in Chapter 11. Taking a historical perspective, O'Dwyer demonstrates how the approach to a long-term care policy for older people bears all the hallmarks of neo-liberal government, in which the state has ceded provision of services to the private home and residential care sector, whilst retaining a regulatory role through bodies such as the Health Information and Quality Authority (HIQA). As she argues, older people's care increasingly hinges on the ability of older people to make 'responsible' ageing choices, 'whereby older people are expected to make the right choice and remain active and independent in old age (the "Third Age"), rather than slide into the Fourth Age of decline and decrepitude' (p. 229). As with so many of the chapters in this section, O'Dwyer's analysis draws attention to the role of the economic domain as a significant context to the development, or otherwise, of governmental aspirations and programmes.

In Chapter 12, Eluska Fernández and Claire Edwards synthesise the main themes of the volume, and provide a broader discussion of the contribution that governmentality-inspired studies can make to our understanding of health and health policy. In particular, they use the chapter as an opportunity to discuss where governmentality-based studies might take us in both methodological and theoretical terms. Cognisant of critiques of governmental analyses, they place a specific emphasis on exploring what, or how, governmentality can contribute to those themes which have so often occupied critical social policy analysts, not least issues of inequality, the role of politics as social relations and the place of contestation and resistance in policy processes. Thus, the chapter seeks to explore how we might write critical politics, and critical policy analysis, back into governmentality studies.

References

Armstrong, D. (1995) The rise of surveillance medicine. *Sociology of Health and Illness*, 17(3): 343–404.

Armstrong, D. (1997) Foucault and the sociology of health and illness: a prismatic reading. IN: Petersen, A. and Bunton, R. (eds) *Foucault, Health and Medicine*. London and New York, Routledge: pp. 15–30.

Armstrong, N. (2005) Resistance through risk: women and cervical cancer screening. *Health, Risk & Society*, 7(2): 161–176.

Armstrong, N. and Eborall, H. (eds) (2012) *The Sociology of Medical Screening: Critical Perspectives, New Directions*. Chichester, Wiley-Blackwell.

Barcelos, C.A. (2014) Producing (potentially) pregnant teen bodies: biopower and adolescent pregnancy in the USA. *Critical Public Health*, 24(4): 476–488.

Barnett, C., Clarke, N., Cloke, P. and Malpass, A. (2008) The elusive subjects of neo-liberalism. *Cultural Studies*, 22(5): 624–653.

Brownlie, J. and Howson, A. (2006) 'Between the demands of truth and government': health practitioners, trust and immunisation work. *Social Science & Medicine*, 62(2): 433–443.

Bunton, R., Nettleton, S. and Burrows, R. (1995) *The Sociology of Health Promotion: Critical Analyses of Consumption, Lifestyle and Risk*. London, Routledge.

Burke, S. (2009) *Irish Apartheid: Healthcare Inequality in Ireland*. Dublin, New Island.

Considine, M. and Dukelow, F. (2009) *Irish Social Policy: An Introduction*. Dublin, Gill and Macmillan.

Dean, M. (1999) *Governmentality: Power and Rule in Modern Society*. Thousand Oaks, Sage.

Dean, M. (2010) *Governmentality: Power and Rule in Modern Society* (second edition). Thousand Oaks, Sage.

Evans, B. and Colls, R. (2009) Measuring fatness, governing bodies: the spatialities of the Body Mass Index (BMI) in anti-obesity politics. *Antipode*, 41(5): 1051–1083.

Faubion, J.D. (2014) Introduction: the use of Foucault. IN: Faubion, J.D. (ed.) *Foucault Now Current Perspectives in Foucault Studies*. Cambridge, Polity: pp. 1–20.

Ferlie, E., McGivern, G. and FitzGerald, L. (2012) A new mode of organizing in healthcare? Governmentality and managed networks in cancer services in England. *Social Science & Medicine*, 74: 340–347.

Fernández, E. (2016) Exploring the story of the smoking ban in Ireland as a neo-liberal project. *Social Theory & Health*, 14(2): 256–274.

Finn, D. (2011) Ireland on the turn? Political and economic consequences of the crash. *New Left Review*, 67: 5–39.

Foucault, M. (1967) *Madness and Civilisation*. London, Tavistock.

Foucault, M. (1973) *The Birth of the Clinic: An Archaeology of Medical Perception*. London, Tavistock.

Foucault, M. (1982) The subject and power. IN: Dreyfus, H. and Rabinow, P. (eds) *Michel Foucault: Beyond Structuralism and Hermeneutics*. Chicago, University of Chicago Press: pp. 208–228.

Foucault, M. (1988) Technologies of the self. IN: Martin, L.H., Gutman H. and Hutton P.H. (eds) *Technologies of the Self: A Seminar with Michel Foucault*. London, Tavistock: pp. 16–49.

Foucault, M. (1991) Governmentality. IN: Burchell, G., Gordon C. and Miller, P. (eds) *The Foucault Effect: Studies in Governmentality (with Two Lectures by and an Interview with Michel Foucault)*. Chicago, University of Chicago Press: pp. 87–104.

Foucault, M. (2007) *Security, Territory, Population: Lectures at the College de France 1977–1978*. Basingstoke, Palgrave Macmillan.

Fullagar, S. (2008) Sites of somatic subjectivity: e-scaped mental health promotion and the biopolitics of depression. *Social Theory & Health*, 6: 323–341.

Gordon, C. (1991) Governmental rationality: an introduction. IN: Burchell, G., Gordon C. and Miller, P. (eds) *The Foucault Effect: Studies in Governmentality*. Chicago, University of Chicago Press: pp. 1–52.

Hacking, I. (2006) Making up people. *London Review of Books*, 28(16): 23–26.

Health Insurance Authority (2016) *A Review of Private Health Insurance in Ireland*. Available at: www.hia.ie/sites/default/files/Final%20Report%20Health%20Insurance%20Authority%202015%2004%2003%2016_0.pdf.

Howson, A. (1999) Cervical screening, compliance and moral obligation. *Sociology of Health and Illness*, 21(4): 401–425.

Huxley, M. (2008) Space and government: governmentality and geography. *Geography Compass*, 2(5): 1635–1658.

Joyce, P. (2001) Governmentality and risk: setting priorities in the new NHS. *Sociology of Health and Illness*, 23(5): 594–614.

Junne, J. and Huber, C. (2014) The risk of users' choice: exploring the case of direct payments in German social care. *Health, Risk & Society*, 16(7–8): 631–648.

Kurunmäki, L. and Miller, P. (2008) Counting the costs: the risks of regulating and accounting for health care provision. *Health, Risk & Society*, 10(1): 9–21.

Kurunmäki, L. and Miller, P. (2011) Regulatory hybrids: partnerships, budgeting and modernising government. *Management Accounting Research*, 22: 220–241.

Larner, W. (2000) Neo-liberalism: policy, ideology, governmentality. *Studies in Political Economy*, 63(Autumn): 5–25.

Legg, S. (2005) Foucault's population geographies: classifications, biopolitics and governmental spaces. *Population, Space and Place*, 11: 137–156.

Lippert, R. and Stenson, K. (2010) Advancing governmentality studies: lessons from social constructionism. *Theoretical Criminology*, 14(4): 473–494.

Lovell, S.A., Kearns, R.A. and Prince, R. (2014) Neoliberalism and the contract state: exploring innovation and resistance among New Zealand Health Promoters. *Critical Public Health*, 24(3): 308–320.

Lupton, D. (1995) *The Imperative of Health: Public Health and the Regulated Body*. London, Sage.

Lupton, D. (2003) *Medicine as Culture: Illness, Disease and the Body in Western Societies* (second edition). London, Sage.

Lupton, D. (2013) *Fat*. London and New York, Routledge.

McDonnell, O. and Allison, J. (2006) From biopolitics to bioethics: church, state, medicine and assisted reproductive technology in Ireland. *Sociology of Health and Illness*, 28(6): 817–837.

McDonnell, O. and O'Donovan, O. (2009) Private health insurance as a technology of solidarity? The myth of 'community' in Irish healthcare policy. *Irish Journal of Sociology*, 17(2): 6–23.

McKee, K. (2009) Post-Foucauldian governmentality: what does it offer critical social policy analysis? *Critical Social Policy*, 29(3): 465–486.

McKinlay, A. and Starkey, K. (eds) (1998) *Foucault, Management and Organization Theory: From Panopticon to Technologies of Self*. London, Sage.

Mercille, J. and Murphy, E. (2015) *Deepening Neoliberalism, Austerity and Crisis: Europe's Treasure Ireland*. Basingstoke, Palgrave Macmillan.

Miller, P. (2001) Governing by numbers: why calculative practices matter. *Social Research*, 68(2): 379–396.

Nettleton, S. (1991) Wisdom, diligence and teeth: discursive practices and the creation of mothers. *Sociology of Health and Illness*, 13(1): 98–111.

Nolan, B. and Wiley, M. (2001) *Private Practice in Irish Public Hospitals*. Dublin, Oak Tree Press.

O'Malley, R. (2008) Governmentality and risk. IN: Zinn, J.O. (ed.) *Social Theories of Risk and Uncertainty: An Introduction*. Oxford, Blackwell: pp. 52–75.

O'Malley, P. and Valverde, M. (2004) Pleasure, freedom and drugs: the uses of 'pleasure' in liberal governance of drug and alcohol consumption. *Sociology*, 38(1): 25–42.

O'Malley, P., Weir, L. and Shearing, C. (1997) Governmentality, criticism, politics. *Economy and Society*, 26(4): 501–517.

Osborne, T. (1997) Of health and statecraft. IN: Petersen A. and Bunton R. (eds) *Foucault, Health and Medicine*. London and New York, Routledge: pp. 173–188.

Petersen, A. and Bunton, R. (2002) *The New Genetics and the Public's Health*. London and New York, Routledge.

Petersen, A. and Bunton, R. (eds) (1997) *Foucault, Health and Medicine*. Abingdon, Routledge.

Petersen, A. and Lupton, D. (1996) *The New Public Health: Health and Self in the Age of Risk*. London, Sage.

Philo, C. (2000) 'The Birth of the Clinic': An unknown work of medical geography. *Area*, 32(1): 11–19.

Porter, S. (1996) Contra-Foucault: nurses, soldiers and power. *Sociology*, 30(1): 59–78.

Rose, N. (1996) The death of the social? Re-figuring the territory of government. *Economy and Society*, 25(3): 327–356.

Rose, N. (2007) *The Politics of Life Itself: Biopolitics, Power and Subjectivity in the 21st Century*. Princeton and Oxford, Princeton University Press.

Rose, N. and Miller, P. (1992) Political power beyond the state: problematics of government. *British Journal of Sociology*, 43(2): 173–205.

Share, M. and Strain, M. (2008) Making schools and young people responsible: a critical analysis of Ireland's obesity strategy. *Health and Social Care in the Community*, 16(3): 234–243.

Teghtsoonian, K. (2009) Depression and mental health in neoliberal times: A critical analysis of policy and discourse. *Social Science & Medicine*, 69: 28–35.

Thomas S., Burke S. and Barry, S. (2014) The Irish health-care system and austerity: sharing the pain. *The Lancet*, 383: 1545–1546.

Tussing, A.D. and Wren, M. (2006) *How Ireland Cares: The Case for Health Care Reform*. Dublin, New Island.

Watson, D. and Williams, J. (2001) *Perceptions of the Quality of Healthcare in the Public and Private Sectors in Ireland*. Dublin, Economic and Social Research Institute.

Weir, L. (2006) *Pregnancy, Risk and Biopolitics: On the Threshold of the Living Subject*. London, Routledge.

Wren, M. (2003) *Unhealthy State: Anatomy of a Sick Society*. Dublin, New Island.

PART I

Constructing health problems and (un)healthy subjects

Governing the future: children's health and biosocial power

Introduction

When Michel Foucault began to develop the concept of biopolitics, he wrote that 'a society's "threshold of modernity" has been reached when the life of the species is wagered on its own political strategies' (1998: 143). More recently, Giorgio Agamben has shown how this threshold is a zone of indeterminacy at the intersection of *zoē*, which is 'bare' metabolic life, and *bios*, or life that has been 'clothed' or cultivated by language and politics, thus amounting to a 'form or way of living proper to an individual or a group' (Agamben, 1998: 9–10). What I want to suggest by way of an introduction is that the 'politicisation of bare life', or 'the entry of *zoē* into the sphere of *the polis*' (*ibid.*: 10) cannot be adequately grasped without examining how the figure of the child came to articulate an idiom of unruly otherness: 'nature', 'animal', 'savage', 'primitive' – these are among the remainders which have been constituted by (and are constitutive of) the modern 'quest for order' (Bauman, 1991). As the embodiment of order's excess, the figure of the child is at times the sign of an innocence or original purity to be preserved or restored (see Faulkner, 2011), at other times the sign of a brutish or savage nature that must be tamed and civilised (Hall, 1911; Sully, 1903). Either way, childhood has long been both a way of projecting the present into the future and a means of making such imagined futures practical and technical. Furthermore, the threshold between *zoē* and *bios* is also the locus of a specific public health strategy that emerged during the nineteenth and twentieth centuries. Grafted to the figure of the child, this was assembled at the intersection of the biological and the social, the medical and the moral, and to this day remains a way of acting through and upon life with a view to governing the future.

This chapter begins by examining the writings of Jean Jacques Rousseau, focusing specifically on how his critical social theory and his normative political theory meet as a conception of childhood that would come into sharper focus during the nineteenth century, largely through the efforts of educationalists and hygienists. This was a social economy (Procacci, 1991) characterised by innovation and also at times by competing strategies, but its anchoring point was the figure of the child which became an analogue to Rousseau's 'state of nature': a way of hitting the reset button; of halting physical and moral decline by returning to the beginning so that the passage from nature to society, from animal to human, from savage to civilised, could be governed. Rousseau marks a beginning (not necessarily *the* beginning) in the story of how childhood has come to articulate a moralised conception of health which is also a medicalised pedagogy. The second part of the chapter tracks this history through the nineteenth and early twentieth centuries by examining reformatory education and public hygiene, focusing specifically on how these strategies were developed and deployed in Ireland. Originating in the problem of delinquency, the scope of these strategies gradually expanded so that by the start of the twentieth century childhood *as such* had become a 'national asset', with the technique of school medical inspection – a form of quality control – tasked with producing healthy, efficient and self-disciplined subjects.

The third and final section looks at how this 'biosocial' apparatus has recently been reconfigured through a policy framework called *Healthy Ireland*, the purpose of which is to 'reduce health inequalities' by 'empowering people and communities'. What this means in effect is that individuals are to take responsibility and make 'right choices', and as was the case in the past, childhood is framed as the key to successful implementation of this strategy. Children are now enmeshed in a networked constellation of instruments, agencies and techniques that measure, monitor and manage the lives of children, and while this network does not exhibit the singularity of a sovereign will or intention, it nevertheless governs by seeking to ensure that one and all participate in what Foucault (2008) described as a neoliberal 'game of inequality'.

Biosocial power and the 'anthropological machine'

Given the context-specific focus of this book (contemporary Ireland), it may seem odd to begin by examining the thoughts of an eighteenth-century French philosopher. My reason for starting with Rousseau is to initiate an analytics of government as this applies to the intersection of childhood and health, and before tackling the question of how this relates to modern Ireland, I first want to plot the main coordinates of a discursive process that would culminate in 'the birth of a subject which a positive science of man could take as its object' (Rose, 1985: 20). Rousseau's writings provide a way of doing this in a reasonably succinct and concise manner, and more importantly, of showing how this subject was constituted in the form of a specific conception of childhood.

Rousseau's *Discourse on Inequality* (published in 1755 and hereafter referred to as the *Discourse*) might be characterised as a 'diagnostics of the present' (Dean, 1999: 6), comparable in fact to the questions Foucault posed through his genealogical studies: How are we constituted as subjects of our own knowledge, as subjects who exercise or submit to power relations, and as moral subjects of our own actions? (Foucault, 1997: 318). Though not expressed in precisely the same way, the questions posed by Rousseau in the *Discourse* are broadly similar, and his way of staging a critical diagnostics utilised what was then a conventional analytical device: the state of nature. However, the way he assembled this device and put it to work marks a departure from convention, and it is this that places Rousseau at the threshold of biopolitical modernity.

According to Rousseau, 'the philosophers who have inquired into the foundations of society have all felt the necessity of going back to a state of nature; but none of them has got there' (2004: 15). What has led them astray, he argues, is an enduring tendency to project 'social man' into the past, thereby neglecting to distinguish what is 'fundamental' to human nature from the 'changes and additions' which have occurred during the long transition from nature to society (2004: 15). Rousseau had studied the works of the naturalists and comparative anatomists, and was aware of the difficulties encountered in discerning what, if anything, distinguished Man[1] from the apes (see Agamben, 2004: 23–27). His solution to this problem was to dispense with conjecture and to commence his discourse on the basis of an assertion which was also a constitutive decision: Man came into the world standing upright, with opposable thumbs, and 'measuring with his eyes the vast expanse of Heaven' (Rousseau, 2004: 17–18). Further to this, he acknowledges the impossibility of actually returning to the state of nature, and so this is to be understood not as a 'historical truth' but as a figure of thought. Within the textual space of Rousseau's *Discourse*, Man emerges in the form of a decision which is anchored in a fiction that functions as a conceptual machine, and this is put to work so that Rousseau can both 'explain the nature of things' and 'form a proper judgement of our present state' (2004: 11–16). Openly oscillating between fiction and fact, fact and judgment, the contingency of this decision rapidly dissolves so that it becomes a solid foundation that supports Rousseau's critical diagnosis.

Returning to the problem of distinguishing Man and animal, Rousseau notes that in the state of nature, 'without industry' and 'without speech', Man 'remained a child' and 'lived the life of an animal limited … to mere sensations' (2004: 38–41). Furthermore, 'every animal has ideas' and it is merely by 'degree that Man differs, in this respect, from the brute' (2004: 23). But there are two faculties that only Man possesses and Rousseau claims that these are beyond dispute: 'free will' and an irrepressible desire for 'self-improvement'. It is this unique combination that spawned speech and language, and this is what enabled 'savage man' to leave the world of the brutes (2004: 23–25). Rousseau admits that he can only speculate on how the transition from voice ('the simple cry of nature') to language occurred, yet somehow it did (2004: 28–31). Here Rousseau seems oblivious to the paradox he creates as a result of this blend of assertion and speculative reasoning, because what he is saying amounts to this: that in the state of nature 'savage man' was merely one animal among others, but at the same time this proto-human was already more than an animal. The *Discourse* might thus be mapped onto Agamben's concept of 'the anthropological machine', in that it produces Man by 'excluding as not (yet) human an already human being from itself, that is, by animalizing the human, by isolating the nonhuman within the human' (Agamben, 2004: 26, 37).

A century before Darwin published his *Origin of Species*, Rousseau wrote this quasi-evolutionary account of Man which culminates as a moral tale of 'degeneracy', a version of the Fall of Man (Rousseau, 2004: 22). As noted already, Rousseau has no answer to the question of why or how language became 'necessary', but once it did there was no turning back. With language came self-understanding, with understanding came knowledge, with knowledge came property and industry, and with the technological revolution in 'iron and corn' came inequalities born from vanity, envy, rivalry and contempt (Rousseau, 2004: 39, 46–50). The *Discourse* concludes on a wholly negative note which, Rousseau insists, is the consequence of self-imposed ignorance: if we had the courage to ask ourselves how we have become what we are, he suggests, then we would be obliged to admit that 'we have nothing to show for ourselves but a frivolous and deceitful appearance, honour without virtue, reason without wisdom, and pleasure without happiness' (Rousseau, 2004: 65). He offers no remedy to this state of affairs in the *Discourse*, but would go on to do so in two later works, one his essay on principles of political right (*The Social Contract*), and the other his treatise on education (*Emile*).

The *Social Contract* is analogous to the state of nature in that it too is a fiction, but it differs in that it articulates a normative ideal. It gestures towards a freedom that comes from willingly submitting to a sovereign power which is stretched between the rule of law and the 'general will', and this is a power that becomes insistent in cases of recalcitrance, so that – as Rousseau phrases it – those who 'refuse to obey the general will shall be constrained to do so by the whole body' (1968: 64). When Rousseau invokes this particular species of constraint, which concerns those who are to be 'forced to be free', he is thinking of cases where individuals are enslaved by passions and thus externalise the general will. Coercion would remind transgressors that the general will mirrored their own free will; that it was in fact nothing other than the collective manifestation of the unique qualities which, as noted in the *Discourse*, distinguishes the 'human machine' from the beasts (2004: 23–25). But there was a far more effective way of ensuring voluntary submission, and this is the significance of *Emile*, which completes Rousseau's triangle in a way that redoubles on itself: first by moving from a critical diagnostics (the *Discourse*) to normative ideal (*The Social Contract*) to remedy (*Emile*), and second by connecting sovereign power to government and to discipline (see Foucault, 1991: 102).

In *Emile*, the sovereign power that orchestrates the transition between the two fictions – the state of nature and the social contract – takes the form of a Tutor, whose sole purpose is to take charge of Emile's education from birth, preparing the boy for the freedom that awaits him upon reaching adulthood. The Tutor anticipates and controls the desires and temptations he knows will lead Emile astray, and he organises everything in such a way that Emile learns without being aware that he is in fact, and at all times, being taught. The indirect and unobtrusive power to which Emile is subject is to be experienced as autonomy, but this is a regulated and supervised freedom which is constitutive of Emile's subjectivity. As he approaches adulthood – with his education about to conclude – Emile entreats his Tutor to continue to 'advise and control us' (1993: 533). 'As long as I live I shall need you', he declares, and at this point, which completes the passage from nature to society, the distance between external control and self-discipline is effaced, so that subjectivity folds into subjection, and the mature Emile willingly embraces – and embodies – the guiding constraint of the general will.

The figure of the child in *Emile* (who represents 'man in general') mirrors the relation between animal–human, voice–language, savage–civilised as examined in the *Discourse*, while the Tutor (representing mandatory education/training) governs the transition from nature to society, thereby restoring what had been lost – Man's natural vigour and independence – while also modifying nature's bounty by engineering a vital and virtuous self-governing subject. Of course Rousseau did not have the last word on these matters, but of greater significance – because this would articulate a whole series of practical innovations – was the enigmatic nature of Man. It was in large part because the answer to this puzzle was, and would remain, so elusive that it could function as a catalyst that fuelled the anthropological machine, and would do so by keeping multiple relations and relays in play: pinning fiction to fact, and fact to norm, it constituted a subject neither entirely animal nor human – a figure representing humanity's infancy that could be acted upon with a view to governing life itself. This then is the subject that 'a positive science of man would take as its object' (Rose, 1985: 20), and it emerged at the threshold of nature–society, animal–human, voice–language, savage–civilised, all of which combined to make the double fiction of natural state and social contract into a technical task. Modern Western childhood was assembled from this series of thresholds, and the figure of the child would become a vehicle for biosocial technologies spanning the physical and the moral, the medical and the pedagogical. The next part of this chapter looks at how the prescriptive thrust of *Emile* was made practical through a pedagogical form of philanthropy (Rose, 1990: 179). More specifically, in Britain and Ireland this was a response to the problem of 'delinquency', which was framed as a 'moral disease' that necessitated publicly funded reformatory schools.

Between the medical and the moral: childhood as a 'national asset'

Reformatory education was a seedbed of innovation during the early decades of the nineteenth century, and among the many experiments were the Rauhe Haus reformatory in Hamburg and the Mettray agricultural colony in France (Barnes, 1989: 21–24). In Britain and Ireland, the initial response to the problem of vagrant, destitute and criminal children took the form of ragged schools, but it was the first industrial feeding school, established in Aberdeen in 1841, that would signal the shape of things to come. Within a decade, a number of prominent individuals – social reformers such as Mary Carpenter – were pressing for legislation to institute a system of publicly funded reformatory and industrial schools. Initially there was no substantive difference between these schools other than in name, and in Carpenter's writings both are subsumed under the heading 'penal reformatory schools', but an emergent distinction was already evident in the way that Carpenter split the problem of delinquency into the two classes of 'dangerous' and 'perishing'. For others this necessitated a dual strategy, so that the reformatory would rebuild the character of children already hardened in criminal habits (hence dangerous), while the industrial school was envisioned as a preventative intervention, targeting the children of the perishing class exposed to the demoralising influence of 'depraved and profligate' parents, and thus destined to become paupers, prostitutes, and criminals (Pim, 1854).[2] Differences aside, the objective was singular: to rescue children from what Carpenter called 'neglect'.

This section begins by examining the origin of these schools, though it should be noted that I will not be discussing their now notorious history or exploring how, in Ireland, they came to be managed by religious orders. Instead the focus will be on the ideas that brought them into existence, and the ways in which these ideas were to be made practical and technical (see Dean, 1999: 18). The second part of this section examines the strategy of public hygiene in the same way, and it may seem as though I am sidestepping the constraints of empirical analysis, and in particular what Ruth Barrington has described as 'the immense influence of the Catholic Church' in shaping the field of public health in Ireland (1987: 2). Though without doubt important, the relationship between church and state, religion and politics, in Ireland has been well documented, but there is still much work to do in examining how the instruments of power that govern through care, control and correction, and which operate both at the level of individuals and population, have been assembled around the figure of the child, and this is what I wish to focus on in approaching the present.

Reformatory education: the school as a 'moral hospital'

The reformatory movement cohered around the view that the existing system of punishment was wholly inadequate. Statistical societies were proliferating at that time: forums where prominent public figures – doctors, civil servants, barristers, philanthropists – presented papers to each other in what they claimed was the impartial language of 'facts'. The science of statistics was the imbrication of 'social economy' and 'social medicine', that is, vital statistics and criminal statistics conversed across the boundary of physical and moral health (Joyce, 2003: 26–29). In Ireland members of the Dublin Statistical Society (established in 1847) accumulated evidence on recidivism rates, which provided ammunition in arguing for the efficacy of prevention over retribution (Hancock, 1860; Haughton, 1850, 1857; Pim, 1854; Wilson, 1857). In identifying education as a solution to crime, reformers insisted that young offenders ought to be treated *as children* in special reformatory institutions *for children* (see Barnes, 1989: 24–26; Miller, 2013). Parkhurst prison on the Isle of White, where young convicts awaited transportation to the penal colonies, was seen to exemplify the problem because – in the words of Carpenter – it attempted 'to fashion children into machines instead of self-acting beings, to make them obedient prisoners within certain iron limits, not men who have been taught how to use their liberty without abusing it' (1851: 321–322). Punishment, whether by hanging, imprisonment or transportation, was deemed to be wasteful. To rescue, on the other hand, was to restore and refashion, so that the lives that were saved could be made useful, hence the salience of the medical register of disease and cure: if the delinquent child was perceived as a 'moral patient', and if delinquency was understood to be a 'moral disease', then the reformatory could be convincingly framed as a 'moral hospital' or 'moral infirmary', which would restore those exhibiting criminal propensities to good moral health (Carpenter, 1851: 15–16, 81, 366; Lentaigne, 1885: 35). In this way life would not be wasted, and society could make use of those it cured. Analogous to Rousseau's argument that those who deviate from the general will should be brought back into line, delinquent children would be forced to be free by placing them in a purpose-built environment that would instil 'habits of industry, regularity and good conduct' (Pim, 1854: 17).

According to Carpenter, delinquency was marked by a prematurely developed muscular strength and a will that was unrestrained by authority and reason, so that among the children of the perishing and dangerous classes, 'the governing faculty of the mind' became 'subservient to the gratification of animal desires' (1853: 296–297). At once an adult in the guise of a child and an animal in human form, the delinquent child was seen to invert the natural order of things, but the anthropological machine did not falter, and the activists driving the reformatory movement insisted that the principal cause of delinquency was social rather than inborn, the result of demoralising associations and influences, particularly as a result of parental 'neglect', meaning inadequate supervision and training. Taken together, this combination of symptom and cause converged in the argument that delinquency was a contagious disease, a moral plague, and the source of an infection that would – if left unchecked – blight the 'social body' (Carpenter, 1851: 344–346; also Pim, 1854: 7). In this discourse of reformatory education can be seen echoes both of Rousseau's diagnosis and his envisioned remedy: the figure of the child remained at the threshold of animal–human, nature–society, while the search for a solution to the problem of Man in society saw the school folded into the prison and the hospital. What enabled this internally complex apparatus to cohere was the technique of moral treatment.

At the end of the eighteenth century, Philippe Pinel and William Tuke had pioneered the technique in treating insanity, while several decades later in North America the principle of 'moral management' was organised into the architectural and administrative fabric of the penitentiary model of correctional punishment (Foucault, 1965, 1977; Rothman, 1971).[3] By the middle of the nineteenth century, moral treatment functioned as a sort of technical-epistemic relay between medicine and law, and the strategy of reformatory education expanded the scope of the practice. As a hybrid of school, hospital and prison, the reformatory aimed not only to cure delinquency by reforming the character of young criminals, but also to subject the incipient delinquent to a course of treatment that mirrored the figure of the Tutor in Rousseau's *Emile*. It would tackle the problem at its source by training the child in the arts of a regulated and supervised freedom, so that children would come to embody the power they were initially subjected to, thereby translating external control into self-restraint. Furthermore, though delinquency was the specific target of reformatory education, the vision was far more ambitious and shared with Rousseau the goal of rescuing society from its own excesses.

Both in terms of design and strategic objective, the penal reformatory school exemplified biosocial power in that it was deployed as a social technology to refashion life that had been deformed by social circumstances. The reach of the strategy was distinctly limited, however, for it could act only upon the actions of those children who crossed the threshold of the law and, as a result, could be forcibly removed from the space of the family. More specifically, the strategy was limited by the way it

replicated the prison in combining school and hospital as an insular institution that operated through exclusion from the wider society. By the end
of the nineteenth century, however, a far more encompassing apparatus
was taking shape, and, importantly, this did not replace the reformatory and industrial schools. Instead it incorporated them, together with
the principle of exclusion, into a strategy of public hygiene that targeted
the normal child so that all children would be within reach of biosocial
interventions.

The strategy of hygiene

One of the major disagreements articulated by the discourse of public health
in Ireland (as elsewhere) concerned the meaning of prevention, which could
be operationalised in the form of environmental measures such as the
improvement of housing, sewerage and drinking water, but also in the form
of eugenic interventions to prevent the birth of children who – according
to the science – would grow into 'degenerate' and 'defective' adults. For
contextual reasons examined by Greta Jones (1992), eugenics failed to gain
any real traction in Ireland, but that does not mean that it did not play a
part in shaping the strategy of hygiene. At the 1911 Congress of the Royal
Institute of Public Health for example, held that year in Dublin, the section
devoted to Child Study and Eugenics examined ways to 'encourage the
breeding of the fit, and discourage the breeding of the unfit' (*Irish Independent*, 1911a, 1911b; *Freeman's Journal*, 1911a, 1911b, 1911c).[4] Eugenicists
and environmental hygienists sometimes met as antagonists, but the strategies were by no means mutually exclusive, and they aligned on the terrain
of 'infant life protection'. This was a field of discourse shaped initially by
concerns over 'baby farming' and infanticide, and it was codified by a series
of legal reforms that commenced in 1872 and culminated in the Children
Act of 1908 (more on this below). Moreover, it also gained traction through
an emerging science of childhood.

   The British Child Study Association, led by James Sully, was established
in 1894 (Cunningham, 1991: 198). Though the organisation's influence had
already waned by the start of the First World War, it paved the way for
professionally trained psychologists to lay claim to a science of childhood
and education, and part of what made this possible was the idea of racial
'degeneration' or, in the case of Britain, 'national deterioration' (see Pick,
1989). In some respects echoing Rousseau's account of the Fall of Man,
this framed the relation between animal–human, nature–society, savage–
civilised as a battle staged on the terrain of evolution: between the 'fit' and
those deemed to be physically, intellectually and morally 'defective'. Influenced by Ernst Haeckel's biogenetic law (whereby ontogeny is seen to
recapitulate phylogeny), the child-study experts believed that human evolution was recapitulated by the child, and this afforded the means of

scientifically ascertaining the 'raw material of morality' (Sully, 1903). In Sully's words (1903: 8, 325), the 'wild untamed nature' of the child could be 'subdued' by education, but only if the child was educable, and it was this concern that was taken up by school hygiene activists.

Ireland was at this time lagging behind international trends in school medical inspection, the aim of which, according to Theophilus Kelynack (1910: iii) – a Fellow of the Royal Society of Medicine and consultant to the National Association for the Feeble-Minded – was 'to secure the prevention of all disorder and disease in early life'.[5] By 'all' Kelynack meant – quite literally – everything, for the method was to leave nothing unaccounted for. To this end, the procedure entailed disassembling both school and scholar so that each element could be scrutinised, whether physical and mental indicators of disease and defect (eyes, ears, teeth, skin, scalp, speech, 'mental condition'), biometric parameters (age, weight, height), biographical details (personal and family history), environmental factors (heat, air, light), and the arrangement of physical objects and equipment (size and positioning of desks, chairs, windows), with each item meticulously examined and recorded by a panoptic medical gaze (see Howarth, 1910; Reid and Priestly, 1910). Why was this extensive labour to be carried out? There was more than one way of answering that question, but there was also widespread agreement that the future of state and nation hinged on the 'efficiency' of the rising generation (Gogarty, 1912; Moffat, 1911; Story, 1911, 1912; Thompson, 1913).

This notion of efficiency relates to a very specific instrument that warrants attention here: the norm. Nikolas Rose has examined the normalisation of childhood in detail, showing how the idea of developmental milestones – norms against which individual children are measured, and hence also a developmental schedule that children are expected to be able to keep pace with – is essentially a fiction made possible through the interpenetration of school and clinic (1990: 140–143). Such norms were derived by measuring the minds and bodies of individual children grouped together on the basis of relatively arbitrary criteria, such as age, and by aggregating this data. But once transformed into an instrument to evaluate physical or mental functioning, then the measure of normality would no longer necessarily correspond to any particular child, which is why Rose insists that 'normality is not an observation but a valuation' (1990: 131). The purpose of school medical inspection was to 'discover' those children who 'presented some deviation from the normal' – those of a 'low mental grade' who would not benefit from 'ordinary day schools' – and yet practitioners could be quite candid about the lack of consensus in determining the cut-off point between the normal and the abnormal (Howarth, 1910: 36–40; Moffat, 1911: 32). Analogous to Rousseau's theory of Man, the discovery of defect proceeded on the basis of a decision anchored in a fiction, and as with the notion of delinquency, defect was a moral judgement. Among the symptoms

and signs of abnormality were mischievousness, disobedience, angry out-
bursts and deceitfulness. This was taken as evidence not simply of individual
defect, but also inadequate parenting, which was seen to necessitate the
extension of the technique from school to home, so that parents could be
supervised and homes placed under medical surveillance (Moffat, 1911;
Story, 1911; Thompson, 1913). It is here that the practice of medical inspection can be seen to augment the penal reformatory school and connect up
with the discourse of infant life protection.

When viewed retrospectively, the Children Act of 1908 can be taken as
a milestone in a long process that, via the Geneva Declaration of the Rights
of the Child adopted by the League of Nations in 1924, culminated in the
UN Convention on the Rights of the Child (UNCRC). At the time, the
Children Act (or Children's Charter as it was known) was referred to as a
'great charter of the helpless' that would 'recognise the rights of children'
and secure 'the protection of infant life' (Lawson, 1919; Millin, 1912,
1917). The Act consolidated existing statutes and amending laws dealing
with infant life protection, including laws on neglect and cruelty (Barnes,
1989: 86–87), and in many respects simply enlarged the scope of the reformatory strategy. But in creating the instrument of the Juvenile Court it also
proved to be a major innovation in the way it cemented the relation between
law and norm, care and control, prevention and correction. As argued by
Rose (1985: 171), the Juvenile Court 'established the linkage between
familial scrutiny and moralisation on the one hand and the penal system
on the other which remains until today, providing "voluntary" interventions into the lives of families and children with the coercive back-up necessary for them to operate'.

The instruments and techniques of infant life protection extended well
beyond the problems associated with (and attributed to) diseased, malnour-
ished and delinquent children. Assembled through the interpenetration of
school, hospital and prison, and at the intersection of the biological–social,
medical–moral, pedagogical–penal, this was a technology of government
that had already begun to envelop childhood *as such* by the time the Irish
Free State was established, and the strategic objective was to govern both
the *quantity* and the *quality* of life.[6] It was in this sense that childhood was
framed as a 'national asset' to be harnessed with a minimum of waste. This
was to be accomplished by monitoring 'the numbers of our children, their
physical fitness, and their mental development', and by ensuring that each
and every child underwent a combination of treatment and training, thereby
minimising 'the manufacture of criminals and paupers' whilst maximising
the numbers equipped to serve the nation as healthy and efficient workers
(Crichton, 1925: 302–305; Lawson, 1919: 497; Millin, 1917: 316; Ryan,
1917). What I want to examine in the final section below is how policy in
Ireland today is instituting very similar objectives under the rubric of 'reducing health inequalities'.

'Healthy Ireland': governing through inequality

On 13 June 2011, Dr James Reilly, then-Minister for Health, and Frances Fitzgerald, then-Minister for Children, jointly launched a new initiative called *Your Health is Your Wealth*. Reilly explained that 'it's up to us as individuals to take responsibility for our life choices and it's also up to us as a society to make our environment safer and the right choices easier to make' (DoH, 2011). Two years later, following a period of public consultation, the framework was published under the title *Healthy Ireland* which is set to run until 2025 (DoH, 2013). Presented as a policy innovation, *Healthy Ireland* attempts to facilitate a 'shift towards a broader, more inclusive approach to governance for health' (DoH, 2013: 8). What this means is that the Department of Health (DoH) as well as non-state actors with a stake in the health sector are to work in partnership with 'other areas of Government and public services concerned with social protection, children, industry, food safety, education, transport, housing, agriculture and the environment' (DoH, 2013: 8). Moreover, the vision is presented as a 'whole system approach' to governance, meaning that this is an attempt to mobilise and coordinate the 'whole-of-Government' and the 'whole-of-society' (DoH, 2013: 8, 13). Viewed historically, it could be argued that these broad conceptions of health and governance are continuous rather than discontinuous with the past, and so is the way the new strategy prioritises children, which it does. In terms of operationalising the long-term objective, which is about reducing expenditure on 'sickness benefits' while increasing 'productivity and contributions to the exchequer', *Healthy Ireland* reads like the latest phase of a long iterative process: 'The creation of healthy generations of children ... is critical to the country's future' (2013: 12). As was the case in the past, childhood is framed as a strategically important asset: a means of governing the future.

Continuities notwithstanding, it is crucial to note the extent to which the focus on children has intensified in recent years. Also significant is an apparent tension between words and actions. Among the key objectives (or 'targets') to be achieved during the lifetime of *Healthy Ireland* is to reduce health inequalities by 'empowering people and communities' (2013: 24). Viewed in terms of the actions, instruments and agencies tasked with hitting this target, what this means in effect is that one and all must participate in the neoliberal game of inequality. Before drilling deeper into the *Healthy Ireland* framework, I first want to take a closer look at Foucault's analysis of neoliberalism.

The 'enterprise society' as a game of inequalities

In his lectures on the *Birth of Biopolitics*, Foucault examines how neoliberal thought began to take shape during the post-war period and – more specifically – how this took the form of a body of ideas that Foucault interprets as 'state-phobia' (2008: 116, 187). The German ordoliberals for example argued against the idea that the state should steer and manage the market in order to correct or ameliorate its negative social effects (such as unemployment and poverty). Instead, the state should be placed under the supervision *of* the market. In contrast to nineteenth-century laissez-faire liberalism, the ordoliberals did not perceive competition to be a 'given of nature'. Instead, competition was conceptualised as a mechanism or machine that would have to be 'carefully and artificially constructed' (*ibid.*: 118–121). Furthermore, for the machinery of competition to function correctly, there would have to be fluctuation within what Foucault refers to as a 'game of differentiation'. In other words stimulating competition would necessitate inequality among equals, which is why Foucault describes neoliberalism a 'formal game between inequalities' (*ibid.*: 141–143). Neoliberalism is thus more than the policies and mechanisms through which competition is generalised – privatisation, the introduction of new markets, deregulation and so forth – because it also requires instruments of control to manage how the game of inequality is played. These instruments of control measure and monitor the performance of the players, thereby ensuring that as many as possible stay in the game (Donzelot, 2008) while also trying to regulate the behavioural excesses that inevitably accompany intensified competition.

This fusion of competition and control is well established in Ireland, most visible perhaps in the public sector, which has undergone a lengthy process of restructuring through a combination of neoliberal reforms and the introduction of performance management systems (see Lynch, Grummell and Devine, 2012). But this is not just about remodelling the state, and the trend is more accurately captured by Foucault's thoughts on the 'enterprise society' (2008). The enterprise society institutes the principles codified by the *Healthy Ireland* framework, that is, individual responsibility and choice, so that competition and control interface as a governmentality that governs through the subject of enterprise. As Peter Miller and Nikolas Rose point out, the enterprised self, as the embodiment of a regulated autonomy, is 'enjoined to bring the future into the present, and is educated in the ways of calculating the future consequences of actions as diverse as those of diet and home security' (2008: 215). In Ireland this combination of enjoining and educating – which is the 'how' of 'empowering people and communities' envisioned by *Healthy Ireland* – is currently being orchestrated through a 'life cycle' approach to policy, evident in the way that *Healthy Ireland* stipulates that 'supporting people to enjoy a healthy and active life, starting in the womb and continuing through childhood, adolescence, adulthood and older age, is a fundamental goal of this policy Framework' (DoH, 2013: 14). At the same time, and echoing the focus of the reformatory and hygienist strategies examined above, the long-term success of *Healthy Ireland* is seen to hinge on early intervention: 'The most effective time to intervene in terms of reducing inequalities and improving health and wellbeing outcomes is before birth and in early childhood' (DoH, 2013: 14). Bearing in mind that *Healthy Ireland* is premised on a 'whole system approach' (also known as HiAP, or Health in All Policies), it can be conceptualised as a biosocial technology that governs two axes of life: one that extends along the life cycle, and a second that encompasses the entirety of childhood and which is codified in Ireland by the idea of the 'Whole Child'.

Governing the future

Instituted through the *National Children's Strategy* (National Children's Office (NCO), 2000), which ran from 2000–2010,[7] the Whole Child approach to policy recognises that children have the 'capacity' to 'shape their own lives as they grow, while also being shaped and supported by the world around them' (see also DoHC, 2007; DCYA, 2011: 17). Children and young people in Ireland are now regularly consulted as part of the policymaking process,[8] and this conception of children – as active subjects rather than passive objects to be acted upon by authoritative adults – dovetails with (and explicitly defers to) Article 12.1 of the UNCRC, ratified by Ireland in 1992, which stipulates that children should be consulted in matters that affect them (NCO, 2000: 6, 30).[9] This is important to note because the Whole Child meshes with the Whole-of-Government approach to policy, both of which combine as a technology of government which exhibits a strong resemblance to the figure of the Tutor in Rousseau's *Emile*. In other words, this attempts to act *upon* children's actions by structuring the field of possible action, thereby governing *through* their capacity for action.

The Whole Child and the Whole-of-Government together articulate a multi-stranded strategy of surveillance, services, supports and interventions that simultaneously enables and constrains in response to emerging social trends and particular situations, so that the biological and social processes that combine as child development can be monitored and managed through a full spectrum of preventive and remedial measures (see Figure 2.1).

Among the problems that are seen to necessitate intervention are the harmful effects that result from the 'pressure to compete and succeed' (NCO, 2000: 6), and in the *National Children's Strategy* it is noted that not all children have the resilience required to withstand such pressures, which may be exacerbated by poverty and homelessness (linked to drug use and prostitution), or racism and discrimination; may become manifest in harmful behaviours such as smoking, alcohol and drug use (in turn associated with crime and 'anti-social behaviour'); and may culminate in unplanned pregnancy and early school leaving, both of which are detrimental to future employability (NCO, 2000: 6–7). This complex web of situational contingencies is seen to necessitate systematic surveillance, which is

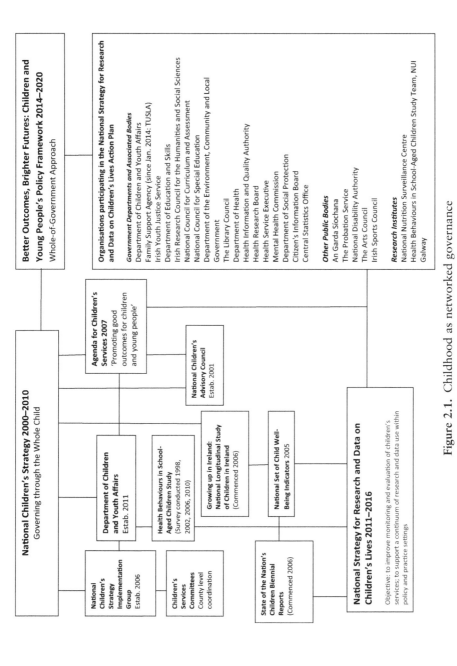

Figure 2.1. Childhood as networked governance

the purpose of the *National Strategy for Research and Data on Children's Lives*. Scheduled to run until 2016, and framed as a 'strategic approach to knowledge about children's lives' that will serve to identify 'the most effective ways to intervene in their lives' (DCYA, 2011: v), this is an innovation that scales-up the technique of school medical inspection.[10] In fact the *Research and Data* strategy is but the latest addition to a series of similar initiatives targeting young life in Ireland, including the *Health Behaviours in School-Aged Children* study (conducted since 1998 by the Health Promotion Policy Unit at the National University of Ireland Galway); the *National Longitudinal Study of Children in Ireland* (which commenced in 2006); and the *State of the Nation's Children Biennial Reports* (which also commenced in 2006; Figure 2.1). The translation of life into data via research is now central to the aims and means of governing childhood, because this is how the lives of those who are to compete in the neoliberal game of inequality are to be measured, monitored and managed. Moreover, when it comes to dealing with problem and risky behaviours, this biosocial apparatus continues the shift from exclusion to inclusion examined above with respect to the strategies of reformatory education and public hygiene. Governing through inclusion today entails ensuring – as far as this is possible – that one and all can withstand 'the pressure to compete and succeed'. There are to be no exceptions, because this is about ensuring an equality of inequality (Foucault, 2008: 142–143). In short, the neoliberal version of egalitarianism dictates that no child be excluded from the opportunity to compete in a race where one's relative position is – apparently – a matter of taking personal responsibility and making the 'right' choices.

Part of a comprehensive networked apparatus, the *Research and Data* strategy collects and stores information on children's lives which is made practical and technical in the form of supports and interventions which act through and upon the actions of children: health services, child welfare and protection, education, juvenile justice, family support, sports council, nutritional surveillance, all of which (in theory at least) combine as 'a continuum of research and data use within policy and practice settings' (see right-hand side of Figure 2.1). It is important to underline what is being proposed here in this idea of a networked apparatus. In the introduction I suggested that this does not exhibit the singularity of a sovereign will, and here I would add that it should not be confused with a 'system' in the Parsonian sense of that word. It is instead an example of what Foucault had in mind when he suggested that power relations are 'intentional' but 'non-subjective'. Non-subjective intentionality is a tactical and strategic game that produces this type of networked apparatus, but as Foucault points out, 'the logic is perfectly clear, the aims decipherable, and yet it is often the case that no one is there to have invented [it]' (Foucault, 1998: 94–95). Otherwise put, this is orchestrated, coordinated and steered as a grid of intentions, but the many actors who participate in this tactical and strategic game need not be singing in chorus or pursuing identical objectives. Friction is in part what enables this type of apparatus to cohere, but to cohere at all it must have an anchoring point, and this is what the figure of the Whole Child accomplishes. Replicating the eighteenth-century fiction of Man, the Whole Child is a biosocial construct assembled from the modern history of childhood: the discourses, the forms of knowledge, the techniques that spiral back in time through the hygienist movement, the strategy of preventive and reformatory education, to the birth of the modern anthropological machine. But if the anthropological machine was originally assembled at the threshold of human and animal, civilised and savage, it now operates solely on the basis of a distinction between those who can and will play the game of inequality from those who cannot or will not keep up with the accelerating pace of competition. This then is what it means to reduce (health) inequalities in the enterprise society, and so this chapter ends where it began, with the supervised and regulated autonomy once envisioned by Rousseau, because in twenty-first-century Ireland, children are routinely forced to be free.

Notes

1 In Rousseau's writings the word 'man' is at times gendered, while at other times it signifies humanity. Here I use it only in the latter sense, and capitalise it to underscore this usage.

2 This distinction was codified by the Reformatory Schools Act 1854 and the Industrial Schools Act 1857.

3 The principle of moral treatment was organised into the first public asylums and penitentiaries in Ireland (see Reuber, 1999).

4 Two years later, following the passage of the Mental Deficiency Act, eugenicists lobbied for the legislation to be extended to Ireland (Dawson, 1913; Jones, 1992: 87).

5 In 1919, the Public Health (Medical Treatment of Children) (Ireland) Bill empowered local authorities to undertake medical inspection and treatment of children in national schools, but there would be no compulsion to do so. Irish Unionist MPs as well as nationalists demanded that the provision be made mandatory, and when government acceded, this became 'the only mandatory public health service on the Irish statute book' (Barrington, 1987: 80, 102).

6 Due to limitations of space, I have presented only a partial sketch of how this was instituted in Ireland. A more thorough account would include both a more detailed discussion of legislation (see Barrington, 1987) as well as the work of the Women's National Health Association of Ireland founded by Lady Aberdeen in 1906, which laid the groundwork for a range of measures to reduce infant mortality, including public health nurses, services for mothers and babies, and school medical inspection (see Keane, 1999).

7 The second phase of this strategy was launched in April 2014 under the title *Better Outcomes, Brighter Futures*, which is very explicit in identifying

children as a national asset. Quoting from the current government's *Medium-Term Strategy for Growth*, the foreword by the Minister for Children and Youth states that 'Our increasing child and youth population is a significant resource for our country … Ensuring the best possible outcomes for this group is therefore an important element in our future economic planning' (DCYA, 2014: viii).

8 A list of National Consultations conducted with children and young people since 2004 is available on the DCYA website: www.dcya.gov.ie/viewdoc.asp?fn=%2Fdocuments%2FChildYouthParticipation%2FNational_Consultations.htm&mn=chiv&nID=5.

9 The wording of Article 12.1 is as follows: 'States Parties shall assure to the child who is capable of forming his or her own views the right to express those views freely in all matters affecting the child, the views of the child being given due weight in accordance with the age and maturity of the child.'

10 The Research and Data Strategy was launched in 2011, the same year as a new Department of Children and Youth Affairs was established, which might be seen as the culmination of a reform processes going back to 1997 when the DoH become the DoH and Children.

References

Agamben, G. (1998) *Homo Sacer: Sovereign Power and Bare Life*. D. Heller-Roazen (trans.). Stanford, Stanford University Press.

Agamben, G. (2004) *The Open: Man and Animal*. K. Attell (trans.). Stanford, Stanford University Press.

Barnes, J. (1989) *Irish Industrial Schools, 1868–1908: Origins and Development*. Dublin, Irish Academic Press.

Barrington, R. (1987) *Health, Medicine, and Politics in Ireland 1900–1970*. Dublin, Institute of Public Administration.

Bauman, Z. (1991) *Modernity and Ambivalence*. New York, Cornell University Press.

Carpenter, M. (1851) *Reformatory Schools for the Children of the Perishing and Dangerous classes*. London, G. Gilpin.

Carpenter, M. (1853) *Juvenile Delinquents, Their Condition and Treatment*. London, W. & F.G. Cash.

Crichton, B. (1925) Infant mortality in Dublin. *Irish Journal of Medical Science*, 4(7): 302–305.

Cunningham, H. (1991) *The Children of the Poor*. Oxford, Blackwell.

Dawson, W.R. (1913) The Mental Deficiency Bill and its proposed extension to Ireland. *The Dublin Journal of Medical Science*, 136(3): 161–167.

DCYA (2011) *National Strategy for Research and Data on Children's Lives 2011–2016*. Dublin, DCYA.

DCYA (2014) *Better Outcomes, Brighter Futures. The Children and Young People's Policy Framework 2014–2020*. Dublin, DCYA. Available from: www.dcya.gov.ie/viewdoc.asp?Docid=3140&CatID=13&mn=&StartDate=1+January+2014.

Dean, M. (1999) *Governmentality: Power and Rule in Modern Society*. London, Sage.

DoH (2011) Your health is your wealth: a policy framework for a healthier Ireland 2012–2012. Press release. Dublin, DoH.

DoH (2013) *Healthy Ireland: A Framework for Improved Health and Wellbeing 2013–2025.* Dublin, DoH.

DoHC (2007) *The Agenda for Children's Services: A Policy Handbook.* Dublin, DoHC.

Donzelot, J. (2008) Michel Foucault and liberal intelligence. *Economy and Society,* 37(1): 115–134.

Faulkner, J. (2011) Innocents and oracles: the child as a figure of knowledge and critique in the middle-class philosophical imagination. *Critical Horizons,* 12 (3): 323–346.

Foucault, M. (1965) *Madness and Civilization: A History of Insanity in the Age of Reason.* New York, Vintage.

Foucault, M. (1977) *Discipline and Punish: The Birth of the Prison.* London, Penguin.

Foucault, M. (1991) Governmentality. IN: Burchell, G., Gordon, C. and Miller, P. (eds) *The Foucault Effect: Studies in Governmentality.* Chicago, University of Chicago Press: pp. 87–104.

Foucault, M. (1997) What is enlightenment? IN: Rabinow, P. (ed.) *Essential Works of Foucault 1954–1984 Volume 1: Ethics, Subjectivity and Truth.* New York, The New Press, 303–320.

Foucault, M. (1998) *The Will to Knowledge: The History of Sexuality Volume 1.* London, Penguin.

Foucault, M. (2003) *Society Must be Defended: Lectures at the Collège de France 1975–1976.* New York, Picador.

Foucault, M. (2008) *The Birth of Biopolitics: Lectures at the Collège de France 1978–1979.* Basingstoke, Palgrave Macmillan.

Freeman's Journal (1911a) Public health congress. 11 August, p. 3.

Freeman's Journal (1911b) Child study and eugenics. 17 August, p. 5.

Freeman's Journal (1911c) Position of the state in regard to eugenics. 18 August, p. 4.

Gogarty, O. (1912) The need for medical inspection of school children in Ireland. *The Dublin Journal of Medical Science,* 132(6): 409–420.

Hall, G.S. (1911) *Adolescence its Psychology and its Relation to Physiology, Anthropology, Sociology, Sex, Crime, Religion and Education.* New York and London, D. Appleton and Company.

Hancock, W.N. (1860) The Aberdeen industrial schools contrasted with Irish workhouses. *Journal of the Statistical and Social Inquiry Society of Ireland,* 3: 6–19.

Haughton, J. (1850) Statistics of crime. *Journal of the Statistical and Social Inquiry Society of Ireland,* 2: 3–14.

Haughton, J. (1857) Education the surest preventive of crime, and the best safeguard of life, property, and social order. *Journal of the Statistical and Social Inquiry Society of Ireland,* 1: 324–334.

Howarth, W.J. (1910) Organisation and administration of the medical examination of scholars. IN: Kelynack, T.N. (ed.) *Medical Examination of Schools and Scholars.* London, P.S. King & Son Orchard House: pp. 33–62.

Irish Independent (1911a) The public health. 16 August, p. 4.

Irish Independent (1911b) Papers at the congress. 18 August, p. 7.

Jones, G. (1992) Eugenics in Ireland: the Belfast Eugenics Society, 1911–15. *Irish Historical Studies*, 28(109): 81–95.

Joyce, P. (2003) *The Rule of Freedom*. London, Verso.

Keane, M. (1999) *Ishbel: Lady Aberdeen in Ireland*. Newtownards, Colourpoint Press.

Kelynack, T.N. (ed.) (1910) *Medical Examination of Schools and Scholars*. London, P.S. King & Son Orchard House.

Lawson, W. (1919) Infant mortality and the notification of births Acts, 1907, 1915. *Journal of the Statistical and Social Inquiry Society of Ireland*, 13: 579–597.

Lentaigne, J. (1885) The treatment and punishment of young offenders. *Journal of the Statistical and Social Inquiry Society of Ireland*, 8: 31–40.

Lynch, K., Grummell, B. and Devine, D. (2012) *New Managerialism in Education: Commercialization, Carelessness and Gender*. Basingstoke, Palgrave Macmillan.

Miller, I. (2013) Constructing moral hospitals: childhood health in Irish reformatories and industrial schools, 1851–1890. IN: MacLellan, A. and Mauger, A. (eds) *Growing Pains: Childhood Illness in Ireland 1750–1950*. Dublin, Irish Academic Press, pp. 105–122.

Miller, P. and Rose, N. (2008) *Governing the Present: Administering Economic, Social and Personal Life*. Cambridge, Polity.

Millin, S.S. (1912) The duty of the state towards the pauper children of Ireland. *Journal of the Statistical and Social Inquiry Society of Ireland*, 12: 249–262.

Millin, S.S. (1917) Child life as a national asset. *Journal of the Statistical and Social Inquiry Society of Ireland*, 13: 301–316.

Moffat, D.M. (1911) The medical inspection of schools. *The Dublin Journal of Medical Science*, 132(1): 27–38.

NCO (2000) *National Children's Strategy: Our Children – Their Lives*. Dublin, National Children's Office.

Pick, D. (1989) *Faces of Degeneration*. Cambridge, Cambridge University Press.

Pim, W.H. (1854) On the importance of reformatory establishments for juvenile delinquents. *Journal of the Statistical and Social Inquiry Society of Ireland*, 3: 3–20.

Procacci, G. (1991) Social economy and the government of poverty. IN: Burchell, G., Gordon, C. and Miller, P. (eds) *The Foucault Effect: Studies in Governmentality*. Chicago, University of Chicago Press: pp. 151–168.

Reid, G. and Priestly, J. (1910) Organisation and administration of the medical examination of schools. IN: Kelynack, T.N. (ed.) *Medical Examination of Schools and Scholars*. London, P.S. King & Son Orchard House: pp. 12–32.

Reuber, M. (1999) Moral management and the 'unseen eye': public lunatic asylums in Ireland, 1800–1845. IN: Jones, G. and Malcolm, E. (eds) *Medicine, Disease and the State in Ireland 1650–1940*. Cork, Cork University Press: pp. 208–233.

Rose, N. (1985) *The Psychological Complex: Psychology, Politics and Society in England, 1869–1939*. London: Routledge and Kegan Paul.

Rose, N. (1990) *Governing the Soul: The Shaping of the Private Self*. London and New York, Routledge.

Rothman, D. (1971) *The Discovery of the Asylum: Social Order and Disorder in the New Republic*. Boston, Little, Brown and Company.

Rousseau, J.J. (1968) *The Social Contract*. Harmondsworth, Middlesex: Penguin.

Rousseau, J.J. (1993) *Emile*. London, J.M. Dent: Everyman.

Rousseau, J.J. (2004) *Discourse on Inequality*. Whitefish, Montana, Kessinger.

Ryan, F.W. (1917) The preparation of national school pupils for technical training and industrial life. *Journal of the Statistical and Social Inquiry Society of Ireland*, 13: 399–418.

Story, J.B. (1911) Medical inspection of schools and school children. *The Dublin Journal of Medical Science*, 131(4): 241–253.

Story, J.B. (1912) Medical inspection of schools and school children. *Journal of the Statistical and Social Inquiry Society of Ireland*, 12: 523–545.

Sully, J. (1903) *Studies of Childhood*. New York, Longmans Green and Co.

Thompson, W. (1913) Medical inspection of school children. *The Dublin Journal of Medical Science*, 136 (3): 161–173.

Wilson, J.M. (1857) Statistics of crime in Ireland 1842–1856. *Journal of the Statistical and Social Inquiry Society of Ireland*, 2: 91–121.

3 Michelle Share and Perry Share

Doing the 'right thing'? Children, families and fatness in Ireland

Introduction

On 10 February 2014, the high-circulation *Irish Independent* newspaper carried 'The Big Issue'. This 'health and living' supplement carried no fewer than 16 articles on the issue of childhood weight, health, activity and diet – framed by the organising concept of the 'growing childhood obesity crisis'. Terms such as 'frightening', 'terrifying', 'chilling' and 'potentially life-threatening' accompanied the inevitable (presumably rhetorical) question, 'is this the generation which will die before their parents because of their weight?'

This supplement, with its highly emotive language, was (and is) by no means untypical. As a growing number of critical writers have observed, construction of the contemporary global 'obesity epidemic' has adopted a similar set of tropes wherever it has emerged. By contrast, 'obesity research critics' question the popular and political consensus that the threat of ever-increasing obesity rates, especially amongst children, is real and urgent. They point to the socially constructed nature of the concept of obesity itself; the vested interests that underpin the medical, scientific and media discourses that surround it; the unintended consequences of the operation of these discourses; and question the very existence of the so-called 'epidemic'.

This chapter analyses recent Irish interventions into the 'obesity' discourse from this critical stance. It focuses on evidence from the first (and increasingly influential) longitudinal study of children in Ireland – *Growing Up in Ireland (GUI)* – and how its findings have entered the media and policy arenas. The analysis is based on secondary documentation, including published reviews of childhood obesity prevalence and *GUI* reports. It builds on earlier research into the framing of children and obesity (and overweight) in Ireland (Share and Strain, 2008).

A governmental discourse operates in Ireland to quantify, individualise and responsibilise the phenomenon of 'obesity', while supporting processes of state and individual (self-)surveillance. This discourse elides complex societal factors and ignores emergent data on children and obesity that point to the *reduced* prevalence of childhood obesity. *In toto* it helps to sustain the myth of a 'childhood obesity epidemic' in Ireland in a way that is potentially damaging to broader issues of public health.

Obesity – a global health and lifestyle issue

Excess bodyweight, adiposity or 'obesity', is considered a major contemporary health and lifestyle issue and 'everyone's concern'. No longer problematic only for industrial countries, increasing obesity is reported across many middle-income and developing nations (WHO, 2014) and has become a key global health issue. In early 2014 the London-based Overseas Development Institute captured global headlines when it revealed over a third of the world's adults to be 'obese or overweight', with the fastest increase (a percentage tripling from 1980 to 2008, or 250 to 904 million people) in the developing world (Keats and Wiggins, 2014). Finucane *et al.* (2011) report that mean BMI (a common if problematic indicator of 'obesity') has increased globally amongst adults since 1980. While under- and malnutrition remain the world's major food policy challenge, affecting an estimated 840 million people (FAO, 2013), the health and economic implications of fatness have come to significantly influence the policies and practices of international organisations and of national governments and health services – including those in Ireland.

This framing of a global obesity 'crisis' occurs alongside an acknowledgement among the research and policy communities that the phenomenon is multifactorial and extends beyond simplistic 'energy-in, energy-out' explanations (Campos *et al.*, 2006). Nevertheless, much research, policy and media reporting continues to mask this complexity. It blurs and oversimplifies issues and draws conclusions and policy recommendations not founded on the facts reported. Such mismatches between available evidence and consequent policy and practice recommendations are not unusual (see Buckingham, 2011: 108 on similar processes for TV advertising and children) but they can have real negative consequences for health policy and practice and for the ostensible targets (in particular, children) of policy and practice interventions (Evans *et al.*, 2008).

A considerable literature has emerged that challenges the mainstream obesity discourse (for example: Oliver, 2006; Coveney, 2006, 2008; Evans *et al.*, 2008; Gard and Wright, 2005; Gard, 2011; Gilman, 2008; Julier, 2008; McCullough and Hardin, 2013; *Critical Public Health*, 2013). It even questions the critical approaches that have emerged from the alternative food movement, such as the work of Michael Pollan (Guthman, 2011). Nevertheless, there is little evidence that mainstream obesity policy or interventions have addressed the issues raised in the critical literature (Moffat, 2010). Public health and social marketing campaigns continue to recirculate overly simplistic and often self-defeating conceptualisations of obesity (Lupton, 2014: 41–42).

Children and obesity

Although the incidence of obesity is highest amongst the adult population of high-income countries (Finucane *et al.*, 2011; Farley, 2015) the policy focus is strongly on children and, often, their mothers (Zivkovic *et al.*, 2010; Friedman, 2015). As Coveney (2008: 203) points out, childhood has 'become a major point of engagement on the war on fat. This extends into areas of children's and families' lives in contexts such as feeding, parenting and sickness where practices can be framed in terms of what is "good" or "bad"'. For Maher, Fraser and Wright (2010: 244) this is reflective of broader societal changes in relation to gender: 'emotions around women's changing roles are mobilised through fears about children's flesh'.

Western societies have long-projected their worries, ideals and concerns for the future onto children (Cross, 2004; Kinchin and O'Connor, 2012; Lee *et al.*, 2014). Gilman (2008: 45) points out that 'childhood obesity comes to hold a special role in defining the dangers to society as a whole'. Evans *et al.* (2008: 15) link the concern with childhood obesity to Victorian 'child saving' movements:

> it has generated something of a moral crusade in which children, perceived as under-socialised into correct ways of eating and exercising, become regarded as maladjusted or pathological, identified as a population 'at risk' of developing obesity and, therefore, in need of 'saving'.

Evans and colleagues are interested in how such 'body-centred talk' impacts on the 'health and embodied subjectivities of young people' themselves (2008: 3). In focusing on and giving voice to those young people susceptible to being labelled as 'obese or overweight', it becomes evident that this perspective is all too rare in the discussion of obesity.

The obesity discourse and its critics

In response to the 'discovery' of the 'obesity epidemic' in the late 1980s (Oliver, 2006; Gilman, 2008: 16) and its subsequent embrace by the media, governments and the medical establishment, a substantial critical counter-discourse has emerged. A significant element of this critique, as we will see, can be couched within a governmentality perspective. Critiques of mainstream obesity discourse concern such issues as: the validity of BMI as a measure; conflation of the terms 'overweight' and 'obesity'; inappropriate use of the term 'epidemic'; critiques of the simplistic 'energy-in, energy-out' formula and of other 'truth claims' made by health professionals, governments and commercial operations; policy and practice responses; neglect of fundamental social factors; the political economy of the food system; and the extension of the clinical gaze and of surveillance of the everyday-life practices of eating and exercise.

Key contributors, from a variety of social scientific perspectives, include Coveney (2006, 2008), Evans *et al.* (2008), Gard and Wright (2005), Gard (2011), Guthman (2011), Gilman (2008), Julier (2008) and McCullough and Hardin (2013) as well as those represented in *Critical Public Health* (2013). The critique includes sustained analyses of how media, government and sectors of the scientific and medical communities socially construct specific public understandings of 'obesity and overweight' in specific ways. Nevertheless, Lupton (2014: 40–41) argues that this extensive counter-discourse has yet to have a significant impact on the hegemony of the mainstream obesity discourse: 'the "truths" of "obesity" science as they are accepted by mainstream public health are re-articulated without any suggestion that there may be a more complex and contentious background to these truths'. Some of these critiques are sketched below, while the reader is directed to the sources for a comprehensive analysis.

'Energy-in, energy-out' and other truth claims

Scientific accounts of obesity are highly complex, volatile and highly contested. If there was a simple agreed explanation for what is seen as excessive weight gain (and its satisfactory resolution) we would no doubt have heard of it by now. This does not prevent numerous actors – from obesity scientists, to dieticians, to diet and fitness gurus of every type – from proclaiming one or other simple answer to the obesity conundrum (e.g. Harcombe, 2012). In reality the links between diet, weight and disease are complex and fraught with numerous 'socionatural entanglements' (Guthman, 2011: 43) across the biological, social, environmental, psychological, political, economic and philosophical fields.

The 'energy-in, energy-out' calorific equation nevertheless retains salience as a starkly simple and attractive explanation (and thus solution) to the problem of excessive weight. It suggests a rational (and thus amenable to governance) 'cause' for obesity. As a spokesperson from the US Department of Agriculture (cited in Guthman, 2011: 91) puts it, 'people eat too much too often, too much of the wrong things, and exercise too little … it's pretty simple'. Even mainstream obesity science recognises that the notion of 'energy balance' is simplistic, rather than simple. Similar warnings apply to the posited linear causative connections between obesity and diabetes, premature death, cancer and other conditions.

The concept of BMI

For Foucault (cited in Henderson, 2015: 327) 'biopower (refers to) the techniques of power that bring "life and its mechanisms into the stream of explicit calculation ... [making] knowledge-power an agent of transformation of human life"'. The obesity discourse rests on a simple calculation: the standard measure of 'obesity' is the BMI – a ratio defined as an individual's body mass divided by the square of their height: expressed as kg/m^2. BMI has been widely adopted internationally, as an indicator – and definer – of 'obesity'. As Ian Hacking, key philosopher of the historical/social role of enumeration and quantification, notes, 'quantification has an intrinsic tendency to generate new classifications of people' (Hacking, 2007: 308) – the category of 'obese' requires a definitional measurement: BMI. In terms of the governmentality of health and everyday life, BMI has come to provide an excellent mechanism, expressed through a single index, for 'identification, classification, ordering and control' (Huff, 2006), in an analogous way to IQ (for 'intelligence') or cholesterol level (as a measure of cardio-vascular health). As Evans and Colls (2009: 1062) suggest, 'the status of the BMI in anti-obesity policy is indicative of the status afforded numbers in governmental practices'.

Nevertheless, it has been recognised that as a measurement tool BMI is severely limited (Guthman, 2011: 26–45), particularly when used for individual diagnostic purposes. It does not take into consideration, for example, gender or ethnic differences, nor different body types and differential distribution of fat and lean mass. It has been identified as an inaccurate measure of 'obesity' in black males, in particular (Cawley, 2013), and of specific population groups such as athletes and older people. Ernsberger (2012) makes the startling point that BMI may be a relatively good indicator of health risk, but that excessive lean tissue, not fat, is the problematic issue. In some cases BMI calculation is now complemented by additional measurements such as skin-fold and waist circumference; but these types of data are considerably more time-consuming and expensive to gather than height and weight (Guthman, 2011: 27) and so remain comparatively underused in epidemiological studies and public health campaigns.

BMI is even less satisfactory as a measure of childhood 'obesity'. It is well recognised that the measurement and classification of obesity in children and adolescents are complex, owing to the effects of age, sex and stage of maturity (Kipping, Jago and Lawlor, 2008; Dinsdale, Ridler and Ells, 2011; NICE, 2013). Duncan et al. (2014: 1) note that 'BMI is not normally distributed in children and thus, when used in statistical analysis, assumptions of normality are violated and inferences made cannot be trusted'. Given the high level in variability in children, the BMI figure itself cannot be used diagnostically at an individual level, therefore children are measured and referred to the statistical distribution of BMI across the relevant population, using special charts. BMI thus becomes a measure of relationship to the norm and not meaningful in any diagnostic sense. This is not to say that specific morbidity-related issues associated with levels of adiposity in some children cannot be detected (Duncan *et al.*, 2014) – but in itself BMI is a very crude and often misleading indicator of current or future medical issues.

This begs the question, Why is BMI so widely used? Its attractiveness lies in the power of a singular index to represent a complex and poorly understood reality (Evans and Colls, 2009). In this it reflects a technology of power through quantification. In terms of individual 'diagnosis' it can (like IQ) be used to evaluate the 'worth' of an individual in relation to a population as a whole. When expressed for a population or segment of a population (such as the people of inner city Dublin, or 'black women') it can be mobilised as an evaluative and moral critique. As Young (2013: 2) notes in relation to cognate research on 'problem gambling', how we 'identify, define and measure [a] problem is intrinsically a socio-political process rather than an objective revelation of an underlying naturalistic phenomenon'. In the discourse of the pathological gambler prevalence study, notes Young, 'politically it does not matter how accurate [the indicators] actually are … having an imperfect instrument plays the same role as a perfect one'. A similar observation can be made for BMI: its increasingly contentious status as a 'health indicator' has not diminished its power as it is circulated and recirculated through traditional and social media (such as the RTÉ television/radio/online product *Operation Transformation*, or newspaper 'health' supplements such as that referred to earlier). For Evans and Colls (2009: 1054) BMI in itself 'constitutes a mechanism of biopower'.

Conflation of overweight and/or obesity

A feature of the obesity crisis literature is that the terms 'obese/ity' and 'overweight' are often linked or – arguably – conflated (Moffat, 2010: 6–7). Even in terms of the measurement of BMI (problematic as it is) they have very different meanings and sets of implications for health and well-being. Nevertheless, as Gard (2011: 12) points out,

> when most people talk about the obesity epidemic they usually do so … in a way that collapses these two categories, thereby greatly increasing the number of people who actually meet the technical definition of obesity. In fact it is doubtful whether the idea of an obesity epidemic would exist at all without this conceptual slippage.

As we will see, childhood obesity rates in Ireland (as defined) appear at within a range of 4% to 7% of the population. It is regularly reported in Western countries, including Ireland, that between a quarter and a third of children are 'overweight or obese' – clearly a much more dramatic figure:

one that might stimulate prompt media interest, medical intervention or government action. Such conflation has been described as 'all too common' in the obesity debate (McNaughton, 2013a) and it is of further concern that these terms themselves are now frequently conflated with others such as 'Type 2 diabetes' in such a way that implies a simple connection between them (McNaughton, 2013b).

Use of term 'epidemic'

The term 'epidemic' has been widely (if controversially) used, in the scientific and medical literature, in political and policy discourse, and in the media, to label the recent increase in observed rates of obesity (Mitchell and McTigue, 2007). In this regard the use of the term 'epidemic', as the 'rampant and widespread occurrence of a disease at a particular time' (as described by the *Oxford English Dictionary*), may be considered inaccurate and sensational. Guthman (2011: 32), critical of the current obesity discourse, disapproves of the use of this word, which she considers loaded: 'the epidemic language is somewhat cruel, simultaneously minimising the violence of serious plagues and overstating the association of corpulence with death'.

For Gilman (2008: 14–43) the notion of 'epidemic' gels with that of 'moral panic'. It is associated with ideas of contagion, infection and fear and supports the demonisation of a group of 'infected persons we openly disdain' (*ibid*.: 21). The categorisation of a cohort of morally suspect, medically (and socially) threatening individuals serves to perpetuate practices that we might otherwise find threatening or intrusive, such as mandatory weighing (and public shaming) of children: controlling actions that are not without consequence but, as Evans *et al.* (2008: 33) argue, can be 'ultimately deeply damaging to some young people's health'. The language of 'epidemic' aligns with a governmentality discourse in which 'everyone' is at risk (Henderson, 2015) and thus open to exceptional levels of social control. When it comes to children, mothers in particular must be seen to exercise prudence and 'good' mothering through the management of self and children for the public good – otherwise they risk attracting personal culpability (Maher, Fraser and Wright, 2010; Friedman, 2015) for their children's adiposity.

Children, overweight and obesity in Ireland: the data

In Ireland, as in most other Western countries, there has been increasing public concern with overweight and obesity in children and young people. Until relatively recently there has been limited measurement data on children's height and weight; Layte and McCrory (2011: 14) note that such data in an Irish context is 'comparatively rare' while Keane *et al.* (2014) point out that 'trends in childhood overweight and obesity in the Republic of Ireland have not been examined in the last decade [i.e. since 2002]'.

Baseline evidence on children's height and weight was made available through the 1948 *Irish Nutrition Survey*, with no further data collection until 1970 (Perry *et al.*, 2009). As the public health issue of 'overweight and obesity' has become more prominent, research into child weight in Ireland has increased, particularly over the last decade. There is now some record of data collection and this reveals a consistent picture over time: a significant increase in average height and a (disproportionate) increase in average weight of Irish children from the period immediately after the Second World War to the early years of this millennium (Perry *et al.*, 2009), followed by a stabilisation and subsequent reduction in childhood obesity rates.

In 2002 Whelton and colleagues (Whelton *et al.*, 2007) compiled information on a sample of 17,499 children in the Republic of Ireland, aged 2 to 16 years. They reported that 28% of girls and 23% of boys were overweight, within which 7% of girls and 6% of boys were obese. The Irish Universities Nutrition Alliance (IUNA, 2005, 2008) reported studies (conducted in 2003–2004 and 2005–2006) of 5–12 year-olds ('children') and 13–17 year olds ('teens'). Amongst the children 17.4% were overweight and 6.7% were defined as obese. Amongst the 'teens', 15.2 % of boys and 14.7% of girls were overweight and 2.7% of boys and 3.2% of girls were obese. A 2007 study (Barron, Comiskey and Saris, 2009) of the height and weight of 969 children aged 4.5 to 13.5 years in Co. Kildare found 17.6% of girls and 17.8% of boys to be overweight, whereof 7.1% of girls and 6.6% of boys were defined as obese. The findings from these studies are summarised in Table 3.1. They reveal consistent patterns of overweight and obesity among Irish children.

Most recently a systematic review of fourteen relevant studies of Irish primary school-aged children in the period 2002–2012 (Keane *et al.*, 2014) has indicated 'a slight decrease in obesity prevalence over the period' with no significant trend in 'overweight'. National-based studies over a similar period show a decline in obesity rates from 7% to 4% (*ibid.*: 12). The latest report from the Childhood Obesity Surveillance Initiative (Heinen *et al.*, 2014) shows that from 2008 to 2012, rates of obesity declined from 4.7% to 2.2% for 7-year-old boys; for similarly aged girls the rate dropped from 7.5% to 5.5%. These are significant declines in childhood obesity rates.

This data is consistent with an OECD report (2012) that points to stabilisation in childhood obesity rates in England, France, Korea and the USA. In the case of Liechtenstein, Kühnis and Erne (2012) also report on a stabilisation of child overweight and obesity during a six-year observation period (2004–2010) using cross-sectional data for children aged 5–14 and report on other evidence of such stabilisation in Switzerland, France and

Table 3.1 Overweight and obesity amongst Irish children and young people

	Boys overweight %	Girls overweight %	Boys obese %	Girls obese %
IUNA (2005) 5–12 yrs (n=594)	17.4		6.7	
Whelton et al. (2007) (n=17,499)	23	28	6	7
Barron et al. (2009) (n=969)	17.6	17.8	6.6	7.1
IUNA (2008) 13–17 yrs (n=440)	15.2	14.7	2.7	3.2

Sweden. Gard (2011: 37–68) observes a stabilisation of obesity rates in a range of societies that includes the USA, the UK, New Zealand and Canada.

Ogden et al. (2014) of the US Centre for Disease Control indicate that obesity rates amongst US children aged two-to-five years have declined by a substantial 43% during the previous decade. This report reinforced earlier findings in the UK (HSCIC, 2013) that indicated evidence of a recent reversal of the trend towards higher levels of childhood 'overweight or obesity'. These reports are further evidence of a general plateauing of the incidence of obesity (not just amongst children) in Western societies (Gard, 2011: 37–68).

The inescapable conclusion is that over the first decade of the millennium, childhood obesity rates in Ireland, as in a number of other Western societies, have *not* increased; rather they have started to stabilise and even to considerably decline.

Irish state response to obesity: the *Taskforce* report

At the mid-point of this stabilisation in childhood obesity (2005), the *Irish Taskforce on Obesity* issued an extensive report that contained a number of recommendations for policy and practice in relation to the management of obesity (DoHC, 2005). The *Taskforce* comprised twenty members, representing medicine, dietetics, health promotion, food safety, sports science and the food industries – all of whom have strong vested interests in the obesity phenomenon. Its terms of reference required it to develop a strategy to halt the rise and to reverse the prevalence of obesity.

In a review of the *Taskforce* report Share and Strain (2008) observed that while it did acknowledge the multifaceted and complex nature of the obesity issue, its subsequent recommendations ultimately reflected a specific and limited governmentality discourse. In particular, it favoured personal and familial responses over structural change, and saw the education sector as the primary locus of action, as opposed to other potential areas, such as 'high-level government' or 'food, commodities, production and supply'. Where it did suggest 'appropriately targeted practical action' this applied predominantly to the education and health sectors; by contrast only broad-based recommendations were outlined for the government and food sectors. In this it focused on horizontal strategies of governmentality, rather than vertical structures of governance (Huff, 2006).

In particular the *Taskforce* specifically recommended techniques whereby schools and individuals would participate in health promotion activities and surveillance of weight status. Families and children were to be responsibilised to protect against the risks of overweight and obesity through educational and lifestyle interventions. Schools, a key site for such interventions, were viewed as 'level playing fields' and broader social, economic, cultural and institutional forces and inequalities were not considered (Share and Strain, 2008). For Koopman (2014: 103) such an approach to 'public health' becomes a 'biopolitical project' for 'making live' at the level of population, as well as having disciplinary power at the level of the individual.

Since publication of the *Taskforce* recommendations, the issue of child overweight and obesity has continued to occupy a significant position in relation to the health and welfare of Irish children. An interim progress report on the implementation of the recommendations (DoHC, 2009) was critical of the minimal observed impact on policy and practice. Subsequent failure to progress many of the recommendations of this interim report has also been critically noted (Layte and McCrory, 2011). Nevertheless, the desire for the Irish government to 'do something' continues: for example as expressed at the launch of a multimedia campaign to 'take on childhood obesity' by Minister for Health James O'Reilly TD (Irish Member of Parliament) and Minister for Children Frances Fitzgerald TD on 21 October 2013 (Safefood, 2013).

Growing Up in Ireland – a new data source on children in Ireland

The work of the *Taskforce* was constrained by the perceived paucity of information on Irish people. Figures for the incidence of obesity and overweight had to be crudely extrapolated from UK data. Subsequently, the emergence of data from the National Longitudinal Study of Children, *Growing Up in Ireland* (*GUI*), has provided an enhanced knowledge base in relation to children and families and the contexts in which they live their lives.

Data from such longitudinal studies is a relatively recent arrival on the Irish social scientific scene, though these are well established in other western states. Given their expense and scale, such studies are typically conducted by state or state-sponsored bodies: *GUI* is conducted by the Economic and Social Research Institute in partnership with Trinity College Dublin and funded by the Department of Children and Youth Affairs in association with the Department of Social Protection and the Central Statistics Office. It is arguable that such longitudinal studies, as a specific type of statistical construct, are an increasingly significant governmental technique, segueing as they do from processes of data collation to those of normative discourse: from what 'is' to what 'should be' by virtue of compelling narratives of what is 'normal' at the national level. Nevertheless, there has been little critique of such longitudinal studies in terms of governmentality: such commentary as exists has tended to focus on established ethical issues such as beneficence and healthcare provision, informed consent, privacy, distributional justice and sustainability (Carrel and Rennie, 2008; WHO, 2015).

GUI aims at a holistic understanding of Irish children, conducted within Bronfenbrenner's ecological framework. It seeks 'to provide evidence for the creation of effective and responsive policies and services for children and families' (Greene *et al.*, 2010: 28), based on its primary objective, 'to describe the lives of Irish children, *to establish what is typical and normal* as well as what is atypical and when it is problematic' (Greene *et al.*, 2010: 5 – emphasis added). In its claim to represent the reality for *all* Irish children the project represents a key normalising process, especially given the unprecedented scale of the exercise. The first wave of data collection involved two cohorts of children and their primary caregivers: 10,000 9-month-olds and their primary caregiver (Infant Cohort) and 9,000 9 year olds and their primary caregiver (Child Cohort). Children from the first wave have so far been followed up at three and five years, and the 9 year olds at thirteen years.

As part of the broad remit to understand Irish children's health and well-being over time, a number of reports have been released that specifically address children's health and well-being, including weight issues:

- *Overweight and Obesity among 9-year-olds* (Layte and McCrory, 2011)
- *Nine-year-olds on their Health and Well-being* (Child Cohort Qualitative Key Findings 2, 2011) (*GUI*, 2011a)
- *Key Findings Infant Cohort (at Age 3). No. 1 The Health of Three-year-olds* (*GUI*, 2011b)
- *Children's Physical Growth from Birth to Age 3* (Infant Cohort Wave 2 Key Findings 4, 2012) (*GUI*, 2012a)
- *Physical Activity and Obesity among 13-year-olds* (Child Cohort Wave 2 Key Findings 2, 2012) (*GUI*, 2012b)
- *Well-being, Play and Diet among Five-year-olds* (Infant Cohort Wave 3 Key Findings 3, 2013) (*GUI*, 2013)
- *Development from Birth to Age Three* (Williams *et al.*, 2013)

Table 3.2 Obesity: *GUI* and prior studies compared

Study	% defined as 'obese' at age in years							
GUI (2011–2013)	*3 years*		*5 years*		*9 years*		*13 years*	
	boys	girls	boys	girls	boys	girls	boys	girls
	5%	6%	5%	6%	5%	8%	5%	8%
Whelton *et al.* (2007)	n/a	n/a	5%	7%	9%	9%	4%	5%
IUNA (2005)	n/a	n/a	*5–12 year olds*				*13–14 year olds*	
			6.7%				boys	girls
							5.3%	3.2%

When we compare the data from these reports with earlier studies of Irish children's overweight and obesity, we find a similar profile to that identified in the studies of a decade earlier (Table 3.2), with *no* recorded increase in obesity rates. The *GUI* data (Williams *et al.*, 2013) shows that 5% of boys and 6% of girls were obese at age 3. At ages 5, 9 and 13, a consistent 5% of boys were obese; girls showed a greater diversity: at 5 years old 6% were defined as obese, while 8% of both 9 and 13 year olds were obese.

The *GUI* findings reflect cross-sectional reporting, but we can also see patterns in the longitudinal data collected by the study. In relation to *overweight* data for the Infant Cohort, 19% of 3 year olds were classified as overweight – 19% of girls and 18% of boys (Williams *et al.*, 2013: 35). Two years later, at age 5, 17% of girls and 13% of boys were overweight: a small decline (*GUI*, 2013: 5). At age 3, 5% of boys and 6% of girls were obese (Williams *et al.*, 2013: 35) and by the time they were 5 years old this proportion remained exactly the same (*GUI*, 2013).

There is a similar picture with the Child Cohort: 17% of boys and 22% of girls in the 9-year-old cohort were described as 'overweight' (Layte and McCrory, 2011: 14); four years later these same children at age 13, had virtually unchanged rates of 'overweight' – 18% for boys and 22% for girls (*GUI*, 2012b: 4). At age 13, the rate of obesity for boys and for girls remained constant at 5%, and 8% respectively (*GUI*, 2012b: 4).

The data from the *GUI* longitudinal study support a strong argument *against* the proposition that childhood obesity (or overweight) is on the increase. *GUI* reports that the substantial majority of children in all age cohorts (3, 5, 9 and 13 years) were *not* overweight (76%; 80%; 75%; 74%, respectively). Furthermore, though we have noted the apparent stability of overweight and obesity across the age cohorts, the *GUI* study also documents where children have moved between weight categories. While overweight from age 9 to 13 has remained virtually unchanged, the *GUI* study has reported a decline for some groups of children who were previously categorised as overweight or obese.

Thus, 89% of non-overweight 9 year olds were still not overweight at age at 13, while 10% had moved into the overweight category, and just 1% had become obese. At the same time, while just over half of those identified as overweight at aged 9 remained so at 13, a third had become non-overweight (with 11% becoming obese). For those who were obese at age 9, half remained in the same category while 40% had become over-weight and 11% were non-overweight – in other words over half of the 9 year olds defined as 'obese' had moved out of this category by the age of 13: hardly cause for panic.

A similar picture emerges from ages 3 to 5 for the Infant Cohort. Although it conflates overweight and obesity in its reporting, the report (*GUI*, 2011b: 5) states that '24% of *GUI* children were overweight or obese at three years, while at five years this figure has dropped slightly to 20%, due to a drop among those who were overweight'. In addition, nine out of ten children (91%) who were in the non-overweight category at age 3 remained so at age 5. Again, as with the Child Cohort, there is evidence of stabilisation of obesity: the rate remained the same at 5% between ages 3 and 5. Furthermore, there is evidence of children moving between catego-ries. For example, while 38% of those who were obese at age 3 were still obese at age 5, 37% moved to the overweight category and 25% moved into the not-overweight group. Thus, the majority of 'obese' 3 year olds were no longer obese at age 5: a finding that might call for some positive response.

We report these figures in some detail, as they fly directly in the face of the public rhetoric in relation to childhood obesity. The previously men-tioned *Irish Independent* childhood obesity supplement claims that 'more and more children are facing potentially life-threatening health problems' (Health & Living supplement, 10 February, 2014: 4); in one article Dr Donal O'Shea, prominent Irish anti-obesity campaigner, is quoted to the effect that we are witnessing 'an obesity epidemic that is killing thousands of people and harming children psychologically and physically' and that 'we're in a disaster situation' (*ibid.*: 12–13).

Contrary to Whelton *et al.* (2007: 8), who claim to 'provide further compelling evidence on the emergence of the obesity epidemic among chil-dren in Ireland', the *GUI* longitudinal data provides evidence of a stabilisa-tion of childhood overweight and obesity and, in some instances, a reversal of trends. Analysis of relevant *GUI* data has the potential to provide a clearer understanding of overweight and obesity among Irish children, in particular in terms of its multifaceted complexity, from which policy may be developed.

This is not what has happened. Rather, the 'headline' figures from the *GUI* study have become part of the established 'obesity epidemic' discourse in Ireland: for example the specific finding and wording (Layte and McCrory, 2011: 20) that 'a quarter of [Irish] children at four years of age are overweight or obese', was repeatedly (pp. 5, 6, 11 and 18) reproduced if unattributed (though on one occasion (p. 18) erroneously to 'Safefood') in the *Irish Independent* supplement mentioned earlier. Publication of the *GUI* report on 'overweight and obesity among 9-year-olds' (Layte and McCrory, 2011) has (whatever the intent of its authors) provided an undoubted stimulus to the emergence of a more sustained 'obesity epidemic' discourse. The provision of numerical data from an Irish population has allowed for specific claims in relation to obesity to be made: though *not* in terms of one of the key findings of the study: that of a stabilisation or even reduction in obesity incidence amongst children (e.g. Fig. 2.4 on p. 16 of Layte and McCrory, 2011 indicates a slight reduction in childhood 'overweight and obesity' from 2002 to 2007).

We could legitimately ask, where is the 'obesity epidemic' so readily propagated by the Irish media, medical profession, researchers (including representatives of the state-funded *GUI* project) and advocacy groups – and, furthermore, how and why is it being so promoted? This is not only a matter of inevitable cherry-picking of data by media outlets keen to reflect news values of negativity (Hartley, 2013: 78; Boero, 2013) but is also found in the 'scientific' literature. For example, the first sentence of the report by Heinen *et al.* (2014: 3) – a report that reveals a substantial *decrease* in Irish childhood obesity – states, 'the prevalence of obesity in children is rapidly rising'. The rates of childhood 'obesity and overweight', which we now know have declined, are described by a senior Health Service Executive (HSE) manager in the introduction to the same report (*ibid.*: 2) as an 'alarming statistic'. In whose interests is it to maintain the existence of the 'epidemic' and to frame our understanding of childhood obesity in this negative way? How might this powerful medicalised discourse impact on Irish children and young people and on the broader population? What is the impact of a discourse about children's health that is repeatedly expressed in terms of risk and threat?

Framing overweight and obesity

As we have shown, the evidence on children's weight strongly indicates that overweight and obesity is *not* a cause for concern amongst the substantial majority of children in Ireland. Over time there is evidence of a general plateauing and subsequent decline in overweight and obesity, in line with that experienced in other comparable countries. We now consider some examples of how child fatness nevertheless continues to be framed as a pervasive and urgent issue in Irish society: operating as a form of potentially oppressive biopower, specifically aimed at children and young people and their parents/caregivers – primarily mothers. First, we examine how the *GUI* research frames children's overweight and obesity in terms of its reporting and policy recommendations. We then illustrate media responses to the issue.

Growing Up in Ireland

So far we have observed that the *GUI* findings in relation to children's weight indicate that for the substantial majority of children in Ireland, fatness is not a cause for concern, and is certainly not the 'epidemic' that is regularly reported. The data on children's weight is in line with other studies that show that obesity is not on the increase, but is declining. Moreover, the *GUI* data shows that across age cohorts it is possible for a reversal of trends: overweight and obese children can, and do, become non-obese and non-overweight: obesity is not a 'life sentence'.

The *GUI* study is interested in understanding the multidimensionality of children's lives in order to comprehend what is typical and atypical – what we can be persuaded to understand as 'normal'. It uses a multidisciplinary relational model that

> adopts a dynamic systems perspective founded on five multidisciplinary insights from different disciplines: ecology, dynamic connectedness, probabilism, period effects and the active role or agency of the child in the developmental process. The bioecological model of Urie Bronfenbrenner is a key tool in constructing this conceptual framework. (Greene *et al.*, 2010: 28)

The bioecological model emphasises that to understand children's development we must examine the 'proximate' and 'distal' contexts in which they live, to include family, friends, local community and wider sociocultural environment. According to the WHO (2002: 13), 'proximal factors act directly or almost directly to cause disease, and distal causes are further back in the causal chain and act via a number of intermediary causes'. As *GUI* has a specific goal to produce research evidence to inform the development of government policy, it is useful to examine how it frames overweight and obesity and to consider how 'proximate' and 'distal' contexts inform the study findings and policy recommendations.

Policy implications identified in *GUI* report

Some policy implications for child overweight and obesity are identified in the *GUI* reports for 3 year olds (Williams *et al.*, 2013) and 9 year olds (Layte and McCrory, 2011). The report on the 3 year olds states,

> *Evidence of the early emergence of an overweight and obesity problem:* The finding that a quarter of three-year-olds are already overweight or obese is a major concern. Although more acute in the most socio-economically

Table 3.3 Conflation of overweight and obese in *GUI* reports

3 year olds	5 year olds	9 year olds	13 year olds
'One in four three-year-old children were overweight or obese' 'Of greater concern is the proportion of these very young children who are already overweight or obese – approximately one in four'	'One-in-five five year olds was overweight or obese'	'A quarter of nine-year-old children in the GUI study are defined as being overweight or obese'	'One in four were either overweight or obese'
GUI, 2011a; Williams et al., 2013	*GUI*, 2013	Layte and McCrory, 2011: 20	*GUI*, 2012b

disadvantaged group, it is a problem across all levels of society and further work is needed to identify the pathways that are leading to what is now being termed an 'epidemic' in some circles. (Williams *et al.*, 2013: 22)

We can observe that by conflating overweight and obesity this statement serves to exaggerate the issue. This pattern of conflation can be found across the reports (Table 3.3).

Despite reference to a particularly 'acute' incidence of 'overweight and obesity' amongst 'socio-economically disadvantaged' groups (an issue known to be highly complex), the report nevertheless echoes an 'everyone-at-risk obesity discourse' that is manifested as an 'epidemic': more work is to be done – by all of us.

In the report (Layte and McCrory, 2011) on the 9 year olds, which specifically addresses issues of overweight and obesity, six areas are identified for policy action:

1. Identification of overweight and obesity
2. Promoting behavioural change
3. Dealing with underlying disadvantages
4. Current government initiatives
5. Health promoting environments
6. Promoting healthy weight without stigmatisation

Of these areas, the report makes specific statements with policy implications for just the first three. In relation to the others, statements are limited to a reiteration of the research findings, and a description and critique of current government initiatives without specific recommendations or implications for policy.

The call for *identification of overweight and obesity* favours individual-istic health promotion and a medicalised response to obesity. It focuses on the role of parents, who

> need to be better informed about the healthy weight for their child, while stigmatisation of being overweight should be avoided, given the problems this can produce. Accurate parental perception of child weight would be helped if the heights and weights of children were routinely measured when they visit their GP and the parents informed of the child's BMI and its implications for their current and future health. (Layte and McCrory, 2011: 56)

This section goes on to recommend that if such a service was provided as part of the General Medical Service contract parents could also receive their BMI at the same time, though there is no indication that this offer/intrusion would serve any particular purpose.

This medicalised response through the assessment of child BMI extends to the education sector:

> The child's school offers another opportunity to measure weight status. Child vaccination and dental and optical checks are already part of the public health nurse routine in Irish schools (PHN). Consideration should be given to the inclusion of height and weight measures in this routine. Unlike visits to GPs, checks in schools would not automatically include parents, but nurses could subsequently make contact with patients if appropriate resources were pro-vided. (Layte and McCrory, 2011: 57)

Again, reflecting a governmentality discourse, the approach is individual-ised and does not comprehend any level of societal or even institutional change: rather it embraces a primitive 'technology of the self' (as reflected in the ubiquitous image of the lo-tech tape measure in obesity-related texts). There is a simplistic assumption that knowledge of weight, height and BMI in itself will lead to positive behavioural outcomes. It neglects to consider the negative social and psychological impact of such processes in schools, for children of both 'normal' and deviant weight status. This issue has been little explored, but is assessed in very critical terms by Evans *et al.* (2008). Evaluation of the impact of the UK Child Measurement Programme (Syrad *et al.*, 2014) suggests that such programmes are inef-fective in bringing about desired behaviour change amongst children and their parents.

Policy implications that favour *behavioural change* reflect an individual-ised 'energy-in, energy-out' response to the prevention of overweight and obesity. While Layte and McCrory (2011: 58–59) acknowledge that not all sport takes place in schools, they do have a particular focus on the role of the education sector in promoting sport and exercise. Also within a behav-ioural change context they make a strong statement that suggests that parent education about child activity and diet can impact positively on behaviour:

> Evidence from England suggests that the upward trend in obesity has pla-
> teaued among more socially advantaged groups. Studies are ongoing, but this
> may have occurred because parents heeded public health warnings and inter-
> vened to change their own and their children's behaviour. This would suggest
> that the upward trend in Ireland is not immutable and that education cam-
> paigns among parents on issues around diet, physical activity and sedentary
> activities may be effective as long as parents are given concrete guidelines
> about children's activities. (Layte and McCrory, 2011: 57)

As is obvious, there is a lot of speculation here, on a number of levels, as to any social mechanisms that may be at play.

The third area that outlines some policy implications, *dealing with underlying disadvantages*, emphasises that the risk factors for obesity have a pronounced socio-economic distribution; this is a conclusion also arrived at by Keane *et al.* (2014) and Heinen *et al.* (2014). What is proposed responsibilises lower socio-economic schools and the delivery of further targeted interventions through the Delivering Equality of Opportunity in Schools Programme (DEIS). The report does acknowledge (Layte and McCrory, 2011: 58) that the DEIS programme does require broader cross-sectoral government leadership to address wider socio-economic factors. But it is possible that the renewed focus on 'disadvantaged' children will, in practice, reinforce a 'child saving' discourse (Smith, 2014: 172) rather than a focus on the complex factors that contribute to body size for this or any category of children.

The *GUI* reports (in particular the full-length 'Research Reports' pub-lished by the programme) do provide considerable amounts of data to illustrate the proximal and distal factors relevant to understanding over-weight and obesity. But the above analysis suggests that consequent policy implications tend to centripetally revert to individualistic health promotion with suggestions for new initiatives that are not evidence-based. In this they reflect the Australian anti-obesity social marketing campaigns critiqued by Lupton (2014). In spite of the acknowledged difficulties of reporting research and policy implications (a stated aim of *GUI*), and the pressures that researchers face in presenting statements of direction for governments (Glasby, 2011), such reporting reverberates in media and policy and becomes embedded in 'truth claims' about childhood obesity. In the following section we briefly examine the media reporting of the *GUI* findings.

Media reporting of *GUI* obesity data

As might be expected, when launched, *GUI* reports receive substantial media attention. They are normally launched by a government minister, most often the Minister for Children, whose own department co-funds and oversees the study. Although the full *GUI* reports do arguably consider the multidimensionality of children's lives, when statements or recommendations are made that relate to policy implications, they tend to stray from the study framework towards simplistic responses that responsibilise individuals to adopt lifestyle change and engage in medicalised management of weight.

Despite the presentation of findings that indicate positive trends, there is a tendency to present a view of all children being 'at risk' of obesity, reflective of pervasive discourses that construct the 'riskiness' of childhood and adolescence (France and Utting, 2005; Smith, 2014: 189). For example, though the report of findings on 13 year olds (*GUI*, 2012b) indicates that few of those who were non-overweight at age 9 became overweight at age 13, it still claims that 'child overweight and obesity are increasing' (*GUI*, 2012b: 1). It is not clear what evidence – if any – supports this claim.

How the *GUI* presents its findings might contribute to the sensationalist media reporting as demonstrated by the *Irish Independent* health supplement discussed earlier. While *GUI* reporting tends to endorse responsibilisation of children and parents, the extent to which *GUI* 'is responsible' in its approach to framing child overweight and obesity requires some consideration. Images used in the *GUI* reports, such as *Overweight and Obesity among 9-year-olds*, further support simple and reductionist responses to obesity: a tape measure frames the first chapter of the report and an image of a child standing on a weighing scales frames the second chapter (indeed the ubiquitous tape measure appears in Safefood childhood obesity campaigns and on the cover of the Childhood Obesity Surveillance Initiative report). Almost identical visual devices are used in the Australian social marketing campaigns described by Lupton (2014), presaging the broader trend towards the 'quantified self' and the 'participatory biocitizen' (Swan, 2012). One could argue that more useful images might be those of the boardrooms of major global food corporations; the machinery used to add additional sweeteners to industrial food; or the heavy vehicular traffic that keeps many children indoors.

At a *GUI* conference on 27 November 2013 in which findings from ages 3 to 5 were publicly released, media coverage continued to present the 'alarming' fact that one fifth of Irish children were overweight or obese (O'Sullivan, 2013, in the *Irish Examiner*) – not that obesity rates had remained stable. Similarly Sheehan in the *Irish Independent* (of the same date) quoted the study's principal investigator as follows: 'Although in overall terms their health is very good, overweight and obesity continue to be a major concern at five years of age.' Sheehan goes on to state that 'the report shows that 20 percent of five-year-olds are overweight or obese, though that was down from 25 percent at age three'. While it is welcomed that the downward trend was reported, there has, it would seem, been little effort made on the part of the study itself or those who report it in the media, to frame a positive picture of stabilisation and a possible downward trend in obesity.

At the launch of the Safefood childhood obesity campaign mentioned earlier, the media reported on references to overweight and obesity and Irish children by the government ministers involved, drawing on *GUI* data. For example,

> Minister for Children Frances Fitzgerald said some statistics on the weight of Irish children pointed to an appalling vista for some children: 'I can still remember the shock I felt when I heard from the Growing Up in Ireland study that 25 per cent of our three-year–olds were obese or overweight'. Research showed that 6 per cent of three year olds were obese. (Healy, 2013, in *The Irish Times*)

In the same reportage, Healy quotes then-Minister for Health, James Reilly, a medical doctor, who makes the sensationalist statement, 'If we don't tackle our problem with childhood obesity we are in danger of becoming the first generation to bury our children.' In the first case, as we have seen, the Irish childhood obesity rate of 6% has not substantially altered in over a decade of data-collection; in the second there is no evidence to support the claim: it is in fact what Gard (2011: 7) has described as a 'rhetorical virus' – 'spread for no other reason than [its] sheer dramatic effect'.

Media reporting about *GUI* and its 'obesity' data mimics the study findings and reflects an uncritical acceptance of the dominant obesity discourse. Despite mounting evidence to the contrary, this pervasive discourse places 'everyone at risk': all people (and especially parents) are exhorted to 'do the right thing' and engage in efforts to protect against fatness. Such a response, in which there is an uncritical acceptance of the need for children and families – indeed ultimately all individuals – to engage in efforts to address obesity, extends and supports governmental techniques in which individuals are responsibilised to participate in self-surveillance to ward against future risks, even when the evidence suggests otherwise.

Conclusion

The framing of childhood obesity illustrates how 'governmentality works by positioning or representing a problem in particular ways' (Coveney, 2008: 210). This chapter sought to undertake an analysis of Irish childhood obesity discourse and, in particular, how the *GUI* study has been mobilised to construct a specific reality of this phenomenon. The social construction of this 'myth' of the 'childhood obesity crisis' can be understood through a governmentality analysis that draws attention to the impact and the techniques of quantification; processes of normalisation;

responsibilisation of individual children and their families; and the endorsement of techniques of surveillance and self-surveillance. It also points to the longitudinal study as a technique of governmentality: one that would repay further analysis.

The influential role of *GUI* is clear. As an explicitly rational, quantitative and 'scientific' statement of what is 'typical' and 'atypical' it establishes, within both social scientific and public policy discourses, the limits of accepted variability in child body size. It deploys quantified 'biopolitical data' to identify groups of children who deviate from the desired 'rational' body-weight norm. It also links specific measurements to (negative) social and health consequences, linking personal responsibility for weight management to public social and fiscal responsibility. It has perpetuated a discourse of normalisation and responsibilisation that was evident in prior Irish public policy documents (Share and Strain, 2008). In symbolic terms, the ubiquitous image of the tape measure is a metaphor for both the process of quantification and the domestication of the issue – every house in Ireland has (or can easily get) one.

We have shown that in Ireland, childhood obesity, as detailed in the *GUI* study, is not 'epidemic' or even on the increase. In common with many other Western countries, Ireland is witnessing a stabilisation and evidence of a decline of obesity among children. Notwithstanding this evidence from the influential and officially sanctioned *GUI* study, dissemination of the research by the researchers themselves, and subsequent responses from policymakers and the media, fails to highlight or even to recognise this challenge to the dominant discourse of 'everyone' – particularly children – being 'at risk' of obesity. By contrast, there is a consistent focus on individual responsibility and, in particular, the role of mothers and schools to protect against future health risks. We observe an uncritical acceptance across the Irish research and policy communities that childhood weight is an issue for all children and their parents and that individualised responses in families, in schools, on sports fields and in medical clinics are required.

Even when there is counterfactual evidence in relation to the 'childhood obesity epidemic', political actors (such as the Irish government ministers for children and for health) and the mainstream media, such as the *Irish Independent* and RTÉ (through its *Operation Transformation*), urge such individualised actions: rather than state action or intervention, except for largely symbolic exercises such as the use of devices such as measuring tapes and scales. We would contend that such efforts are misguided at best, and may be more serious in deflecting attention from other issues of child health and well-being – such as poverty and inequality. There is a need for critical and honest reflection amongst the Irish research and policy community about what we know and should do about childhood obesity. An analytical approach informed by a governmentality frame can assist in such a reflection.

References

Barron, C., Comiskey, C. and Saris, J. (2009) Prevalence rates and comparisons of obesity levels in Ireland. *British Journal of Nursing*, 18(13): 799–803.

Boero, N. (2013) Obesity in the media: social science weighs in. *Critical Public Health*, 23(3): 371–380.

Buckingham, D. (2011) *The Material Child: Growing Up in Consumer Culture*. Cambridge, Polity.

Campos, P., Saguy, A., Ernsberger, P., Oliver E. and Gaesser, G. (2006) The epidemiology of overweight and obesity: public health crisis or moral panic? *International Journal of Epidemiology*, 35(1): 55–60.

Carrel, M. and Rennie, S. (2008) Demographic and health surveillance: longitudinal ethical considerations. *Bulletin of the World Health Organization*, 86: 612–616. Available from: www.ncbi.nlm.nih.gov/pubmed/18797619. Accessed 24 February 2016.

Cawley, J. (2013) The economics of obesity. *NBER Reporter 2013/4*. Cambridge, MA, National Bureau of Economic Research. Available from: www.nber.org/reporter/2013number4/cawley.html. Accessed 24 February 2016.

Coveney, J. (2006) *Food, Morals and Meaning: The Pleasure and Anxiety of Eating*. London, Routledge.

Coveney, J. (2008) The governance of girth. *Health Sociology Review*, 17(2): 199–213.

Critical Public Health (2013) Special issue – obesity discourse and fat politics: research, critique and interventions. 23(3).

Cross, G. (2004) *The Cute and the Cool: Wondrous Innocence and Modern American Children's Culture*. New York, Oxford University Press.

Department of Education and Science (2005) *DEIS: (Delivering Equality of Opportunity in Schools) An Action Plan for Educational Inclusion*. Department of Education. Available from: www.education.ie/en/Publications/Policy-Reports/deis_action_plan_on_educational_inclusion.pdf. Accessed 24 February 2016.

Dinsdale, H., Ridler, C. and Ells, L. (2011) *A Simple Guide to Classifying Body Mass Index in Children*. Oxford, National Obesity Observatory. Available from: www.noo.org.uk/uploads/doc/vid_11601_A_simple_guide_to_classifying_BMI_in_children.pdf. Accessed 24 February 2016.

DoHC (2005) *Obesity: The Policy Challenges. The Report of the National Taskforce on Obesity*. Dublin, DoHC.

DoHC (2009) *Report of the Intersectoral Group on the Implementation of the Recommendations of the National Task Force on Obesity*. Dublin, DoHC. Available from: www.thehealthwell.info/node/773742. Accessed 24 February 2016.

Duncan, M., Martins, C., Silva, G., Marques, E., Mota, G. and Aires, L. (2014) Inverted BMI rather than BMI is a better predictor of DEXA determined body fatness in children. *European Journal of Clinical Nutrition*, 68: 638–640.

Ernsberger, P. (2012) BMI, body build, body fatness, and health risks. *Fat Studies: An Interdisciplinary Journal of Body Weight and Society*, 1(1): 6–12.

Evans, B. and Colls, R. (2009) Measuring fatness, governing bodies: the spatialities of the Body Mass Index (BMI) in anti-obesity politics. *Antipode*, 41(5): 1051–1083.

Evans, J., Rich, E., Davies, B. and Allwood, R. (2008) *Education, Disordered Eating and Obesity Discourse*. London, Routledge.

FAO (Food and Agriculture Organization of the United Nations) (2013) *The State of Food Insecurity in the World 2013* [Executive summary]. Rome, FAO. Available from: www.fao.org/docrep/018/i3458e/i3458e.pdf. Accessed 24 February 2016.

Farley, T. (2015) The problem with focusing on childhood obesity. *New York Times*, 18 December, p. A39.

Finucane, M., Stevens, G., Cowan, M., Danaie, G., Lin, J., Paciorek, C., Singh, G., Guitterez, H., Lu, Y., Bahalim, A., Farfadzar, F., Riley, L. and Ezzati, M. (Global Burden of Metabolic Risk Factors of Chronic Diseases Collaborating Group (Body Mass Index)) (2011) National, regional, and global trends in body-mass index since 1980: systematic analysis of health examination surveys and epidemiological studies with 960 country-years and 9.1 million participants. *Lancet*, 377: 557–567.

France, A. and Utting, D. (2005) The paradigm of 'risk and protection-focused prevention' and its impact on services for children and families. *Children and Society*, 19: 77–90.

Friedman, M. (2015) Mother blame, fat shame, and moral panic: 'obesity' and child welfare. *Fat Studies*, 4: 14–27.

Gard, M. (2011) *The End of the Obesity Epidemic*. London, Routledge.

Gard, M. and Wright, J. (2005) *The Obesity Epidemic: Science, Morality and Ideology*. London, Routledge.

Gilman, S. (2008) *Fat: A Cultural History of Obesity*. Oxford, Polity.

Glasby, J. (ed.) (2011) *Evidence, Policy and Practice: Critical Perspectives in Health and Social Care*. Bristol, The Policy Press.

Greene, S., Williams, J., Layte, R., Doyle, E., Harris, E., McCrory, C., Murray, A., O'Dowd, T., Quail, A., Swords, L., Thornton, M. and Whelan, C. (2010) *Growing Up in Ireland National Longitudinal Study of Children: Background and Conceptual Framework*. Dublin, Office of the Minister for Children and Youth Affairs.

GUI (2011a) *Nine-year-olds on their Health and Well-being. Child Cohort Qualitative Key Findings 2*. Available from: www.growingup.ie/index.php?id=62. Accessed 24 February 2016.

GUI (2011b) *Key Findings Infant Cohort (at Age 3). No. 1 The Health of Three-year-olds*. Available from: www.growingup.ie/index.php?id=61. Accessed 24 February 2016.

GUI (2012a) *Children's Physical Growth from Birth to Age 3. Infant Cohort Wave 2 Key Findings 4*. Available from: www.growingup.ie/index.php?id=61. Accessed 24 February 2016.

GUI (2012b) *Physical Activity and Obesity among 13-year-olds. Child Cohort Wave 2 Key Findings 2*. Available from: www.growingup.ie/index.php?id=62. Accessed 24 February 2016.

GUI (2013) *Well-being, Play and Diet among Five-year-olds. Infant Cohort Wave 3 Key Findings 3*. Available from: www.growingup.ie/index.php?id=61. Accessed 24 February 2016.

Guthman, J. (2011) *Weighing In: Obesity, Food Justice and the Limits of Capitalism*. Berkeley, University of California Press.

Hacking, I. (2007) Kinds of people: moving targets. Paper read to British Academy, 11 April. Available from: www.britac.ac.uk/events/archive/hacking-ba.cfm. Accessed 24 February 2016.

Harcombe, Z. (2012) *The Obesity Epidemic*. Public lecture at Cardiff Metropolitan University, 7 February. Available from: www.youtube.com/watch?v= ysoScJ2Q5RQ. Accessed 24 February 2016.

Hartley, J. (2013) *Understanding News*. London, Routledge.

Healy, A. (2013) Minister calls for action to tackle clear danger of childhood obesity. *The Irish Times*, 22 October.

Heinen, M., Murrin, C., Daly, L., O'Brien, J., Heavey, P., Kilroe, J., O'Brien, M., Scully, H., Mulhern, L., Lynam, A., Hayes, C., O'Dwyer, U., Eldin, N. and Kelleher, C. (2014) *The Childhood Obesity Surveillance Initiative (COSI) in the Republic of Ireland: Findings from 2008, 2010 and 2012*. Dublin, HSE.

Henderson, J. (2015) Michel Foucault, governmentality, health policy and the governance of childhood obesity. IN: Collyer, F. (ed.) *The Palgrave Handbook of Social Theory in Health, Illness and Medicine*. London, Palgrave Macmillan.

HSCIC (Health and Social Care Information Centre) (2013) *National Child Measurement Programme (NCMP) England 2012/13 School Year*. Available from: www.hscic.gov.uk/catalogue/PUB13115/nati-chil-meas-prog-eng-2012–2013-rep.pdf. Accessed 24 February 2016.

Huff, R. (2006) Governmentality. IN: Bevir, M. (ed.) *Encyclopedia of Governance*. Thousand Oaks, California, Sage: pp. 389–391.

IUNA (2005) *National Children's Food Survey*. Available from: www.iuna.net/?p=27. Accessed 24 February 2016.

IUNA (2008) *National Teen's Food Survey*. Available from: www.iuna.net/?p=29. Accessed 24 February 2016.

Julier, A. (2008) The political economy of obesity: the fat pay all. IN: Counihan, C. and van Esterikj, P. (eds) *Food and Culture: A Reader*. London, Routledge.

Keane, E., Kearney, P., Perry, I., Kelleher, C. and Harrington, J. (2014) Trends and prevalence of overweight and obesity in primary school aged children in the Republic of Ireland from 2002–2012: a systematic review. *BMC Public Health*, 14: 974.

Keats, S. and Wiggins, S. (2014) *Future Diets: Implications for Agriculture and Food Prices*. London, Overseas Development Institute. Available from: www.odi.org.uk/ sites/odi.org.uk/files/odi-assets/publications-opinion-files/8776.pdf. Accessed 24 February 2016.

Kinchin, J. and O'Connor, A. (2012) *Century of the Child: Growing by Design 1900–2000*. New York, Museum of Modern Art.

Kipping, R., Jago, R. and Lawlor, D. (2008) Obesity in children. Part 1: epidemiology, measurement, risk factors, and screening. *British Medical Journal*, 337(7675): 922–927.

Koopman, C. (2014) Michel Foucault's critical empiricism today: concepts and analytics in the critique of biopower and infopower. IN: Faubion, J. (ed.) *Foucault Now: Current Perspectives in Foucault Studies*. Cambridge, Polity.

Kühnis, J. and Erne, S. (2012) Stabilisation in the prevalence of childhood overweight in Liechtenstein between 2004 and 2010. *Schweizerische Zeitschrift für 'Sportmedizin und Sporttraumatologie'*, 60(1): 4–7. Available from: www.sgsm.ch/

fileadmin/user_upload/Zeitschrift/60–2012–1/Stabilisation_1_2012_Kuehnis. pdf. Accessed 24 February 2016.

Layte, R. and McCrory, C. (2011) *Growing Up in Ireland National Longitudinal Study of Children: Overweight and Obesity among 9-year-olds*. Dublin, Government Publications.

Lee, E., Bristow, J., Faircloth, C. and MacVarish, J. (2014) *Parenting Culture Studies*. Basingstoke, Palgrave Macmillan.

Lupton, D. (2014) 'How do you measure up?' assumptions about 'obesity' and health-related behaviors and beliefs in two Australian 'obesity' prevention campaigns. *Fat Studies: An Interdisciplinary Journal of Body Weight and Society*, 3(1): 32–44.

Maher, J., Fraser, S. and Wright, J. (2010) Framing the mother: childhood obesity, maternal responsibility and care. *Journal of Gender Studies*, 19(3): 233–247. Available from ro.uow.edu.au/cgi/viewcontent.cgi?article=2070&context=edupa pers. Accessed 24 February 2016.

McCullough, M. and Hardin, J. (eds) (2013) *Re-constructing Obesity: The Meaning of Measures and the Measure of Meanings*. Food, Nutrition, and Culture Series, vol. 2. New York, Berghahn.

McNaughton, D. (2013a) 'Diabesity' and the stigmatizing of lifestyle in Australia. IN: McCullough, M. and Hardin, J. (eds) (2013) *Re-constructing Obesity: The Meaning of Measures and the Measure of Meanings*. New York, Berghahn: pp. 71–86.

McNaughton, D. (2013b) 'Diabesity' down under: overweight and obesity as cultural signifiers for Type 2 diabetes mellitus. *Critical Public Health*, 23(3): 274–288.

Mitchell, G. and McTigue, K. (2007) The US obesity 'epidemic': metaphor, method, or madness? *Social Epistemology*, 21(4): 391–423.

Moffat, T. (2010) The 'childhood obesity epidemic': health crisis or social construction? *Medical Anthropology Quarterly*, 24(1): 1–21.

NICE (National Institute for Clinical Evidence) (2013) *Managing Overweight and Obesity Among Children and Young People: Lifestyle Weight Management Services*. Public health guidance, PH47. Available from: publications.nice.org. uk/managing-overweight-and-obesity-among-children-and-young-people-lifestyle-weight-management-ph47/recommendations. Accessed 24 February 2016.

OECD (2012) *OECD Obesity Update 2012*. Paris, OECD. Available from: www.oecd.org/health/49716427.pdf. Accessed 24 February 2016.

Ogden, C., Carroll, M., Kit, B. and Flegal, K. (2014) Prevalence of childhood and adult obesity in the United States, 2011–2012. *Journal of the American Medical Association*, 311(8): 806–814.

Oliver, J. (2006) *Fat Politics: The Real Story behind America's Obesity Epidemic*. New York, Oxford University Press.

O'Sullivan, C. (2013) 'Growing Up in Ireland' links screen time to child behavioural difficulties. *Irish Examiner*, 27 November.

Perry, I., Whelton, H., Harrington, J. and Cousins, B. (2009) The heights and weights of Irish children from the post-war era to the Celtic tiger. *Journal of Epidemiology and Community Health*, 63: 262–264.

Safefood (2013) Safefood launches campaign to take on childhood obesity. Press release. Available from: www.safefood.eu/News/2013/safefood-launches-campaign-to-take-on-childhood-ob.aspx. Accessed 24 February 2016.

Share, M. and Strain, M. (2008) Making schools and young people responsible: a critical analysis of Ireland's obesity strategy. *Health and Social Care in the Community*. Special edition on health and social care needs of children and young people. 16(3): 234–243.

Sheehan, A. (2013) Children from poorer homes 'watch more TV and eat fattier foods'. *Irish Independent*, 27 November.

Smith, K. (2014) *The Government of Childhood: Discourse, Power and Subjectivity*. Basingstoke, Palgrave Macmillan.

Swan, M. (2012) Health 2050: The realisation of personalized medicine through crowdsourcing, the quantified self, and the participatory biocitizen. *Journal of Personalized Medicine*, 2: 93–118.

Syrad, H. *et al.* (2014) Health and happiness is more important than weight: a qualitative investigation of the views of parents receiving written feedback on their child's weight as part of the National Child Measurement Programme. *Journal of Human Nutrition and Dietetics*, 28(1): 47–55.

Whelton, H., Harrington, J., Crowley, E., Kelleher, V., Cronin M. and Perry, I. (2007) Prevalence of overweight and obesity on the island of Ireland: results from the North South Survey of Children's Height, Weight and Body Mass Index, 2002. *BMC Public Health*, 7: 187.

WHO (2002) *The World Health Report 2002*. Geneva, WHO.

WHO (2014) *Health Topics: Obesity*. Available from: www.who.int/topics/obesity/en. Accessed 24 February 2016.

WHO (2015) *Global Health Ethics: Key Issues*. Geneva, Global Network of WHO Collaborating Centres for Bioethics, WHO. Available from: apps.who.int/iris/bitstream/10665/164576/1/9789240694033_eng.pdf. Accessed 24 February 2016.

Williams, J., Murray, A., McCrory C. and McNally, S. (2013). *Growing Up in Ireland National Longitudinal Study of Children: Development from Birth to Age Three*. Research report, wave 2, report no. 5, Executive summary. Dublin, The Stationery Office.

Young, M. (2013) Statistics, scapegoats and social control: a critique of pathological gambling prevalence research. *Addiction Research and Theory*, 21(1): 1–11.

Zivkovic, T., Warin, M. Davies M. and Moore V. (2010) In the name of the child: the gendered politics of childhood obesity. *Journal of Sociology*, 46(4): 375–392.

32 and 37 inches – the healthy body and the politics of waist circumference: a governmental analysis of the *Stop the Spread* campaign

> We believe, in any event, that the body obeys the exclusive laws of physiology; and that it escapes the influence of history, but this too is false. The body is molded by a great many distinct regimes; it is broken down by the rhythms of work, rest, and holidays; it is poisoned by food or values, through eating habits or moral laws; it constructs resistances. (Foucault, 1984 [1971]: 87)

Introduction

In a novel departure in Irish public health promotion, in 2011 250,000 free measuring tapes were distributed via pharmacies throughout Ireland to encourage people to measure their waists. This was part of the *Stop the Spread* (STS) campaign which sought to change people's perception of a healthy and normal waist size. Its central message was that a waist circumference above 32 and 37 inches for women and men, respectively is overweight and an indicator of particular health risks. By distributing free measuring tapes the campaign urged people to measure their waists to assess how they fared against these thresholds. This gifting of measuring tapes was part of a larger media campaign, including television and radio commercials and a website with videos, tools and other resources related to body size, weight and diet aiming to encourage people to lose weight, reduce their waist circumference and thus reduce their risk of diseases indicated by waist measurements above the prescribed limits. The campaign also sought to highlight the fact that almost two thirds of people in Ireland exceeded the recommended waist circumference measurements. Using an ominous horror film aesthetic in its first of two television advertisements, the controversial campaign cast the problem of being overweight as a virus spreading within communities to unsuspecting individuals whose notion of normal waist size is erroneously shaped by what they see as the average or normal waist size in their obesogenic social networks as opposed to a biologically based norm. At first glance the campaign can be located within the larger policy concern about obesity which has been part of the international public health agenda since the early 2000s and which is Share and Share's central concern in Chapter 3. In this chapter I suggest that such campaigns are equally important for how they construct and what they tell us about obesity's presumed opposite, namely the healthy body and healthy body size. In particular the chapter aims to analyse how one's waist has become political, or how the construction and regulation of healthy body size, specifically the size and shape of one part of the body, the waist, has become a biopolitical concern.

As Foucault documented the body has, since the 'birth of the clinic' and the accompanying clinical gaze, been the centre of power relations. Such relations rest on the construction of the normal and the abnormal body through particular truths and norms, rooted in the dominance of biomedical knowledge of the body and the proliferation of disciplinary and regulatory techniques of power in the treatment of disease and the pursuit of health. By the end of the twentieth century, what might be called the late modern clinic sees biomedicine shift and expand its gaze from disease to health and from cure to risk (Vaz and Bruno, 2003). Consequently biomedical knowledge and scrutiny spreads in diverse ways beyond the site of the clinic (Howson, 2013). In particular, health promotion policy has become the vehicle by which governments have used biopedagogical strategies, a term used to use to conjoin biopower and pedagogy, to construct and regulate the healthy body (Wright, 2009; Harwood, 2009). Biopedagogy includes the tactics used to educate people about their health, of how they should understand their corporeality, the signs and coordinates of both the healthy and unhealthy body, and the strategies to enable people to work on themselves and engage in practices and regimes to strive for a healthy body. Biopedagogical discourses fuse together biomedical, socio-economic and moral discourses to inform and cajole individuals about nutrition and physical activity. Specific prescriptions about what to eat and in what quantity, as well as exercise, how much and how often, and advocations to monitor both, are, in more recent health promotion policy, being augmented by specific attention to the monitoring of body size through techniques that calculate the size of the body and offer categories that correlate body size with health and disease. In this regard the *STS* campaign reflects a shift in biomedical discourse from calculations based on BMI–waist circumference. This is underpinned by a raft of research findings that suggest that waist circumference is a more reliable correlate of central adiposity or abdominal fat distribution and a risk indicator of a range of illnesses such as Type 2 diabetes, cardiovascular disease and certain cancers (WHO, 2000, 2011). In this chapter I suggest that this campaign illustrates a change in biopedagogical instructions and techniques in health promotion. Therefore, in addition to the more established focus on health-promoting *behaviour* as a sign or indicator of health, this shift emphasises the *appearance* of the body. Moreover the shift involves not only the appearance of the body or body size as a whole, but specific body parts, instating a reductive and highly visible register of what and who is healthy or unhealthy, normal or abnormal.

This emphasis on bodily appearance and bodily composition in terms of where and what types of fat are located in the body is, in turn, reflective of what Novas and Rose (2000) have termed 'somatic individuality'. This is a concept indicative of the particular way in which we are governed, relate to and modulate our bodies in the late twentieth and early twenty-first centuries. As defined by Rose (2007a: 96), it is

> the tendency to define key aspects of one's individuality in bodily terms, that is to say to think of oneself as 'embodied', and to understand that body in the language of contemporary biomedicine. To be a 'somatic' individual, in this sense, is to code one's hopes and fears in terms of this biomedical body, and to try to reform, cure, or improve oneself by acting on that body ... it involves understanding troubles and desires in terms of the interior 'organic' functioning of the body ...

Seeing STS as an instrument of governance or the making of somatic individuals also helps to illuminate the increasing invasiveness of neoliberal governmentality. Typically neoliberal governmentality amplifies individualised forms of government, privileging the individual and their ability to exercise freedom, choice and responsibility as the means of change. Bio-power is thus manifested in ways that, as Rose (1999) puts it, obliges us to be free. Campaigns such as STS, in their move from a focus on health-promoting activities to a notion of healthy bodily appearance, tighten or restrict the ways in which, to reword Rose's formulation, we are obliged to be healthy. They mark increasingly invasive interventions in terms of how we think about our bodies and work on them, revealing the gap between neoliberalism's belief in individual freedom and its readiness to encroach on and mould that freedom with increasing precision. In this regard STS is critically examined in the light of recent debate, which to a degree was anticipated by Foucault (2008) in his brief remarks on neoliberalism in the 1970s, on understanding neoliberalism and neoliberal government. Such debate pays more attention to how neoliberalism can in practice be particularly directive and interventionist in its use of techniques and strategies to make people fit for the market (Peck, 2010; Cahill, Edwards and Stilwell, 2012). Thus in the case of understanding health promotion under contemporary neoliberal governmentality, norms and behaviour are steered with increasing specificity, while health and its determinants remain within a highly individualised frame of reference.

The chapter therefore seeks to make three core points about the STS campaign. It highlights it as a shift in terms of biopedagogies to a more restrictive, reductive and increasingly visible register of health; it links this shift with the concept of somatic individuality and governing the body in this sense; and finally it examines the particular ways in which it is indicative of contemporary manifestations of a more invasive neoliberal governmentality. In order to examine the campaign across these three lines of inquiry the chapter is structured as follows. First, a cluster of conceptual tools coming from Foucault's work on power, in particular his discussions of disciplinary power, biopower and governmentality and his brief remarks on neoliberalism, is outlined for the purposes of broadly locating *STS* within a Foucauldian conceptual framework. This discussion also draws on some recent Foucauldian scholarship in order to extend the relevance of such concepts to twenty-first-century movements in biopolitics and neoliberalism, and in order to set out an analytical framework by which *STS* can be analysed. To ground the analysis the chapter then makes use of a set of a questions offered by Rabinow and Rose (2006) in their discussion of biopower as a plane of actuality, and elaborated on by Harwood (2009) in her outline of an analytical approach to biopedagogy. Thus, *STS* is analysed in terms of three elements: truth, power and subjectification. The first refers to truth produced about life, that is, the biopedagogical message the campaign asserts about health and waist size. The reference to power brings into focus the power relations the campaign effectuates in terms of bodies and health and the ways in which the campaign uses tactics indicative of a more invasive neoliberal governmentality. Finally the focus on subjectification entails analysis of the campaign in terms of how it encourages people to think about and work on themselves, and how somatic individuality is constituted, but also resisted, through bodily composition and waist size.

Foucault, biopolitics and the body

As Koopman (2014: 108) observes, Foucault's work offers both conceptual and analytical resources for what he calls a 'critical empiricism', which 'is a form of critique whereby we can engage how we are conditioned today, in all our complexity and contingency'. The concepts of biopower and governmentality are central to this critical empiricism. In a nutshell, biopower, as Foucault (2003: 241) put it, refers to the power to '"make" live and "let" die'. He deployed it to mean a generative or productive power, concerned with how people actually lived and the administration of their health, security and well-being, upon which the security of the state, including its economic and military security, rests. Foucault contrasted biopower with sovereign power. Characteristic of premodernity, the more absolute, negative nature of the power of the sovereign meant that 'he can, basically, either have people put to death or let them live', in short, 'take life or let live' (Foucault, 2003: 240, 241). While sovereign power is in marked contrast with biopower, disciplinary power, in a chronological sense at least, can be located between the dominance of sovereign power and the rise of biopower. Moreover it is not to be seen directly contrasting with biopower, but, as Foucault puts it, 'dovetailing' with it. In the seventeenth and eighteenth centuries the proliferation of disciplinary power could be seen in 'the emergence of techniques of power that were essentially centred on the body, on the individual body' and included 'a whole system of surveillance, hierarchies, inspections, bookkeeping, and reports' (Foucault, 2003: 242) in order to increase the productive force of individual bodies. Such techniques were made possible by the spread of institutions, such as schools, asylums and prisons, as sites that allowed for panoptic relations and the observation, ordering and disciplining of bodies at close hand. By the second half of the eighteenth century Foucault suggests that 'a new technology of power', namely biopower, can be seen emerging. Crucially he does not see it as displacing disciplinary power but merging with it. Biopower thus

> does not exclude disciplinary technology, but it does dovetail into it, integrate it, modify it to some extent, and above all, use it by sort of infiltrating it, embedding itself in existing disciplinary techniques. This new technique does not simply do away with the disciplinary technique, because it exists at a different level, on a different scale, and because it has a different bearing area, and makes use of very different instruments. (Foucault, 2003: 242)

To distinguish their scale and techniques Foucault (2003: 243) referred to the latter as an individualising power – 'an anatomo-politics of the human body' – and the former as a massifying power, concerned with the quality and characteristics of the population as a whole. While disciplinary power was built upon knowledge and surveillance of individual bodies, biopower operates with such knowledge scaled to population level in order to regulate its productive force. Made possible or brought into being by the 'avalanche of printed numbers' (Hacking, 1982: 281),

> the mechanisms introduced by biopolitics include forecasts, statistical estimates, and overall measures. And their purpose is not to modify any given phenomenon as such, or to modify a given individual in so far as he is an individual, but, essentially, to intervene at the level of their generality. The mortality rate has to be modified or lowered; life expectancy has to be increased; the birth rate has to be stimulated. (Foucault, 2003: 246)

The common ground between both disciplinary and biopower, as Foucault notes, is the focus on the body. Moreover both types of power operate with reference to norms, in particular medical norms. Foucault therefore suggested that by the nineteenth century medical knowledge is,

> if not the most important element, an element of considerable importance because of the link it establishes between scientific knowledge of both biological and organic processes (or in other words, the population and the body), and because, at the same time, medicine becomes a political intervention-technique with specific power effects. ... [T]here is one element that will

> circulate between the disciplinary and the regulatory, which will also be
> applied to body and population alike, which will make it possible to control
> both the disciplinary order of the body and the aleatory events that occur
> in the biological multiplicity. The element that circulates between the two is
> the norm. The norm is something that can be applied to both a body one
> wishes to discipline and a population one wishes to regularise. (Foucault,
> 2003: 252–253)

At this point, then, it becomes apparent that we can analyse *STS* as a campaign which is targeted at both the individual body, through techniques such as the measuring and monitoring of waist size at the individual level, and the population, through the regulatory techniques the campaign uses to spread the word about the dangers or 'epidemic' of overweight and oversized waists. The medically derived norms for waist size, or the numbers 32 and 37, are at the core of the campaign and circulate between its two levels: the proportion of the population with oversized waists and supposedly at heightened risk of particular diseases, and, at an anatamo-political level, each individual who needs to be made aware of and apply the norm to their own bodies. However, the disciplinary techniques of *STS* at the anatamo-political level are not dependent on direct institutional measuring, recording and monitoring, but on individual measuring and monitoring and what Foucault called techniques of the self. For this reason it is necessary to locate biopower and its two poles within Foucault's later work on governmentality, power and the self, and subsequent scholarship on neoliberal governmentality.

Foucault's interest in what he termed governmentality served in part to reorient his interest in biopower. In this regard, he noted how it was important to look at how power, or government, a term with which he gradually replaced his reference to power, was problematised and rationalised in its own right. Thus he traced how both state and non-state actors pondered what he called the 'art of government' (Foucault, 2000a: 201) from the sixteenth century onwards. Returning to the distinction between sovereign power and biopower, Foucault tied the latter to questions of how to govern and how best to govern. Whereas sovereign power was and is about the imposition of the law such that obedience to law could be seen as an end in itself and a reflection of the power of the sovereign,

> with government it is a question not of imposing law on men but of disposing things: that is, of employing tactics rather than laws, and even of using laws themselves as tactics – to arrange things in such a way that, through a certain number of means, such-and-such ends may be achieved. (Foucault, 2000a: 211)

The emphasis on tactics and arrangements meant that for Foucault the focus of analysis is not on the state itself but on the dispersal of power, down to the level of individuals and how individuality is shaped and patterned. The use of tactics to shape individuality is at the heart of Foucault's concept of governmentality, which in short he described as an exercise of power based on 'a "conduct of conducts" and a management of possibilities' (Foucault, 2000b: 341) or 'a set of actions upon other actions' (*ibid.*: 341). In this, the power relationship in the conduct of conducts is not one of violence or direct action on the body: 'a relationship of violence acts upon a body or upon things; it forces, it bends, it breaks, it destroys, or it closes off all possibilities' (*ibid.*: 340). On the contrary the exercise of power as the conduct of conducts

> incites, it induces, it seduces, it makes it easier or more difficult, it releases or contrives, makes more probable or less; in the extreme, it constrains or forbids absolutely, but it is always a way of acting upon one or more acting subjects by virtue of their acting or being capable of action. (*Ibid.*: 341)

From here it is a short step to Foucault's subsequent interest in subjectification and the actions of individuals on themselves: 'the way a human being turns him- or herself into a subject' (Foucault, 2000b: 327). The conduct of conducts therefore opened up new ways of looking beyond discipline and bioregulation, to ways in which individuals modified and transformed themselves, through what Foucault (1993: 203) called 'techniques of the self'. With this Foucault added another layer of complexity to understanding power and the body. This meant revising his earlier emphasis on discipline in which he had 'investigated subjectivity primarily with a view to "docile bodies"' (Lemke, 2001: 203) and instead holding within the concept of government the complex ways in which different types of power work on the body and on the self. For Foucault (1993: 203), therefore, one

> has to take into account the interaction between these two types of techniques – techniques of domination and techniques of the self. He has to take into account the points where the technologies of domination of individuals over one another have recourse to processes by which the individual acts upon himself. And conversely, he has to take into account the points where the techniques of the self are integrated into structures of coercion or domination. The contact point, where individuals are driven by others is tied to the way they conduct themselves, is what we can call, I think, government.

The biopolitics of the *STS* campaign can be located at this contact point between techniques of domination or discipline and techniques of self. The campaign may therefore be seen as a form of government which aims to discipline and regulate body shape / waist size. It does this not by direct clinical monitoring and intervention but by a social marketing campaign which deploys a set of tactics to encourage individuals to act on their bodies in particular ways, and to problematise themselves as subjects of health in terms of their body size against the medical norm of a healthy waist. This 'contact point' must moreover be set within the wider matrix of neoliberal governmental rationality.

In *The Birth of Biopolitics*, Foucault (2008), in a rare moment of writing about the present, made acute observations on neoliberalism as an 'ambient problematic' and defined neoliberalism not as a minimal state but as a market-regulating state. In doing so, he did not, as Miller (2014: 194) notes, 'fall for the *canard* that it sought to withdraw the state from economic activity'. Thus, Foucault (2008: 121) suggested that the free, competitive market 'is produced by an active governmentality. … [O]ne must govern for the market, rather than because of the market'. If from its beginnings biopower has been about fashioning bodies for the economic security of the state and securing their productivity, under neoliberal governmental rationality, biopower is about the making of bodies fit for the market. The relationship between social policy and neoliberal governmentality, as Foucault suggested, is such that

> the society regulated by reference to the market … is a society in which the regulatory principle should be not so much the exchange of commodities as the mechanisms of competition … The *homo economicus* sought after is not the man of exchange or man the consumer; he is the man of enterprise and production. (*Ibid.*: 147)

Social policy elaborated under neoliberal governmentality thus does not rest on the principle of freedom as non-interference but 'neoliberalism implies continuous corrective or ameliorative interventions upon societies and upon individuals to make them fit for competition as market societies and entre-preneurs of the self' (McFalls and Pandolfi, 2014: 173). Foucault drew this point from his case study of ordo-liberalism, the German version of social liberalism that promotes a strong role for the state to ensure the market works effectively according to market principles such as competition. Turning to American neoliberalism, he saw more radical relations between state and market. Here neoliberal governmentality looks for 'the generalisa-tion of the economic form of the market … throughout the social body and including the whole of the social system not usually conducted through or sanctioned by monetary exchange' (Foucault 2008: 243). The state which regulates the market thus must also be subject to the type of market prin-ciples it is trying to produce. As Foucault (2008: 247) puts it, the call that governments 'respect the form of the market and *laissez-faire*' under clas-sical liberalism is, under neoliberalism, transformed into a call to become 'a *do-not-laissez-faire* government, in the name of a law of the market which will enable each of its activities to be measured and assessed'. This in turn means that governmental action or intervention is carried out in market-approving, or seemingly non-interventionist, ways. Thus as Miller (in Flew 2012: 47) pithily states, the 'grand contradiction of neo-liberalism [is] its passion for intervention in the name of non-intervention'. *STS* as a social marketing campaign fits this bill. It is highly directive and specific in its biopedagogical messages about waist size, yet relatively non-interventionist in its actions. The agent of change is the individual, who is coaxed, via the distribution of free measuring tapes and other marketing techniques, to 'stop the spread' and to think about and act upon themselves and their bodies in seemingly precise, biomedical terms.

There remains the question of how to empirically ground what Rabinow and Rose (2006) admit were Foucault's rather sketchy outlines of the concepts of biopower and governmentality unlike, for example, his work on disciplinary power. Rabinow and Rose (2006: 197) suggest that biopower can be empirically interrogated or be treated as 'a plane of actuality' along three elements: truth or 'truth discourses about the "vital" character of living human beings'; power, or 'strategies for intervention upon collective existence in the name of life and health'; and subjectivity, or 'modes of subjectification, through which individuals are brought to work on themselves'. Taking up these three elements in relation to analysing biopedagogy, Harwood (2009: 24) suggests a number of questions which can be asked in respect of each element; for truth discourse: 'what are the instructions that are being given?' and 'what are the biopedagogies of truth, and who tells them?' For the second, 'what strategies are in place to ensure that living beings can indeed become objects to be worked on, to be pedagogized. ... [W]hat power relations make the strategies of speaking the truth possible?' (*ibid.*: 25). With regard to subjectification we can ask,

> what disciplinary techniques are used on the individual that individualise him or her, and what exercises do these provoke? What techniques of regularisation used on the population affect the subjectification of true discourses? How are these to be understood at the level of the population, at the level of the individual? (*Ibid.*: 25–26)

Or in other words, how does the campaign work in terms of 'individualising and collectivising subjectifications' (Rabinow and Rose, 2006: 215)? The remainder of the chapter aims to explore the points sketched about *STS* within Foucault's framework by looking in more detail at the core components of the campaign along these three elements and using Harwood's questions as a broad guide.

STS, vital norms and truth discourses

STS is in part reflective of how biological facts about the body have amassed over time as advances in technology yield increasingly meticulous and complex knowledge about the composition of the human body, biological processes, illness and disease. Yet such facts or 'vital norms' (Canguilhem in Rose 2010) about the body do not stand on their own or speak for themselves. As Hacking (1982: 292) puts it, 'you can't just print numbers. You must print numbers of objects falling under some concept or other.' In this way the human sciences 'which are thought to have to do with finding out facts,... are also engines for making up people' (Hacking, 2006: 24). In the case of *STS* two numbers become the facts and signs on the female and male body by which it is decided whether one is categorised as having a healthy weight or is overweight. In looking at how such numbers become norms central to the biopedagogical message of health promotion campaigns, the point is not necessarily to treat the underlying biophysical phenomenon of central adipose tissue and its correlation with particular health problems as a scientific fabrication. Rather it is to look at how such data is used to make up healthy and unhealthy people and instate modes of governing bodies that focus on body measurement and the normalisation of particular body shapes and waist sizes. As such waist-circumference numbers may be considered what Guthman (2013: 265) calls 'fatuous measurements' or a product of 'artifactual constructivism' which denotes 'the techniques, laboratory practices, conventions, observational methods, instrumentation and measurements that produce scientific facts and in that way bring the material world into being'. This is not to suggest that waists have not got bigger but to look at how tools which measure waists and visualise the fat that lies beneath become central to how health and healthy bodies are conceptualised and 'can paint the picture in ways that may over-dramatize some elements and under-specify others and can also foreclose other problem conceptualizations' (*ibid.*: 263).

Measurement of waist size belongs to the discipline of anthropometry, the measuring of human morphology, including both surface and internal dimensions of the body and body organs. Particularly since the nineteenth century when anthropometry became increasingly prevalent as a way of quantitatively formalising biological differences, the discipline became a central element of biopower and the categorisation and regulation of bodies. Cranial measurements dominated early anthropometric practice and were used to produce racial hierarchies, reflecting biopolitical concerns with racial purity. The use of anthropometry to measure and record differences in stature was a parallel concern. In this case the measurement reflected apprehension about the physical vigour of populations, and their military and economic might, with height in the army, navy and wider working stock of the population being of particular concern (Ulijaszek and Komlos, 2010). While the norms and ways of 'making up people' generated by use of anthropometric measurements in theories of race and eugenics are no longer conferred truth status, by the late nineteenth and twentieth centuries anthropometry became a cornerstone of public health practice, involving the measuring of weight, stature, circumference and skinfold thickness in ascertaining the overall health status of a population and populations groups, particularly children. Such practices were also frequently combined with a social liberal from of governmentality (Frandsen and Triantafillou, 2011; Faubion, 2014).

Although, as Ulijaszek and Komlos (2010) note, anthropometric methods have remained practically unchanged since the nineteenth century, other instruments used to quantify and assess body size and composition have changed. The technologisation of medicine (Rose, 2007a), as demonstrated by developments in molecular imaging, when combined with anthropometric measurements of the body surface, are at the crux of 'making up' healthy and unhealthy bodies on the basis of the metric of waist size and underlying central adiposity. Traditional techniques to estimate whole body fat involve indirect measurements and calculations. These include the aforementioned measurement of skinfold thickness/subcutaneous fat; the calculation of total body water and total body potassium as an index of body composition; and 'densitometry', a method of determining body composition by way of measuring whole-body density through, for example, underwater weighing (Lukaski, 1987). By the end of the twentieth century far greater precision and new ways of seeing the body were afforded by molecular imaging, which is 'the visual representation, characterization, and quantification of biological processes at the cellular and subcellular levels within intact living organisms' (Massoud and Gambhir, 2003: 545). Technological innovations including computerised tomography (CT scans) and magnetic resonance imaging (MRI scans) allowed the production of two-dimensional images, and more recently three-dimensional images, of the underlying anatomy of the area of the body being scanned, or indeed the whole body. In the case of body fat, these means of seeing fat in the body were also taken to denote more accurate results than the more error-prone traditional methods. Such techniques permitted in-body visualisation, allowing us to see fat residing within the depths of the body, to measure its volume and to distinguish between different types of fat depending on its location in the body (Robinson *et al.*, 2005). In particular the new technologies enabled the visualisation and measurement of deep abdominal or visceral fact, lying behind the abdominal wall and between abdominal organs. This not only permitted greater knowledge about fat in terms of body composition, but also the qualities of fat molecules in different parts of the body, so that measurement and localisation of fat become significant in diagnosis of risk of disease rather than disease per se. Research from the 1980s onwards found correlations between visceral fat and risk of cardiovascular disease, Type 2 diabetes and cancers such as colorectal cancer (Seidell, Hautvast and Deurenberg, 1989). These research findings suggested that at least some fat in the body is not simply excess energy waiting to be used, but is biologically active and involved in the alteration of hormonal balances and the production of biochemicals with harmful effects for insulin resistance and blood pressure (Després, 2001).

Such knowledge paralleled the shift in medicine from a focus on disease to 'the assessment and government of "risk", and the maintenance and optimisation of the healthy body' (Rose, 2007b: 10). Specifically, the translation of techniques to measure visceral fat and the research findings which posed it as a disease risk factor into 'vital norms' about waist size, was taken up by public health bodies by the late 1990s, including the WHO in its 1997 consultation on obesity. The consultation proposed alternative anthropometric measures besides BMI to indicate disease risk, including waist–hip ratio and waist circumference (WHO, 2000). The WHO drew attention to the issue of distribution of fat in the body, suggesting that obesity needs to be understood in a way that recognises the different effects of fat in the body depending on its location and that 'excess abdominal fat is as great a risk factor for disease as is excess body fat *per se*' (WHO, 2000: 6). Waist circumference was highlighted as a 'simple and practical method of identifying overweight patients at increased risk of obesity-associated illness due to abdominal fat distribution' (WHO, 2000: 7). As an indication of how waist-size cut-off points were linked to risk of disease, the WHO suggested that, for Caucasians, 94 cm for men and 80 cm for women could be taken as the point at which there is considered to be 'increased risk' of metabolic complications, and 102 cm for men and 88 cm for women for 'substantially increased' risk of metabolic complications. By its 2011 report of an expert consultation on waist circumference and waist–hip ratio, its review of practice across the world found that several countries were using cut-off points from either the WHO (the most popular authority), the United States Cholesterol Education Programme or the International Diabetes Federation (WHO, 2011). It was, however, cautious of the use of single cut-off points. The consultation suggested that further research was needed to recommend suitable thresholds or norms for clinical screening of different populations and of different types of disease risk, and that this might result in the use of multiple sets of cut-off points.

The use of cut-off points in public health campaigns and the way they are portrayed in obliging us to be healthy is not quite so subtle, demonstrating the 'power of the single figure' (Miller, in Rose 1999). In *STS* 32 and 37 inches (the imperial conversion of the WHO's 94 cm and 80 cm) act as 'inscription devices' (Rose, 1999: 198) and become a singular technical, factual boundary between health and risk and disease. The campaign was launched in May 2011 with a particularly striking and emotive television advertisement. Utilising a pedagogy of fear, the advertisement conveyed its message about waist size in the style of a horror film, using a sombre male voice-over, grainy images and sinister, tense background music. The advertisement was scripted as follows:

> *We're all in the grip of an epidemic. Most of us already have it and we're rapidly passing it on to others, giving them a higher risk of developing heart disease, diabetes and cancer. It's overweight. And it's spreading. To find out if it's spread to you just measure around your middle and if the number is bigger than 32 inches for women or 37 inches for men it probably has. Stop*

the Spread at safefood.eu. Safefood. Be safe, be healthy, be well. (Author's
transcription of advertisement, Safefood, 2011)

The message quickly shifts from a massifying to an individualising one.
In its opening lines the entire population is problematised; *'we'* and *'most
of us'* are elided *'in the grip of an epidemic'*. With that opening purposively
intended to shock, the message is personalised by encouraging individuals
to discover if the 'epidemic' of overweight has spread to them by telling
them to measure their middle. By equating overweight with the notion of
an epidemic the advertisement reflects the transformation of the meaning
of overweight from 'an adjectival descriptor of corpulence, a physical sign
or symptom, and even, in some cultures, a sign of wealth and status' (Jutel,
2006: 2268) to a disease in its own right. However, the advertisement and
the campaign, by pinpointing the waist, shifts the meaning of overweight
and its association with disease from a whole-body phenomenon to the size
of a single part of the body surface. In this way the truth discourse promoted
by the advertisement reflects what Rose (2007b: 11) notes as the 'molecularisation of styles of biomedical thought, judgement and intervention'
following the technological advances of molecular imaging. Understanding
the body and promoting its health shifts from a whole-body, molar level to
a molecular level (*ibid.*). The body is molecularised in how it bears signs of
health or unhealthiness, such that the size of one part of the body and its
underlying risky fat cells, as indicated by a single sex-specific numerical
threshold, is now a sign of disease and risk of disease.

The molecularised biomedical message of the advertisement is complemented by a particular individualised explanation for the spread of the
overweight epidemic: people themselves are presented as carriers, overweight is something *'we're rapidly passing ... on to others'*. The campaign
thus not only promoted a particular truth about health and disease at the
level of the individual, but also posed individuals as unwitting sources of
contagion. The campaign drew on the concept of obesogenicity, which first
emerged in the late 1990s (Swinburn, Egger and Raza, 1999) to describe
environments which made people fat by, for example, facilitating ease of
access to fattening foods and offering little opportunity for physical activity.
However, adapting the concept somewhat, the campaign placed people and
their body sizes at the centre of the obesogenic environment. The visual
message of the advertisement thus suggested that the bulging waistlines of
the majority of the population contribute to an environment which nor-
malises what is actually an oversized waist line. The advertisement portrayed everyday scenes in a sinister air; normal activities are presented with
overtones of danger. However, departing from horror convention, the
horror depicted in the advertisement is not an unnatural, external threat
– it is a horror from within. Individuals on screen were depicted as both
unaware of the lurking risks and that they themselves are the source of

those risks, passing them on to others in their families, neighbourhoods and communities by virtue of their waist size. The advertisement began with having the viewer see through a dark, dimly lit, arched alleyway to people walking along a street. Subsequent scenes in a café, the street outside and within a family home show people in their ordinary interactions passing on the disease of overweight. In the street, four young people stand outside a 'corner shop', their arms are outstretched in greeting each other; the two women in the group greet each other with a kiss, the two men greet by touching each other on the arm. At this point the voice-over is telling us that *'we're rapidly passing it on to others'*. Switching to the spread within families and across generations, the advertisement's final scenes moved to a night-time shot of a housing estate dimly lit. We first see the exterior of a house, partly lit by the street lighting and partly covered by a tree shadow, looming ominously over the house. Through a window pane we see a family sitting down, a mother and father are on a couch and their son and daughter are at their feet, all facing the same direction (presumably looking at a television, although this is not shown) and eating full plates of food which are balanced on their laps (Safefood, 2011). The scenes are significant not only for how they portray the truth discourse of oversized waists as danger-ous and which individuals themselves are unwittingly but dangerously spreading, but also for how they invoke particular power relations and particular strategies to pedagogise and to intervene, which is the focus of the next section.

STS, power and pedagogy

The molecularised knowledge and message of the *STS* campaign follow through in the way that power relations are also molecularised. When the advance of biomedical knowledge is taken together with neoliberal governmentality it leads, as McFalls and Pandolfi (2014: 180) note, to 'radical biopolitical self-government of individual bodies'. What occurs, they suggest, is a deepening of 'the capillarization of biopower from the statistical aggregation of populations down to the genetic minutiae of sub-cellular life' (*ibid.*: 173). In the case of *STS* power is used to ultimately reform the waist and the composition of the body beneath, through acting on the actions of free, willing, self-governing subjects. The means to effect that change is a 'conduct of conducts' through the inciting and contriving of social and digital marketing techniques. Stemming from techniques first used in the commercial sector and now also frequently used by NGOs (French, 2011; Crawshaw, 2012), the use of social marketing to plan and deliver health promotion policy reflects Foucault's (2008) observation that the neoliberal state is judged not only for how it supports the market, but also for how its own activities conform to market principles. Social marketing as a form of intervention involves directing behaviour change and self-management from a distance, including, according to French's (2011) typology, nudging, shoving, hugging, smacking. Of these, the nudge in particular has been elevated in recent policy discourse as an effective and efficient way for government to facilitate individual change (Thaler and Sunstein, 2008).

The distribution of 250,000 free measuring tapes which were made available in pharmacies was a particularly innovative aspect of the campaign, emulating the 'free gift' tactic frequently used by companies to promote their products. The tapes were designed with the cut-off point of 32 inches for women displayed on one side of the tape and the cut-off point of 37 inches for men on the other side. Using the free gift as a nudge tactic to make the possibility of self-measurement more likely to occur, the distribution of measuring tapes conforms to nudge principles of being positive (a positive reward), voluntary, avoidable, passive/easy (requiring little work) and low cost (French, 2011). This strategy is something *STS* had in common with an Australian campaign, *Measure Up*, which offered a tape measure on its campaign website, albeit requiring a bit more 'do it yourself' work than the Irish version. That tape measure could be assembled by downloading a sex-specific measuring tape with instructions to '*cut out 6 sections and stick together to create your very own tape measure*' (Australian Government, 2012). In either case the use of a measuring tape to self-measure has the effect of bringing a particular norm or number to power, checking one's waist size 'tells the truth' and inscribes those numbers on the body, bringing the healthy or unhealthy body and its degree of riskiness into being. The offer of a free measuring tape to enact a technique of the self contrasts with the direct use of disciplinary power in a Japanese campaign on waist size. This involved legislating for the introduction of mandatory waist measurement by companies and local authorities for all adults falling between the ages of 40 and 74, as part of annual health checks. Financial penalties were also introduced for companies and local authorities that failed to meet particular targets as part of an overall drive to reduce the proportion of the population deemed overweight over the following twenty-five years (Onishi, 2008).

The drive to self-measure was followed up with the promotion of a website, adding a digital marketing element to the campaign (Safefood, n.d.a). Here the clinical gaze on the body and the disciplinary power of the clinic are dispersed to the interactivity of a pedagogical website which presents its visitors with two options: '*measure up*' and '*get started*'. Again, engagement is on the basis of free, willing and wilful participants whose desire to be healthy is mobilised by the personalised tools and related information reinforcing the key messages of the advertising arm of the campaign. The '*measure up*' option, which is accompanied with the subscript '2 *in 3 are overweight. How do you measure up?*' allows website users to input their waist measurement. Accurate waist measurement is also a concern of the website which features both textual instructions and a video demonstrating how it should (and should not) be done. The website thus instructs on how to use the everyday object of a measuring tape as an 'instrument of precision' (Rosenberg, 2002) and to reproduce clinical protocol in terms of what part of the body should be deemed the waist for measurement purposes, the correct body pose and the correct procedure. Upon submitting a waist measurement feedback is prompted which tells whether the number submitted equates with being either underweight (a waist size of 21 inches or below for women and 26 inches or below for men),[1] a healthy weight (a waist size of 32 inches or below for women and 37 inches or below for men) or overweight (waist circumferences above 32 and 37· inches for women and men, respectively). As well as categorising the website users' weight, the accompanying feedback stresses the benefits of having a *'healthy lifestyle'*, ranging from the aesthetic and psychological: *'looking good'* and *'feeling our best'*; to the medical: reduced risk in the long term of particular diseases. For those whose feedback is that their waist size means they are overweight, weight loss is advised. Whether one receives the feedback of being a healthy weight or overweight, users are encouraged to visit another Safefood website, 'weigh2live'. This website provides an online weight-loss programme in the interests of taking either preventive action to maintain a healthy weight and low-risk disease status or corrective action in the case of being deemed at risk and overweight (Safefood, n.d.b). The second website option, *'get started'*, appeals to people to *'get ready'* once they have measured their waists by setting a goal, with the suggestion that the loss of 1–2 inches around the middle can be accomplished by weight loss over 6–8 weeks, and to *'go!'*, leading again to the 'weigh2live' website.

In addition to the types of power relations enacted by the measuring tape and the interactive website, the campaign also relies on the power technique of the synopticon. Synoptic power marks a shift from the panoptic power techniques of disciplinary institutions which rest on the surveillance of the many by the few. Synoptic power relations are still visual, but individuals are drawn to co-view and co-surveil in a post-panoptic world where power relations are more mobile and power moves downwards and outwards from the institution to the individual (Gane, 2012). As Gane (2012: 622, 623) suggests, synoptic power reverses the 'logic of the Panopticon, for now the few do not watch the many ... the many watch the many ... as well as watching over themselves'. *STS*'s obesogenic explanation of healthy and unhealthy body size requires this type of seeing and surveillance by the population as a whole. Thus the campaign in its message about the obesogenic causes of overweight, draws attention to our distorted perception of what a healthy waist and body size and shape is, and invites us to not only re-evaluate how we understand our own bodies, but also the waist size and health status of those around us. In normalising a particular waist size with health, it seeks to abnormalise the current waist sizes and body shape of the majority of the population. Thus, to return to the visual tactics of the first advertisement aired in the campaign, as a synoptic abnormalising mechanism the advertisement directs the viewer's gaze to what are portrayed as the abnormal waist sizes of those on screen. The shooting style invokes an act of looking at others; our gaze is directed to individuals who are unaware of being watched and focuses in on their expanded middles. In the café scene of a couple in conversation, our gaze is directed to the man's waist line which bulges slightly over his trouser belt; in the street, the shot draws attention to one of the young people's waists, this time a woman's, displaying her slightly rounded waistline in comparison to the rest of her frame. Similarly in the second advertisement of the campaign, which is described in more detail below, the visual focus on waist size is maintained as scenes depict people concealing or making little of their waist size, from a middle-aged woman pulling her top over her middle, to a young man entering a lift and pulling up his belted trousers, to the belted waistline of a young woman again in a café. The advertisements therefore deploy what Novas and Rose (2000: 487) call a molecular optics, which is a molecularised viewing of the body, including 'the molecular structure of bodily components' in its inciting recognition of the significance of waist size and its association with disease.

STS and modes of subjectification

This molecularisation of knowledge about the body and intervention on the body is also taken up in how the campaign operates as a mode of subjectification and how, in particular, norms and techniques are used to somaticise health and risk as physical body signs and size. The campaign essentially encourages the body to be known and experienced as a set of measurements and risks. The numbers at the heart of the campaign, posed as the threshold between health and unhealthiness, are at the centre of how it subjectifies: 'numbers, and the techniques of calculation in terms of numbers, have a role in subjectification – they turn the individual into a calculating self endowed with a range of ways of thinking about, calculating about, predicting and judging their own activities and those of others' (Rose, 1999: 214). Measuring the waist and assessing the result against 32 or 37 inches brings into being a calculative relationship with our bodies as the riskiness of one's waist size is judged on whether it is the harbinger of too much harmful fat deep beneath the waist surface. However, the type of subjectification engendered simultaneously promotes and blurs the idea of a numeric threshold between health and risk. Whether or not our waists conform to the measurements deemed to indicate a healthy weight in the present, we are asked, in particular through the campaign's website, to consider our longer-term health and risk status; 'in the world of susceptibilities' as Rose (2007a: 96) puts it, 'we are all asymptomatically ill'. Whether we are invoked to take corrective action now, or preventive action for the future, our sense of ourselves is shaped to keep the risks of our waist size at bay and to constantly monitor and modulate our body size and manage our susceptibilities. This management of susceptibilities somaticises risk: it is not only a matter of assessing behaviour – what we eat, what we drink, how we move – as risky or prudent; but is more fundamentally about knowing and monitoring the appearance of our bodies for risky body signs. And in the world of early twenty-first-century biopower, these calculations and forms of somatic individuality are ultimately about maximising our human capital and self-entrepreneurship. This involves the making of lean bodies both fit for and homologised with the notion of the competitive, lean market, and, as wider health promotion policy would have it, 'allow[s] people to live their lives to their full potential, to create the right environment to sustain jobs, to help restore the economy' (Government of Ireland, 2013: 6).

Yet in its attempts to instate a somatic individuality resting upon a biologically based norm for waist size, the notion of the subject in denial is also a central part of the campaign's mode of subjectification. Thus a key message of the campaign centres around denial at the degree of the overweight problem amongst the population which is directed specifically at individuals and their refusal to accept the campaign's message of what actually constitutes being overweight. Concern with denial reflects an emerging theme in neoliberal discourse and the rationale behind nudge-based policy interventions. The rationally calculating neoliberal subject is as, McFalls and Pandolfini observe, assumed to be

> concerned only with maximizing himself, his human capital, as a source of revenue. As entrepreneur of the self, the human capitalist counts, calculates, and deploys his economic, cultural, technical, and physical resources including his body and genetic composition. The latter thus become not a fact or gift of nature but variables to be manipulated. (2014: 172)

However, in contemporary discussion of the arts of neoliberal government, questions are evident about whether the neoliberal subject is wholly a rationally calculating subject who will deploy their resources, including their bodies, to their best entrepreneurial advantage. Recent neoliberal debate and its segueing to a more liberal paternalist rationality as reflected in nudging involves concern about ways in which subjects are not rational, but make decisions and engage in behaviour that also bears less than rational or irrational components (Wilkins, 2013; Whitehead, Jones and Pykett, 2011). Such thinking acknowledges and problematises ways in which 'human decision making does not predominantly follow a "rational" model of contemplative, economically efficient, and self-serving calculation, but is structurally marked by a tendency towards a limited, or "bounded" form of rationality, which could be characterised as irrational' (Whitehead, Jones and Pykett, 2011: 2819). While the concept of nudging and related ways of influencing behaviour are an acknowledgement of this way of thinking and reflect particular tactics of the campaign as already described, techniques of subjectification predicated on 'irrational' thinking about waist size and the harm of being overweight also engage more directly with what and how people think and their faulty or irrational health subjectivities. Although the tape measure might 'tell the truth' of one's waist size, the campaign has to deal with ways of thinking that are a barrier to accepting the truth that the tape measure tells and the reality that waist size reveals. This is in part dealt with on the campaign website which features '5 facts' about the waist sizes above 32 and 37 inches, and 'stories' about people which aim to debunk the idea, in the majority of cases, that particular body sizes or circumstances mean that the waist limits don't apply (Safefood, n.d.a). However, the most compelling way denial is dealt with is in the second television advertisement which aims, it might be said, to get inside people's heads. This brings to mind Foucault's (2000b: 333) likening of modern state power as pastoral power, one of the elements of which is that 'this form of power cannot be exercised without knowing the inside of people's minds, without exploring their souls, without making them reveal their innermost secrets. It implies a knowledge of conscience and an ability to direct it.' Thus after the shock tactics of the first advertisement, the second advertisement took a slightly gentler approach. In seeking to lay open the irrationality of our thinking about body size it engaged with how people interpret and rationalise waist sizes exceeding the prescribed measurements. The sinister effects of the initial advertisement are played down; the background music is a little more upbeat, the male voice-over slightly less sombre, and its authoritative commentary is interwoven with the inner dialogue of the individuals on screen. Remaining rather dimly lit and in soft focus, the advertisement begins with a shot of a middle-aged woman walking along the street who pauses to look at her reflection in a shop window. Contemplating her waist, she pulls the edge of her top down a little and in her inner voice says, 'that's just middle age spread'. The voice-over begins by claiming, to the contrary, that 'although most of us are now overweight, a lot of us still can't accept it'. The scene then switches to a young man, dressed in typical office wear, entering a lift. As he pulls his belt up over a slightly bulging belly we hear him saying to himself that 'it's okay to be a bit bigger at my height'. The voice-over returns and remarks that 'but no matter what you say if your middle measures more than 32 inches for women or 37 for men you probably are, giving you a higher risk of developing heart disease, cancer and Type 2 diabetes'. The scene then switches to a group of people gathered around a café table and the camera focuses on the belted waist of a young woman, who says 'but we're all a bit like this in my house'

(Safefood, 2012). In each scenario, therefore, subjects in denial are countered with the 'expert' biomedical voice, which interacts with and 'acts on the interior of the person' (Miller, in Mckee, 2009: 471), aiming to realign what we think about and how we normalise our waist size with acceptance of how we actually 'measure up'.

Looking at the effects of the campaign and recognising that biopower is not an omnipotent, all-pervasive form of power, we also need to ask, as Harwood (2009: 27) suggests, 'does everyone believe what they are told?' Asking this question is to recognise, as McKee (2009: 474) suggests, that 'subjection is neither a smooth nor a complete project; rather one inherently characterised by conflict, contestation and instability'. The debate and controversy generated by the campaign suggest ample scope for looking at how governmentality also produces resistance and comes against health subjectivities that diverge from the governable subject desired by the campaign. In particular the truth discourses were contested. Media commentators and health advocacy organisations variously drew attention to the spuriousness of obesogenicity as an explanation for body size and weight and to the stigmatising effects of the campaign, and questioned the efficacy of its scare tactics and its narrow definition of what constitutes healthy and unhealthy weight and body size (Houston, 2011a, 2011b; Sheehan, 2011; Horan, 2011). Such questioning was also evident amongst users of Internet fora such as Boards.ie, where discussion about the campaign ranged from agreement with its message to a querying and rejecting of its message about waist size as an indicator of health (Boards.ie, 2011). What discussions such as these suggest is not so much that individuals are in denial and need to be shocked into facing facts, but may equally be 'subjects of doubt' (Clarke *et al.*, in McKee, 2009: 477). While some may accept the message, others react with scepticism, which recalls Guthman's (2013) concept of fatuous measurements. As such they draw on a greater range of understandings of health, which may still be part of a somatic individuality, but one which does not depend on single numbers such as waist size, even as Safefood responded with 'facticity of the figure' (Rose, 1999: 208), reinforcing the notion of concrete evidence and the incontestability of the numbers 32 and 37 (Fogarty, 2011).

Concluding remarks

This chapter has sought analyse *STS* as a form of twenty-first-century biopolitics concentrating on the campaign as an empirical site of biopower and looking at how such power operates in a mutually reinforcing context of molecularised biomedicine and increasingly invasive forms of neoliberal governmentality. Opening up the campaign's exercise of biopower in terms of truth, power and subjectivity, the chapter has attempted to show how the campaign collapses the meaning of health to a restrictive, reductive and increasingly visible register. Individual parts of the body are subject to scrutiny and reform in ways that reflect an anatamo-politics by way of techniques of the self. Individuals are cast with bearing a very precise sign of health on their bodies, and at the same time the visibility of their health or unhealthiness is borne as an explanation for health status at the level of the population, making individuals responsible not only for themselves but for others in society. Yet, as McKee (2009) reminds us, the messy reality of governmentality also needs to be engaged with. As much as the campaign aimed to make people subjects of health in particular ways, it also encountered resistance, which points to the scepticism with which some people at least reacted to its attempts to equate health with a singular, numerical, calculating way of knowing. Despite or perhaps because of the controversy surrounding the campaign Safefood claimed the campaign a success because of the increased levels of awareness about waist size, or this way of knowing about health, following the campaign (Faughnan, 2012). The analysis presented in this chapter, together with the scepticism the campaign engendered, points to the ways in which health is not a given and the importance of asking how health is constructed, governed and a political object. Ultimately it points to how we need to attend to health and the healthy body not only as a fact but as a value, open to diverse ways of knowing and embodiment.

Notes

1   For participants whose waist measurement is deemed an indication of underweight, feedback suggests a number of reasons for being underweight such as being stressed, trying to lose weight or trying to look thin. It is also suggested that for some being underweight is the result of a slender constitution, but for others it may put their health at risk and consulting a GP is advised if the website user feels concerned.

References

Australian Government (2012) Measure Up, tape measures (male and female). Available from: www.measureup.gov.au/internet/abhi/publishing.nsf/Content/tape-measures. Accessed 3 October 2014.

Boards.ie (2011) Stop the Spread!!! Available from: www.boards.ie/vbulletin/showthread.php?t=2056266149. Accessed 16 December 2014.

Cahill, D., Edwards, L. and Stilwell, F. (eds) (2012) *Neoliberalism Beyond the Free Market*. Cheltenham, Edward Elgar.

Crawshaw, P. (2012) Governing at a distance: social marketing and the (bio)politics of responsibility. *Social Science & Medicine*, 75: 200–207.

Després, J.-P. (2001) Health consequences of visceral obesity. *Annals of Medicine*, 33(8): 534–541.

Faubion, J.D. (2014) Introduction: the use of Foucault. IN: Faubion, J.D. (ed.) *Foucault Now: Current Perspectives in Foucault Studies*. Cambridge, Polity: pp. 1–20.

Faughnan, M. (2012) *Stop the Spread Campaign, The Food, Health, Choice and Change Conference*, 6–7 June, University College Cork. Available from: www.safefood.eu/Safefood/media/SafeFoodLibrary/Documents/Professional/Events/MarianFaughnan.pdf. Accessed 15 July 2014.

Flew, T. (2012) Michel Foucault's *The Birth of Biopolitics* and contemporary neo-liberalism debates. *Thesis Eleven*, 108(1): 44–65.

Fogarty, J. (2011) Prevention better than cure. *The Medical Independent*, 2 June. Available from: www.medicalindependent.ie/4507/prevention_better_than_cure. Accessed 17 December 2014.

Foucault, M. (1984 [1971]) Nietzsche, genealogy, history. IN: Rabinow, P. (ed.) *The Foucault Reader*. London, Penguin: pp. 76–100.

Foucault, M. (1993) About the beginning of the hermeneutics of the self: two lectures at Dartmouth (ed. Mark Blasius). *Political Theory*, 21(2): 198–227.

Foucault, M. (2000a) Governmentality. IN: Faubion, J.D. (ed.) *Michel Foucault Power, Essential Works of Foucault, 1954–1984 vol. 3*. New York, The New Press: pp. 201–222.

Foucault, M. (2000b) The subject and power. IN: Faubion, J.D. (ed.) *Michel Foucault Power, Essential Works of Foucault, 1954–1984 vol. 3*. New York, The New Press: pp. 326–348.

Foucault, M. (2003) *'Society must be defended': Lectures at the Collège de France, 1975–1976*. M. Bertani and A. Fontana (eds). D. Macey (trans.). New York, Picador.

Foucault, M. (2008) *The Birth of Biopolitics: Lectures at the Collège de France 1978–1979*. G. Burchell (trans.). Basingstoke, Palgrave Macmillan.

Frandsen, M. and Triantafillou, P. (2011) Biopower at the molar level: liberal government and the invigoration of Danish society. *Social Theory & Health*, 9(3): 203–223.

French, J. (2011) Why nudging is not enough. *Journal of Social Marketing*, 1(2): 154–162.

Gane, N. (2012) The governmentalities of neoliberalism: panopticism, post-panopticism and beyond. *The Sociological Review*, 60(4): 611–634.

Government of Ireland (2013) *Healthy Ireland: A Framework for Improved Health and Wellbeing 2013–2015*. Dublin, Stationery Office.

Guthman, J. (2013) Fatuous measures: the artifactual construction of the obesity epidemic. *Critical Public Health*, 23(3): 263–273.

Hacking, I. (1982) Biopower and the avalanche of printed numbers. *Humanities in Society*, 5(3–4): 279–295.

Hacking, I. (2006) Making up people. *London Review of Books*, 28(16): 23–26.

Harwood, V. (2009) Theorizing biopedagogies. IN: Wright, J. and Harwood, V. (eds) *Biopolitics and the 'Obesity Epidemic': Governing Bodies*. New York, Routledge: pp. 15–30.

Horan, N. (2011) I'm not fat, but 250,000 tapes are telling me I am. *Sunday Independent*, 5 June.

Houston, M. (2011a) Weighing up the obesity campaign. *Irish Medical Times*, 22 August. Available from: www.imt.ie/opinion/2011/08/weighing-up-the-obesity-campaign.html. Accessed 16 December 2014.

Houston, M. (2011b) Shock and awe campaign fails to measure up. *The Irish Times*, 24 May.

Howson, A. (2013) *The Body in Society: An Introduction* (second edition). Cambridge, Polity.

Jutel, A. (2006) The emergence of overweight as a disease entity: measuring up normality. *Social Science & Medicine*, 63: 2268–2276.

Koopman, C. (2014) Michel Foucault's critical empiricism today: concepts and analytics in the critique of biopower and infopower. IN: Faubion, J.D. (ed.) *Foucault Now Current Perspectives in Foucault Studies*. Cambridge, Polity: pp. 88–111.

Lemke, T. (2001) 'The birth of bio-politics': Michel Foucault's lecture at the Collège de France on neo-liberal governmentality. *Economy and Society*, 30(2): 190–207.

Lukaski, H. (1987) Methods for the assessment of human body composition: traditional and new. *American Journal of Clinical Nutrition*, 46: 537–556.

Massoud, T. and Gambhir, S. (2003) Molecular imaging in living subjects: seeing fundamental biological processes in a new light. *Genes and Development*, 17: 545–580.

McFalls, L. and Pandolfi, M. (2014) Parrhesia and Therapeusis: Foucault on and in the world of contemporary neoliberalism. IN: Faubion, J.D. (ed.) *Foucault Now: Current Perspectives in Foucault Studies*. Cambridge, Polity: pp. 168–187.

McKee, K. (2009) Post-Foucauldian governmentality: what does it offer critical social policy analysis? *Critical Social Policy*, 29(3): 465–486.

Miller, T. (2014) Foucault, Marx, Neoliberalism: unveiling undercover boss. IN: Faubion, J.D. (ed.) *Foucault Now: Current Perspectives in Foucault Studies*. Cambridge, Polity: pp. 188–202.

Novas, C. and Rose, N. (2000) Genetic risk and the birth of the somatic individual. *Economy and Society*, 29(4): 485–513.

Onishi, N. (2008) Japan, seeking trim waists, measures millions. *New York Times*, 13 June. Available from: www.nytimes.com/2008/06/13/world/asia/13fat.html?pagewanted=all&_r=0. Accessed 5 September 2014.

Peck, J. (2010) Zombie neoliberalism and the ambidextrous state. *Theoretical Criminology*, 14(1): 104–110.

Rabinow, P. and Rose, N. (2006) Biopower today. *Biosocieties*, 1: 195–217.

Robinson, K., Whelan, P.F., Ghita, O. and Brennan, D. (2005) Measurement and localization of body fat in whole body MRI. IN: Third annual IEI biomedical engineering research award, Dublin, Ireland. Available from: www.rince.ie/~robinsok/pdfs/Robinson_BERA2005a.pdf. Accessed 5 November 2014.

Rose, N. (1999) *Powers of Freedom: Reframing Political Thought*. Cambridge, Cambridge University Press.

Rose, N. (2007a) Governing the will in a neurochemical age. IN: Maasen, S. and Sutter, B. (eds) *On Willing Selves Neoliberal Politics vis-à-vis the Neuroscientific Challenge*. Basingstoke, Palgrave Macmillan: pp. 81–99.

Rose, N. (2007b) *The Politics of Life Itself: Biomedicine, Power, and Subjectivity in the Twenty-First Century*. Princeton, Princeton University Press.

Rose, N. (2010) Normality and pathology in a biomedical age. *Sociological Review*, 57, s2: 66–83.

Rosenberg, C.E. (2002) The tyranny of diagnosis: specific entities and individual experience. *The Milbank Quarterly*, 80: 237–260.

Safefood (2011) Safefood Stop the Spread TV ad. Uploaded 9 May 2011. Available from: www.youtube.com/watch?v=YarpWrLn9Zo. Accessed 17 December 2014.

Safefood (2012) Safefood Stop the Spread. Uploaded 12 January 2012. Available from: www.youtube.com/watch?v=srdQ6iMeUiw. Accessed 17 December 2014.

Safefood (n.d.a) Stop the Spread. Available from: www.safefood.eu/Stop-The-Spread.aspx. Accessed 17 December 2014.

Safefood (n.d.b) weigh2live. Available from: weigh2live.safefood.eu/. Accessed 17 December 2014.

Seidell, J., Hautvast, J. and Deurenberg, P. (1989) Overweight: fat distribution and health risks. Epidemiological observations. A review. *Infusionstherapie*, 16(6): 276–281.

Sheehan, A. (2011) Simplistic obesity ad is scaring people, say experts. *Irish Independent*, 8 June.

Swinburn, B., Egger, G. and Raza, F. (1999) Dissecting obesogenic environments: the development and application of a framework for identifying and prioritizing environmental interventions for obesity. *Preventive Medicine*, 29 (6 Pt 1): 563–570.

Thaler, R. and Sunstein, C. (2008) *Nudge Improving Decisions about Health, Wealth and Happiness*. New Haven, Yale University Press.

Ulijaszek, S. and Komlos, J. (2010) From a history of anthropometry to anthropometric history. IN: Mascie-Taylor, C.G.N. and Ulijaszek, S.J. (eds) *Human Variation: from the Laboratory to the Field*. Boca Raton, CRC Press: pp. 183–197.

Vaz, P. and Bruno, F. (2003) Types of self-surveillance: from abnormality to individuals 'at risk'. *Surveillance & Society*, 1(3): 272–291.

Whitehead, M., Jones, R. and Pykett, J. (2011) Governing irrationality, or a more than rational government? Reflections on the rescientisation of decision making in British public policy. *Environment and Planning A*, 43(12): 2819–2837.

WHO (2000) *Obesity: Preventing and Managing the Global Epidemic Report of a WHO Consultation*. Geneva, WHO.

WHO (2011) *Waist Circumference and Waist–Hip Ratio: Report of a WHO Expert Consultation, Geneva, 8–11 December 2008*. Geneva, WHO.

Wilkins, A. (2013) Libertarian paternalism: policy and everyday translations of the rational and the emotional. *Critical Policy Studies*, 7(4): 395–406.

Wright, J. (2009) Biopower, biopedagogies and the obesity epidemic. IN: Wright, J. and Harwood, V. (eds) *Biopolitics and the 'Obesity Epidemic': Governing Bodies*. New York, Routledge: pp. 1–14.

5 Eluska Fernández

The contemporary self in tobacco control: exploring the introduction of the smoking ban in Ireland

Introduction

This chapter focuses on one of the most well-known episodes in the history of tobacco control in Ireland: the introduction of an overall workplace smoking ban in 2004. In keeping with the overall theme of this edited collection, it aims to tell this story drawing on some key ideas and concepts put forward by governmentality studies. The introduction of the smoking ban in Ireland is considered by politicians, public health and anti-smoking advocates and Irish citizens as one of the biggest success stories in the history of public health policy and tobacco control. However, commentaries and surveys published at the time of the announcement of the ban in January 2003 show that most people thought not only that the ban was too radical a proposal, but that it would be unworkable and difficult to enforce, especially in Ireland, a country often associated with pub culture. Despite vociferous objections to the ban from the hospitality industry and high levels of controversy in the media which followed its announcement, the smoking ban came into effect on 29 March 2004 with little need for coercive enforcement mechanisms. The ban was mainly self-enforced by the public and compliance was remarkably high from the beginning.

Drawing upon Foucault's (1982) definition of 'government' as the 'conduct of conduct', defined here as the power to act and influence the actions of others, this chapter traces *how* government was sought in an effort to transform the view that the smoking ban was unworkable. More specifically, the focus of the chapter is on exploring what types of conduct were embraced and promoted in the context of the debates over the ban, in order to achieve a successful exercise in the 'conduct of conduct'. Informed by the centrality that notions of rational, responsible and civilised selfhood play in contemporary public health and health promotion discourses, it reveals how notions of what came to be promoted as rational, responsible and civilised behaviours, and their flip side, irrational, irresponsible and uncivilised ones, were central to the exercise of power in the context of the ban. This chapter also discusses some of the social and political implications of conducting a governmental analysis by drawing attention to the fact that the regulation of smoking became interlinked with social and moral processes, and exposing how some of these processes played a symbolic role in promoting boundaries between different social groups.

Governmentality, tobacco control and the self

A key element within a Foucauldian understanding of power is that the meaning of government is not seen as necessarily tied to the nation-state. Rather, it is defined as the 'conduct of conduct' (Foucault, 1982), which might be understood to refer to 'a form of activity aiming to shape, guide or affect the conduct of some person or persons' (Gordon, 1991: 2). As developed in our Introduction to this edited collection (p. 6) Foucault's first major point is that power is not something that belongs to anyone, such as the state. Rather, it needs to be understood in terms of the relations between different fields, institutions, bureaucracies and other groups (such as the private media and other businesses) within the state. As a result, governmentality studies extend the scope of political analysis beyond the domain of the state and institutional politics (Rose and Miller, 1992). It also means that within this conceptualisation of government, the political vocabulary structured by oppositions between state and civil society, public and private, government and market, coercion and consent, sovereignty and autonomy and the like, does not adequately characterise the diverse ways in which rule is exercised today (Rose and Miller, 1992; Lupton, 1995; Dean, 1999). Instead, a governmentality study aims to highlight the 'interconnection between "top-down" power (technologies of domination) and "bottom-up" power (technologies of the self)' (Petersen, 2007). Technologies of domination make reference to forms of external government, such as policing, surveillance and regulation. Technologies of the self are defined as techniques that allow individuals to effect change in the forms in which they govern their body, thought and conduct 'so as to transform themselves in order to attain a certain state of happiness, purity, wisdom, perfection, or immortality' (Foucault, 1988: 18). As a result, analysing governmentality processes involves focusing on the 'art of government' as a form of activity which seeks to shape the conduct of people, and more precisely, how people *conduct themselves* (Foucault, 1988). From this perspective, power is not so much a matter of imposing constraints upon citizens as of 'making up' citizens, and personal autonomy is not the antithesis of political power, but a key term in its exercise (Rose and Miller, 1992: 174).

Foucault (1991) was interested in government as a *strategic* activity or practice, what he referred to as the 'art of government', used interchangeably with the term 'rationality of government'. According to Gordon (1991: 3),

> A 'rationality of government' will thus mean a way or system of thinking about the nature of the practice of government (who can govern; what governing is; what or who is governed), capable of making some form of activity thinkable and practicable both to its practitioners and to those upon whom it was practiced.

In the context of undertaking a governmentality study, this means that the emphasis is often placed on revealing the techniques of subjectification which explore the relationships between the government of the state, the government of others and the government of the self. Foucault's focus is on how the subject and its relations to others (self, other persons, state) are constituted and ordered. This focus refuses to position the subject (state, person) as either a pre-existing source or target of negative power or control, but actively constituted through, and positioned within, particular fields of discourse (Kitching, 2013; Fernández, 2016a).

In the context of public health policy, governmentality scholars such as Rose and Miller (Rose, 1989, 1999; Rose and Miller, 2008) have highlighted how the intensification of health promotion strategies developed in the twentieth century, coupled with the rise of private health insurance, have enhanced the obligations that individuals face for monitoring their own health. We have all become active partners in seeking health, and the underlying expectation is that coercion is unnecessary and that rational and responsible citizens will 'freely' govern themselves in ways consistent with expert knowledge. A review of the literature reveals that there are three dominant notions of self that have come to be privileged by prevailing public health and health promotion discourses: these include the 'rational self' (Lupton, 1995, 1997, 1999), the 'responsible self' (Lupton, 1995, 1999, 2008; Poland, 1998) and the 'self-restrained' (Poland, 2000) or 'civilized self' (Lupton, 1995). An example of how particular notions of self are privileged is found in the ways in which, increasingly, notions of consumerism in healthcare contexts tend to assume that lay people act as 'rational' actors. This is reflected in the development of patient-satisfaction surveys, which presuppose a particular conception of the patient as a 'rational evaluator' 'who is willing, wishing and able to judge all aspects of hospital care relatively dispassionately and reasonably reliably' (Meredith, 1993: 599). The 'making up' of the rational subject also involves the construction of the irrational subject; non-compliance with health advice is often portrayed as irrational. The issue of vaccination, for example, has highlighted some of the contradictions within the public health discourse in relation to the rational self: while citizens are encouraged to make an informed and active choice, failing to comply with expert advice is often portrayed as irrational (Blume, 2006). In the context of tobacco control, education and knowledge are often seen as key elements to promote behaviour change: if people are informed about the dangers of smoking, it is argued they will then rationally use this information and act accordingly. The flip side of this perspective is that often, those who fail to give up smoking are constructed as ignorant and lacking knowledge.

Notions of rationality are in turn tied to notions of responsibility. In contemporary discourses of health, new regimes of the body are often 'founded on the assumption that subjects of risk will opt to participate in a self-imposed programme of health and fitness' (O'Malley, 1996b: 199). That is, voluntary participation in risk management has become an essential pre-condition of 'responsible selfhood'. As O'Malley states (1996b: 199–200),

> The rational individual will wish to become responsible for the self ... the responsible individual will take rational steps to avoid and to insure against risk, in order to be independent rather than a burden on others. Guided by actuarial data on risks (e.g. on smoking and lung cancer; bowel cancer and diet, etc.) and on the delivery of relevant services and expertise (e.g. relative costs and benefits of private and public medicine), the rational and responsible individual will take prudent risk-managing measures.

Furthermore, the moral code of health promotion not only implies a distinctive set of civil duties for the individual vis-à-vis the management of one's own risks, but increasingly, also of the risks one poses to others (in terms of second-hand smoking, drunk driving and so on). Recent calls from the anti-tobacco movement include the abolition of smoking in cars where children are being carried. In the context of smoking restrictions in public spaces, Poland's work (1998, 2000) has shown how smoking bans, while legally binding, are rarely enforced by formal authorities. Authorities provide guidelines and mark spaces of permission and prohibition of smoking, but restrictions are mostly self-enforced. His work highlights how 'in new forms of governmentality, rather than the explicit exercise of the law through formal agents of the State, the reflexive self-policing of the responsibilized subject is central to the exercise of power' (Poland, 2000: 2). Enforcement mechanisms do not completely disappear, but increasingly, the conceptual separation between technologies of force and technologies of the self becomes blurred.

Finally, the focus on the self also brings us to the centrality that notions of self-control themselves have played in the context of public health discourses. Lupton (1995) refers to the relevance of the 'civilised self', rational, self-restrained and in control, in the way that health promotional campaigns routinely construct a dualism between the civilised and grotesque body: the grotesque body is represented 'as a horror of flesh-out-of-control: the beer belly, the ugly, wrinkled face, the distorted lip, the helpless, disabled body in the wheelchair, the entrapped addict' (Lupton, 1995: 120). In contrast, the civilised body is that which will be achieved through the regiments of health promotion, with due application to personal control. For example, the analyses of Lupton (2000) and Mennell (1991) have shown how the 'risks' associated with food consumption are not simply health-related, but are influenced by the loss of rationality and self-control, the privileging of the body over the mind, and the associated self-hate and anxiety that eating and appetite bring with them. In the same way that the sight of an obese body, or the thought of oneself as obese, may provoke emotions of revulsion and fear (Bordo, 1993), evidence suggests that smoking and smokers also provoke these same emotions of disgust (Poland, 1998; Brandt, 1998; Tuggle and Holmes, 2003; Corrigan, 2004). These studies also suggest that concerns over second-hand smoke exacerbate the negative stereotypes, as well as the prejudice experienced by smokers (Rozin and Singh, 1999), and that these are influenced by moral objections which go beyond health concerns.

Undertaking a governmental analysis of the Irish smoking ban

As policy is regarded as a form of power which works upon individuals' sense of self, a central concern when undertaking a governmental analysis of the Irish smoking ban was to analyse the processes by which new *forms of conduct* were drawn upon and promoted by government bodies and organisations in the context of its introduction. Specifically, the analysis was undertaken by revealing the multiple identities that were assumed and promoted during the debates over the ban in order to enlist people into its rationale, not only by those advocating the smoking ban, but also by those who resisted official discourses. This study drew on various sets of data: newspaper articles and Letters to the Editor from two national newspapers in Ireland (*The Irish Times* and *Irish Examiner*); official speeches; press releases (official and non-governmental); and social marketing campaigns deployed in the context of the ban. The analysis concentrated on the period between the announcement of the smoking ban on 30 January 2003 and its introduction on 29 March 2014. Applying broad principles of Foucauldian-inspired discourse analysis (see for example, Jäger and Maier, 2009), the analysis of these texts sought to expose two key things: first of all, the key discursive strategies deployed (how did the language and images deployed frame and problematise smoking?); and second, the rhetorical means used (what were the key words, metaphors, analogies and symbols deployed to give effect to particular forms of conduct?). The findings have been organised under three dimensions of analysis, which include the rational self, the responsible self and the civilised self. Each of these sections reveals what types of conduct were promoted, what discursive strategies were used in order to do so and how these particular types of conduct might have been resisted by alternative discourses.

The smoking ban and the rational self

Notions of rationality were central to the debates that took place in the context of the smoking ban in Ireland. The analysis demonstrates that official representatives and public health officials were often promoted as rational actors. These rational identities were reinforced by using a number of discursive strategies. For example, the smoking ban was often presented as evidence-based policy, which left the minister with 'no choice' but to introduce the ban. As the minister himself stated, 'before this consensus was correlated and stated so bluntly, it was possible to temporise, to negotiate, to water down the measures I'd like to have taken … [now] there is no other option open to me other than to take action' (Martin, 2003a). Official actors were constructed as rational actors who were compelled to act by scientific reason. The relevance afforded to rational science and expert knowledge was further re-emphasised by the various key pro-ban medical charities and professional groups that engaged in the debates. In a Letter to the Editor published by *The Irish Times*, Fenton Howell, chairman of ASH Ireland, the most prominent anti-smoking lobby group in Ireland, highlighted that 'every *independent*, *authoritative* scientific body which has examined the evidence has concluded that passive smoking causes many diseases, including lung cancer' (Howell, 2003; emphasis added). Brian Maurer, President of the Irish Heart Foundation also wrote that

> The Irish Heart Foundation, among other *impartial*, *independent*, health-promoting organisations, accepts the scientific evidence that exposure to environmental tobacco smoke is harmful. This evidence has been endorsed by all major *independent* scientific bodies which have considered the question. (Maurer, 2003; emphasis added)

Sears (1991) and Petersen (1999) highlight that public health officials and scientists are typically represented as dispassionate and politically neutral, altruistic and rising above vested interests to serve the community. In their reliance upon scientific expertise and an emphasis on neutrality, the discourses of the various medical charities and health professional groups also relied upon and promoted the notion of a neutral and beneficent state acting in the best interests of the majority and standing above vested interests.

On the other hand, smokers often appeared to be constructed not as rational and autonomous individuals, but as addicts. As Minister Martin highlighted, 'Anybody here who's been a smoker and who has succeeded in giving up cigarettes knows that it sounds easy, but is incredibly difficult. This is an insidious and persistent addiction' (Martin, 2003a). The analysis of the Letters to the Editor shows that the constitution of smokers as addicts, and the smoking ban as a technology which would help them quit their addiction, was also taken up by smokers themselves. As this Letter stated, 'As one who smokes, I say: please bring in the smoking ban. I hate them, but I'm addicted' (Boland, 2003). The analysis reveals that irrational smokers seemed to suffer from a double deficit: knowledge and capacity. For example, a letter highlighted that 'Cigarette smoke contains radioactive polonium and so is a radiation hazard. Very few smokers realise this.' That is, smokers were often constructed as ignorant. This letter concluded by stating 'I call on him [Minister for Environment, Martin Cullen] to quit smoking immediately or resign his Cabinet post' (MacHale, 2003). The suggestion was that Minister Cullen's identity as a smoker made him too irrational to hold a Cabinet post.

Smokers were also constructed as 'victims' of the tobacco industry and their manipulative campaigns to attract, especially, young people. So, for example, the Minister stated,

> It [smoking] has been inculcated – some would say deliberately – in young people, at a time in their lives when they have no sense of mortality ... when, a few years later, they decide to give up cigarettes, they find it is arguably the most difficult life-change they could ever choose to make. That life-change is often complicated by the smoking habits of friends. (Martin, 2003a)

Smokers were presented as weak, susceptible to both tobacco advertising campaigns, when they are young, and later on in life, to peer pressure.

The analysis demonstrates that these notions of rationality were not always shared by every side of the debate. Opponents of the ban also drew upon notions of rationality in order to oppose the smoking ban, but the construction of smokers as irrational and lacking knowledge was strongly contested. In fact, in some letters, it was Minister for Health Micheál Martin who was constructed as ignorant. For example, one letter stated that 'The Minister's new bill is draconian and ignorant of people. Smoking gives an immense number of people immense pleasure, usually in the full knowledge that they are shortening their lives' (Davies, 2003). Some of the constructions of smokers as ignorant and/or dependent and addicted individuals who wished to quit were opposed by the constitution of smoking as a pleasurable activity, and smokers as autonomous selves aware of the damage that smoking does to their health.

Some studies suggest that anti-smoking messages can result in active opposition (Poland, 2000; Thompson, Pearce and Barnett, 2009) and challenge notions of rationality which are linked to the imperative of health in public health and health promotion literature. This challenge was often reflected in the construction of proponents of the ban as irrational:

> The climate of Fagphobia which the Minister and his fellow travellers in the Health Police (they know who they are!) are currently whipping up is dangerously close to Health Fascism (a representative of the Irish Heart Foundation was heard to say on Five Seven Live last week that they wish to 'stamp it out all-together' – in other words, 'we'll make you healthy whether you like it or not!) ... The Law of Unintended Effects rules, as any organisation which has tried to change will testify ... Faghobs beware! (Dunne, 2003)

In this letter, it was the 'Minister and his fellow travellers in the Health Police' who were constructed as irrational and as 'health fascists'. Indeed, rather than as rational 'experts', they were constructed more in religious terms, wishing to convert everyone to their own values ('we'll make you healthy whether you like it or not!'). Another letter also used the analogy of 'religion' to refer to proponents of the ban, in this case by constructing the government officials and health professionals as 'crusaders': 'Unde-terred, the anti-smoking fanatics continue their crusade with a mixture of selective facts, flawed epidemiology and bogus statistics' (Donnelly, 2003).

Proponents of the ban were also produced as irrational in the discursive strategies that sought to highlight the selective concerns with environmental smoke. By highlighting that 'this current uprising against smoking is a joke' (Heaney, 2003), for example, they compared it to the damage that alcohol causes in society. On some other occasions, proponents of the ban were presented as spreading 'fairytales' about passive smoking and contested the construction of smokers as irrational and as victims of the manipulative strategies of the tobacco industry: 'I shall also avoid the tedious brainwash-ing that now passes for public debate in Ireland, not to mention the fairy-tales about passive smoking and the evil machinations of Big Tobacco' (McCarthy, 2003). This perspective suggested that it was not smokers who were irrational, victims of 'Big Tobacco', but rather proponents of the ban, who believed in fairytales.

The smoking ban and the responsible self

Notions of responsible behaviour were also central to the debates over the smoking ban. One of the key identities promoted in this context was the irresponsible smoker, who damages other people's health. As Minister Martin underlined at the announcement of the proposed ban on 30 January 2003, 'Bottom line: you don't have to be a smoker to get cancer from ciga-rette smoking. You can get it if you were never a smoker. You get it from other people's smoke' (Martin, 2003a). Jane Curtin, Communications Manager of the Irish Cancer Society, in a Letter to the Editor published by *The Irish Times* stated, 'Even the most determined of smokers must accept that their habit is damaging to those around them ... Passive smoking kills. We all have a right not to have to inhale other people's smoke and be safe in environments we all frequent' (Curtin, 2003). Michael O'Shea, Chief Executive of the Irish Heart Foundation, in a Letter to *The Irish Times* also stated, 'This is a health issue. We do not have the right to knowingly kill other people or seriously damage their health. Passive smoke kills and harms people' (O'Shea, 2003). The concept of responsibility, in this context, was very closely linked to the idea of selfishness. Smokers were seen as passively irresponsible (they should know about the damage they do to others), or indeed as actively irresponsible and selfish (if they do realise the damage they do and continue to do so).

The construction of smokers as irresponsible was reinforced by a number of discursive strategies. For example, one of them was to draw upon the metaphor of contagion. A press release by the office of the Chief Medical Officer on smoking in the workplace on 21 August 2003, stated that

> Standing in the path of a smoker or their cigarette or being in a room in which there are smokers means being exposed to at least 50 agents known to cause cancer and other chemicals that increase blood pressure, damage the lungs and cause abnormal kidney function. (DoHC, 2003)

Not only were the audience warned that it is dangerous 'being in a room in which there are smokers', but also 'standing in the path of a smoker or their cigarette' (the use of 'or' here merges the 'smoker' with 'their cigarette'). Proximity to smokers in itself was presented as a risk. Corrigan has observed that concerns about contagion are prevalent in smoking, which he argues go beyond fear of exposure to direct pathogens, but also reflect a fear of moral contagion. He argues that this is because 'an epistemological error occurs when people mistake the behaviour for the person' (Corrigan, 2004: 353).

Another one of the strategies for constituting smokers as irresponsible, often selfish, was to refer to the various victims of smokers. The victims of smokers were non-smokers in general, but children in particular. As Minister Martin stated, 'Environmental Tobacco Smoke doesn't just cause cancer. It causes heart disease. It causes respiratory problems. In adults. And in children. It damages the health of children right from the start: for example, it lowers birth weight' (Martin, 2003a). The concern for the impact of second-hand smoke on children (and foetuses) was a key feature of almost all of the social marketing campaigns deployed to enhance government. For example, *Passive Smoking Can Kill*, launched by the Department of Health and Children to highlight how cigarette smoking impacts on the health of those in the company of smokers, showed three cameos: a couple enjoying a drink as the woman is being strangled by her partner's cigarette smoke; a group of builders enjoying a cigarette break in a steel container at the expense of a non-smoker; and a baby snoozing in a buggy whilst being smothered by his mother's cigarette smoke. One of the key features of these ads is the explicit level of violence that is suggested as being perpetuated by those smokers around us. Indeed, blowing smoke in anyone's face is a sign of disrespect and aggression (Oaks, 2000).

The construction of children as victims was also a feature of some of the leaflets deployed by the Office of Tobacco Control and the Irish Cancer Society on Environmental Tobacco Smoke / Passive Smoking. In both cases, children were given a section. The following text belongs to the information sheets developed by the Irish Cancer Society: 'Smoking in the presence of young children can cause them serious illness and may make them more likely to suffer health problems in later life. Their health may be *endangered even before birth*' (emphasis added). In all these leaflets mothers were a clear target of the messages, and protecting the foetus, babies and children was a mechanism to convey the message that smoking affects innocent victims. The construction of the irresponsible mother identity was reinforced by the fact that not only was exposure to environmental tobacco smoke problematised, but also 'smoking during pregnancy'. The moralisation of motherhood in the context of smoking (Weir, 1996) was also reflected in the social marketing campaign *Passive Smoking Can Kill*, as mentioned above. While two of the locations of the ads were set in the workplaces, one of them was in fact set at home (which had nothing to do with the workplace smoking ban). As Oaks (2000) argues, in such campaigns the target population are not solely mothers, but the public in general. All viewers are implicitly urged to increase social pressure on pregnant women and mothers not to smoke.

The identity of the irresponsible smoker was also reinforced by a discourse that constituted smokers as a 'burden' to the state and the economy. From the very outset, the non-smoking workplace ban was linked to 'less absenteeism from smoking-related illness. It reduces the fire hazard. It reduces maintenance and redecoration costs.' This was done in order to encourage publicans to embrace the smoking ban. In the process, smokers were constituted as a financial burden. At a seminar on 'The Costs and Productivity Impact of Tobacco Use' organised by the OTC, the Minister stated,

> As Minister for Health and Children I am fully aware of the *enormous burden* that the consumption of tobacco products directly imposes on our health care system through active and passive smoking ... The State assumes most of the costs of health care and tackling the *tobacco epidemic* is a Government approved public health priority. A significant number of beds in our acute hospitals are occupied by people with tobacco related illnesses. (Martin, 2003b; emphasis added)

These discourses resulted in the construction of smoking, and hence smokers, as irresponsible, because they are seen as an 'enormous burden' to the state, again, reinforced by rhetorical devices such as the analogy of contagion/ infectious diseases by referring to 'the tobacco epidemic', as reflected in the extract above.

While smokers were often presented as irresponsible individuals, the analysis also shows that smokers' cooperation was sought by appealing to a responsible smoker identity. This took place in two specific contexts: first of all, in the context of the constitution of the smoking ban as an opportunity for 'responsible smokers' to quit smoking; and second, by promoting the construction of smokers as 'responsible citizens' in the context of compliance. While the smoking ban was defined primarily as a health and safety measure to protect workers and customers from the harmful effects of Environmental Tobacco Smoke, the smoking ban was also constituted as the ultimate instrument to reduce smoking prevalence in society – 'the health initiative of the century' (Clancy, 2004). The Minister predicted that 'there are many smokers who will use the new smoke-free areas to assist them in their efforts to quit smoking' (Martin, 2003c). A senior medical social worker, in a letter to *The Irish Times*, echoed the Minister's 'sympathetic and encouraging' approach to smokers who wanted to quit smoking. As he stated, 'We should be *sympathetic* and *encouraging* to those smokers who are making every effort to rid themselves of this addiction and protective of our own and other's health when we are being *infected* by those who insist wrongly that smoking is a civil right' (Morris, 2003; emphasis added). This letter makes a clear distinction between responsible smokers (those who are trying to quit) and irresponsible smokers, those who continue to 'infect us'. As such, it creates a distinction between deserving and undeserving smokers. The implications draw on a moral responsibility to be enterprising, to try to give up smoking, or otherwise be subject to social disapproval by being perceived as irresponsible, destructive and 'contagious' (also highlighted earlier).

Second, smokers were also given a responsible identity in the context of compliance and implementation. The Minister stated 'I am confident that people will adapt. Most people are law abiding and responsible and I am confident that the vast majority of employers, employees and the public will respect the new measure' (Martin, 2004a). The responsible smoker identity was also promoted in the context of the debates spurred by some media reports on the tragic murder of a bouncer in New York in April 2003 (Humphreys, 2003). The Vintners Federation of Ireland used this event to highlight the dangers of introducing the smoking ban, drawing upon the construction of smokers as dangerous. In response to vintners' and publicans' concerns, the Minister stated, 'I am confident that the majority of citizens will undertake to respect the rights of workers to a healthy, smoke-free environment' (Martin, 2003d). In fact, according to the Minister, the policing of the smoking ban would not be an issue and 'the public will be the biggest enforcers of all' (Sheahan, 2003).

The smoking ban and the civilised self

Notions of civilisation have been central to the discourses that have come to define the Irish smoking ban as a success (Fernández, 2016b). As a Letter to the Editor published in *The Irish Times* a week after the ban was introduced stated, 'The general drinking public have already decided how to respond to this piece of noble and innovative legislation – that is in a mature, responsible and law-abiding manner as befits *civilised* human behaviour in any *enlightened* society' (O'Brien, 2004; emphasis added). They were also central to the debates that dominated the introduction of the smoking ban. Notions of civilisation were often deployed in the form of ideas about progress. For example, at the announcement of the ban,

Minister Martin stated, 'I believe that in every decade, we are presented with one major choice – a choice where, if we call it right, *we can change the future for the better*. This is one of those choices' (Martin, 2003a; emphasis added). The idea of progress was conveyed by the use of the metaphor of the present as a 'crossroads'. The smoking ban as progress was also strengthened by the use of an analogy of antibiotics. As the Minister stated,

> We nod reverently when we read about the introduction of antibiotics: yes, we think. They made a great impact ... Removing tobacco damage from our lives would have a comparable effect, on individual health and survival. On domestic and workplace well-being. On the nation as a whole. (Martin, 2003a)

The smoking ban was presented as medical progress, that is, what Curtis (2007) refers to as the 'heroic progress' of the science and medicine narrative embedded within medical materialist explanations. Furthermore, the smoking ban was repeatedly referred to by using the adjective 'progressive'. The Minister defined it repeatedly as a 'positive, *progressive* health and safety measure' (emphasis added) and this term was also adopted by the pro-ban lobby groups, such as its most vehement champion, ASH Ireland. In a Letter to the Editor published by *The Irish Times* on 5 August 2003, Valerie Coghlan, ASH Ireland, 'urged the Government to proceed with this ban and not to compromise in any way on this vital and *progressive* health initiative' (Coghlan, 2003; emphasis added).

Another key strategy, drawing on the definition of the smoking ban as progress, was to present and promote Ireland as a leading anti-tobacco player on the world stage. At the announcement of the ban, ASH Ireland stated, 'Ireland can set the trend internationally on this issue – a most positive health issue' (ASH Ireland, 2003a). EU Health Commissioner David Byrne, at the *Promoting Heart Health European Consensus Conference* in Cork, also highlighted how 'in clearing the air of tobacco smoke in Ireland, a beacon of health is being lit that will one day illuminate the whole of Europe' (Shanahan, 2004). The fact that Ireland would be the first country in the world to introduce an overall blanket ban on smoking became a sign of the civilising process of the Irish public body. The analysis suggests that this process of collective civilisation was reinforced by 'othering' the Irish collective body of the past, an older and traditional Ireland (also developed by Fernández, 2016b). Those that opposed the smoking ban also contributed to this 'othering' process. For example, they often lamented the impact that it would have on 'Irish culture' and on the 'traditional social life in Ireland'. This 'perceived destruction of Irish social and cultural values' is also identified by Fahy's (2009: 55) analysis of opinion articles. These discourses also contributed to reinforcing the idea of the smoking ban as progress and moving the country forward. As a letter highlighted, 'I've no doubt that future generations will view public smoking in the twentieth century in the same way that we now look back on practices which were acceptable in the nineteenth century but are now viewed with abhorrence' (Jordan, 2003). That is, smoking was presented as a 'practice' from the past, once 'acceptable' but 'now viewed with abhorrence'. The dictionary defines 'abhorrence' as a feeling of extreme repugnance or aversion; utter loathing; abomination. It is indicative that smoking has become moralised (Rozin and Singh, 1999).

The essence of the smoking ban as progress, and what it meant to Ireland, was captured by well-known Irish journalist David McWilliams, in an article published just the day before the smoking ban was introduced. He stated,

> Take your last drag, pop down to the shops now, get a pack of 20, get into a pub and smoke away – because by midnight tonight, smoking in public will be *a thing of the past*. Tomorrow marks the beginning of *a new smoke-free dawn*. It is also a *revolutionary moment*. Banning smoking in Irish pubs – and the ease with which it has come to pass – tells us an enormous amount about how much our society has changed. (McWilliams, 2004; emphasis added)

Many elements in this article resonate with Minister Martin's speech at the announcement of the smoking ban, exactly fourteen months before McWilliams's piece. Smoking in public here, too, was presented as 'a thing of the past' and the smoking ban as a history-making piece of legislation, 'a new smoke-free dawn', 'a revolutionary moment'. It reflects the significance of the contrast between an Irish collective body of the past and the dominant discourse of Ireland as a leading and innovative country.

Notions of progress were also central in the construction of vintners and the hospitality industry as uncivilised. At the announcement of the proposed smoking ban on 30 January 2003, Minister Martin noted,

> Looking back at issues like asbestos, all of us regard the industries that refused to take action when they knew their product killed workers – we regard those industries as having been *beneath contempt*. They chose not to face up to the facts. They *sacrificed human beings*. And for a long time, they got away with it. (Martin, 2003a; emphasis added)

Being 'beneath contempt' denotes uncivilised behaviour, further reinforced by the use of the term 'sacrificed human beings', with its connotations of uncivilised and primitive behaviour. This rhetorical metaphor was also used to attack the tobacco industry. For example, the Minister also highlighted how the WHO *Treaty on Tobacco Control* (2003) 'will make a significant contribution to protecting future generations from the *predatory practices* of the global tobacco industry' (Martin, 2003b; emphasis added). Again, predatory denotes primate and animalistic features.

Discourses of order and self-control were also central in the making up of an uncivilised smoker identity. My analysis reveals that in the context of the ban, smokers were often presented as lacking self-control. One of the key aspects of the smoking ban was to de-normalise smoking and eradicate, as the Research Director of the Institute of Cancer Research wrote, 'the unholy alliance of smoking and drinking. When people take alcohol, their inhibitions are reduced and this may contribute to smoking' (Armstrong, 2003). The centrality of the discourse of control was also reflected in some of the Letters to the Editor. For example, one letter, in response to a previous letter which described 'the simple enjoyment of a cigarette with a pint at the end of a day's work' as a 'basic human right', stated, 'The problem is that it is not "a" cigarette and a pint that most smokers want, but one damn cigarette after another until the air in the bar is unbreatheable to all except themselves' (Kelly, 2003).

An uncontrolled and disorderly smoker identity was often promoted in the debates that emerged in relation to enforcement. For example, as previously referred to, the media reported that a bouncer had been stabbed by a smoker in New York, the implication of which was that smokers might become uncivilised, potentially violent and dangerous if not allowed to smoke. In July 2004, the Taoiseach came out in support of the smoking ban, and on RTÉ television highlighted that the smoking ban would bring 'decent people' back to pubs. This remark was not lost on smokers, one of whom, in a Letter to the Editor published by *The Irish Times*, stated that 'Micheál Martin has dismissed us a health menace and the Taoiseach has asked us to make way for the "decent people" to enjoy the treats of smoke-free, empty public houses' (O'Donnell, 2004). Players in the hospitality industry, as well as some politicians opposing the ban, also drew upon a potentially disorderly smoker identity, by pointing to the impossibility of enforcing the ban. Senator Eddie Bohan highlighted that 'Publicans will find this too difficult to control' and Noel Davern, Galway Councillor, stated, 'If you have a crowd of young fellows in the corner, would you tell them to stop?' (Hennessy, 2003). In the process, some groups were promoted as dangerous and uncivilised, especially young men.

It must be highlighted, once again, that there were multiple discourses at play, and that the analysis of media discourses shows that there were also contesting voices. For example, rather than viewing it as progress, those opposing the ban saw it as a reflection of the 'Americanisation' of Ireland, which was contrasted with the more 'civilised' European neighbours. These arguments were mostly deployed by members of the public and reflected in Letters to the Editor, but they also emerged from within the government backbenchers. Minister for Environment Martin Cullen (who, as previously highlighted, was often portrayed as an irrational smoker) was reported to say he was 'uneasy about us following what I consider to be political correctness of the United States and would prefer us to be like our European counterparts who are slightly more irreverent'. Referring to wider debates in Irish health policy, he said 'I suppose I'm closer to Berlin than Boston on smoking and obviously like having a couple of cigarettes with a cup of coffee' (quoted in O'Brien and Duffy, 2003). Smoking therefore, rather than disgusting and uncivilised, was constructed as more 'fun' and smokers as more 'irreverent' and 'social'. Again, as Minister Cullen said, 'I have a healthy traditional dislike of over-regulation and being told what to do all the time, particularly now when it becomes part of invading into your social life.' The use of the word 'healthy' in this context could be considered quite ironic. Some of the Letters to the Editor also drew on such notions to warn that they would, if the ban was introduced, be 'spending my holidays, and money, in a *civilised* country such as France or Spain' (McCarthy, 2003; emphasis added).

Conclusion

In this chapter, I have explored the centrality of rational, responsible and civilised selves in debates about smoking restrictions and the role they played in the introduction of the smoking ban in Ireland. In the process, I have also revealed how official and dominant public health discourses may be challenged. Undertaking a governmental analysis of these debates proved revealing in a number of ways: first of all, I was able to expose the ways in which the same terms are often used to support different (and often completely opposing) arguments. For example, 'civilised' can be used as an argument both for smoking and against it; 'hedonistic' experiences can be associated with neglect, self-indulgence and lack of control, or in fact positively, with 'revelry', pleasure and letting go. These findings draw attention to the use of rhetorical strategies in policy debates and expose how certain words and ideas can be intentionally used to influence opinion.

Second, revealing the strategic character of these debates also shed light on how power might be exercised 'through' people, rather than 'on' people, by exploring some of the identities that were assumed and promoted in order to give effect to government. My analysis showed that there were three dominant notions of 'self' which informed the myriad of discourses and technologies deployed in the context of the ban: the 'rational self', the 'responsible self' and the 'civilised self'. These identities were reinforced by a number of strategies: for example, drawing on discursive devices such as the crossroads metaphor of the analogy of antibiotics, the smoking ban was constructed as evidence-based policy and medical progress. In the process, scientists and public health and health-promotion groups were produced as rational actors drawing on a conceptualisation of experts as independent and altruistic. On the other hand, smokers were often constructed as irrational, irresponsible and uncivilised. Some of the strategies deployed to enhance the irresponsible smoker identity included the metaphor of 'contagion' and the deployment of social marketing campaigns in which smokers were explicitly portrayed as choking their loved ones. This identity was further reinforced by discourses that constituted smokers as a burden to the state and the economy. Smokers also emerged as uncivilised in the context of discourses that drew upon notions of progress and disorder.

Third, this study also showed that where there is power, there is also resistance. The construction of smokers as irrational, irresponsible and uncivilised was contested by discourses that presented smoking as rational, pleasurable and fun. Some of these contributions promoted, instead, the construction of proponents of the ban as 'fanatics' and 'puritans', drawing for example on analogies of religion which constructed official actors and public health promoters as 'crusaders'. Giving further credence to the strategic use of language and rhetoric, the analysis shows that in order to promote compliance, proponents of the ban also relied upon the construction of smokers as rational, responsible and civilised actors. For example, in the context of debates over enforcement, smokers were continually referred to as 'responsible and law-abiding citizens'. Indeed, the smoking ban relied upon the self-regulating capacities of subjects, which were enhanced, among other ways, by promoting a responsible smoker identity.

Finally, this chapter has revealed that while the ban was presented as a collective measure, there were also targeted dynamics deployed as part of the ban. For example, discourses often reproduced women as mothers, young people as irrational and young men as dangerous. While these dynamics have not been analysed in detail here, these findings indicate that, perhaps, a governmental analysis might help to expose the unequal effects of discourses and power. Future research should consider looking into how these unequal dynamics may be implicated in debates about smoking and smoking restrictions.

References

Armstrong, J. (2003) Smoking ban. Letter to the Editor. *The Irish Times*, 3 March.

ASH Ireland (2003a) ASH Ireland supports workplace ban. Press release. 30 January. Available from: www.ash.ie/News/Archived_News_2003/Workplace_Ban.html. Accessed 1 July 2013.

ASH Ireland (2003b) ASH Ireland welcomes workplace regulations. Press release. 23 October. Available from: www.ash.ie/News/Archived_News_2003/Regulations.html. Accessed 1 July 2013.

Blume, S. (2006) Anti-vaccination movements and their interpretations. *Social Science & Medicine*, 62(3): 628–642.

Boland, J. (2003) Impending ban on smoking. Letter to the Editor. *The Irish Times*, 13 November.

Bordo, S. (1993) *Unbearable Weight: Feminism, Western Culture and the Body*. Berkeley, University of California Press.

Brandt, A.M. (1998) Blow some my way: passive smoking, risk and American culture. IN: Lock, S., Reynolds, L.A. and Tansy, E.M. (eds) *Ashes to Ashes: The History of Smoking and Health*. Amsterdam, Rodopi: pp. 164–191.

Clancy, L. (2004) Smoking ban can be health initiative of the century. Press release. 18 February. Available from: www.ash.ie/News/Archived_News_2004/Century. html. Accessed 1 July, 2013.

Coghlan, V. (2003) Ban on smoking in pubs. Letter to the Editor. *The Irish Times*, 5 August.

Corrigan, P.W. (2004) Marlboro Man and the stigma of smoking. IN: Gilman, S.L. and Tun, Z. (eds) *Smoke: A Global History of Smoking*. London, Reaktion Books: pp. 344–354.

Curtin, J. (2003) Proposal for complete ban on smoking in pubs. Letter to the Editor. *The Irish Times*, 30 July.

Curtis, V.A. (2007) Dirt, disgust and disease: a natural history of hygiene. *Journal of Epidemiology and Community Health*, 61(8): 660–664.

Davies, H. (2003) Banning smoking. Letter to the Editor. *The Irish Times*, 1 February.

Dean, M. (1999) *Governmentality: Power and Rule in Modern Society*. London, Sage.

DoHC (2003) Statement from the office of CMO on smoking in the workplace ban. Press release. 21 August 2003.

Donnelly, P. (2003) Smoking ban in pubs. Letter to the Editor. *The Irish Times*, 14 July.

Dunne, T. (2003) Smoking ban in pubs. Letter to the Editor. *The Irish Times*, 31 July.

Fahy, D. (2009) The Irish punditocracy as contrarian voice: opinion coverage of the workplace smoking ban. *Irish Communications Review*, 11: 50–62.

Farrimond, H.R. and Joffe, H. (2006) Pollution, peril and poverty: a British study of the stigmatization of smokers. *Journal of Community and Applied Social Psychology*, 16(6): 481–491.

Fernández, E. (2016a) Exploring the story of the smoking ban in Ireland as a neo-liberal project. *Social Theory & Health*, 14(2): 256–274.

Fernández, E. (2016b) No smoke without fire: public health, morality, and the civilized self. *Irish Journal of Sociology*, 24(2): 153–174.

Foucault, M. (1982) The subject and power. IN: Dreyfus, H. and Rabinow, P. (eds) *Michel Foucault: Beyond Structuralism and Hermeneutics*. Chicago, University of Chicago Press: pp. 208–226.

Foucault, M. (1988) Technologies of the self. IN: Martin, L.H., Gutman, H. and Hutton, P.H. (eds) *Technologies of the Self: A Seminar with Michel Foucault*. London, Tavistock: pp. 16–49.

Foucault, M. (1991) Governmentality. IN: Burchell, G., Gordon, C. and Miller, P. (eds) *The Foucault Effect: Studies in Governmentality (with Two Lectures by and an Interview with Michel Foucault)*. Chicago, University of Chicago Press.

Gilmore, N. (2004) *Clearing the Air: The Battle over the Smoking Ban*. Dublin, Liberties.

Gordon, C. (1991) Governmental rationality: an introduction. IN: Burchell, G., Gordon, C. and Miller, P. (eds) *The Foucault Effect: Studies in Governmental Rationality*. Hemel Hempstead, Harvester Wheatsheaf: pp. 1–51.

Goudsblom, J. (1986) Public health and the civilizing process. *The Milbank Quarterly*, 64(2): 162–188.

Heaney, A. (2003) Plan to ban smoking in pubs. Letter to the Editor. *The Irish Times*, 7 February.

Hennessy, M. (2003) FF TDs put pressure on Martin over ban on pub smoking. *The Irish Times*, 29 March.

Holahan, A. (2003) Plan to ban smoking in pubs. Letter to the Editor. *The Irish Times*, 17 February.

Howell, F. (2003) Smoking in public places. Letter to the Editor. *The Irish Times*, 27 February.

Howell, F. (2005) Smoke-free bars in Ireland: a runaway success. *Tobacco Control*, 14(2): 73–74.

Humphreys, J. (2003) Smoking ban concerns raised after US murder. *The Irish Times*, 16 April.

Jäger, S. and Maier, F. (2009) Theoretical and methodological aspects of Foucauldian critical discourse analysis and dispositive analysis. IN: Wodak, R. and Meyer, M. (eds) *Methods of Critical Discourse Analysis*. London, Sage: pp. 34–61.

Jordan, D. (2003) FF division over smoking ban. Letter to the Editor. *The Irish Times*, 13 August.

Kelly, D. (2003) Plan to ban smoking in pubs. Letter to the Editor. *The Irish Times*, 16 July.

Kitching, K. (2013) Governing 'authentic' religiosity? The responsibilization of parents beyond religion and state in matters of school ethos in Ireland. *Irish Journal of Sociology*, 21(2): 17–34.

Kuhling, C. (2004) The smoking ban in Ireland: smoke-free or smokescreen? *Capital and Class*, 28(3): 211–216.

Lupton, D. (1995) *The Imperative of Health: Public Health and the Regulated Body*. London, Sage.

Lupton, D. (1997) Consumerism, reflexivity and the medical encounter. *Social Science & Medicine*, 45(3): 373–381.

Lupton, D. (1999) Developing the 'whole me': citizenship, neo-liberalism and the contemporary health and physical education curriculum. *Critical Public Health*, 9(4): 287–300.

Lupton, D. (2000) Food, risk and subjectivity. IN: Williams, S.J., Gabe, J. and Calnan, M. (eds) *Health, Medicine and Society: Key Theories and Future Agendas*. New York, Routledge: pp. 205–218.

Lupton, D. (2008) 'You feel so responsible': Australian mothers' concepts and experiences related to promoting the health and development of their young children. IN: Zoller, H. and Dutta, M. (eds) *Emerging Perspectives in Health Communication: Meaning, Culture, and Power*. New York, Routledge.

Lupton, D. and Petersen, A. (1996) *The New Public Health: Discourses, Knowledges, Strategies*. London, Sage.

MacHale, D. (2003) Plan to ban smoking in pubs. Letter to the Editor. *The Irish Times*, 4 October.

Martin, M. (2003a) Speech at the launch of the *Report on the Health Effects of Environmental Tobacco Smoke in the Workplace*. 30 January. Available from: www.dohc.ie/press/speeches/2003/20030130.html. Accessed 2 July, 2013.

Martin, M. (2003b) Speech at the opening of the Seminar on the *Costs and Productivity Impact of Tobacco Use*, 2 October.

Martin, M. (2003c) Speech at the opening of *Smokers – Attitudes, Behaviours and Cessation* seminar, 4 March. Available from: www.dohc.ie/press/speeches/2003/20030304.html. Accessed 2 July, 2013.

Martin, M. (2003d) Minister Martin responds to recent comments on the smoking ban. Press release. 28 August. DoHC.

Martin, M. (2004a) Minister Martin TD welcomes the commencement of the Smoke Free at Work Initiative. Press release. 29 March. DoHC.

Martin, M. (2004b) Minister Martin attends the launch of an information campaign prior to the commencement of Smoke Free legislation in Norway. Press release. 25 May 2004. Available from: www.dohc.ie/press/releases/2004/20040525.html. Accessed 2 July, 2013.

Martin, M. (2004c) Speech at the announcement of the commencement date for the smoke-free workplace regulations. 18 February. Available from: www.dohc.ie/press/speeches/2004/20040218.html. Accessed 2 July, 2013.

Maurer, B. (2003) Plan to ban smoking in pubs. Letter to the Editor. *The Irish Times*, 30 August.

McCarthy, H. (2003) 'Political correctness' and the proposed smoking ban. Letter to the Editor. *The Irish Times*, 26 September.

McWilliams, D. (2004) Welcome to the age of wellness. *Sunday Business Post*, 28 March.

Mennell, S. (1985) *All Manners of Food: Eating and Taste in England and France from the Middle Ages to the Present*. Oxford, Blackwell.

Mennell, S. (1991) On the civilizing of appetite. IN: Featherstone, M., Hepworth, M. and Turner, B.S. (eds) *The Body: Social Process and Cultural Theory*. London, Sage: pp. 126–157.

Meredith, P. (1993) Patient satisfaction with communication in general surgery: problems of measurement and improvement. *Social Science & Medicine*, 37(5): 591–602.

Morris, T. (2003) Plan to ban smoking in pubs. Letter to the Editor. *The Irish Times*, 11 October.

Oaks, L. (2000) Smoke-filled wombs and fragile fetuses: the social politics of fetal representation. *Signs*, 26(1): 63–108.

O'Brien, C. and Duffy, C. (2003) Concern growing in FF over ban on smoking in workplace. *The Irish Times*, 12 August.

O'Brien, P.J. (2004) Deasy in the Dail bar. Letter to the Editor. *The Irish Times*, 7 April.

O'Donnell, S. (2004) Banning smoking in pubs. Letter to the Editor. *The Irish Times*, 14 July.

O Fatharta, C. (2014) Time to clear the air over use of e-cigarettes. *Irish Examiner*, 18 March.

O'Malley, P. (1996a) Indigenous governance. *Economy and Society*, 29(3): 310–326.

O'Malley, P. (1996b) Risk and Responsibility. IN: Barry, A., Osborne, T. and Rose, N. (eds) *Foucault and Political Reason: Liberalism, Neo-liberalism and Rationalities of Government*. London, University College London Press: pp. 189–208.

O'Shea, M. (2003) Smoking ban in pubs. Letter to the Editor. *The Irish Times*, 1 August.

Petersen, A. (1999) Public health, the new genetics and subjectivity. IN: Petersen, A., Barns, I., Dudley, J. and Harris, P. (eds) *Postsctruturalism, Citizenship and Social Policy*. London, Routledge: pp. 114–153.

Petersen, A. (2007) *The Body in Question: A Socio-Cultural Approach*. London and New York, Routledge.

Poland, B.D. (1998) Smoking, stigma and the purification of public space. IN: Kearns, R.A. and Gesler, W.M. (eds) *Putting Health into Place: Landscape, Identity and Well-being*. New York, Syracuse University Press: pp. 208–225.

Poland, B.D. (2000) The 'considerate' smoker in public space: the micro-politics and political economy of 'doing the right thing'. *Health & Place*, 6(1): 1–14.

Poland, B.D., Stockton, L., Ashley, M.J., Pederson, L., Cohen, J., Ferrence, R. and Bull, S. (1999) Interactions between smokers and non-smokers in public places: a qualitative study. *Canadian Journal of Public Health*, 90(5): 330–333.

Reilly, J. (2014) Statement on the 10th anniversary of the Workplace Smoking Ban in Ireland. Media release of the DoH, 24 March. Available from: www.dohc.ie/press/releases/2014/20140324.html. Accessed 19 September, 2014.

Rose, N. (1989) *Governing the Soul: The Shaping of the Private Self*. London, Routledge.

Rose, N. (1999) *Governing the Soul: The Shaping of the Private Self* (second edition). London, Free Association Books.

Rose, N. and Miller, P. (1992) Political power beyond the State: problematics of government. *British Journal of Sociology*, 43(2): 271–303.

Rose, N. and Miller, P. (2008) *Governing the Present: Administering Economic, Social and Personal Life*. Cambridge, Polity.

Rozin, P. and Singh, L. (1999) The moralization of cigarette smoking in the United States. *Journal of Consumer Psychology*, 8(3): 321–337.

Sears, A. (1991) AIDS and the health of nations: the contradictions of public health. *Critical Sociology*, 18(2): 31–50.

Shanahan, C. (2004) Byrne rules out EU challenge to smoking ban. *Irish Examiner*, 26 February.

Sheahan, F. (2003) Publicans face jail for failing to ban smoking. *Irish Examiner*, 29 July.

Stallins-Smith, S., Zeka, A., Goodman, P., Kabir, Z. and Clancy, L. (2013) Reductions in cardiovascular, cerebrovascular, and respiratory mortality following the national Irish smoking ban: interrupted time-series analysis. *Plos One*, 8 (4). Available from: http://journals.plos.org/plosone/article?id=10.1371/journal.pone.0062063. Accessed 18 March 2016.

Thompson, L., Pearce, J. and Barnett, R. (2009) Nomadic identities and socio-spatial competence: making sense of post-smoking selves. *Social and Cultural Geography*, 10(5): 565–581.

TNS/MRBI (2003) Smoking ban survey. *Irish Examiner*, 24 July.

Tuggle, J.L. and Holmes, M.D. (2003) Blowing smoke: status politics and the Shasta county smoking ban. IN: Kelly, D.H. and Clarke, E.J. (eds) *Deviant Behaviours: A Text Reader in the Sociology of Deviance*. New York, Worth: pp. 43–56.

Weir, L. (1996) Recent developments in the government of pregnancy. *Economy and Society*, 25(3): 372–392.

Welshman, J. (2004) Smoking, science and medicine. IN: Gilman, S.L. and Tun, Z. (eds) *Smoke: A Global History of Smoking*. London, Reaktion Books: pp. 326–331.

Woods, B. (2003) Smoking ban in pubs. Letter to the Editor. *The Irish Times*, 26 July.

Zdenkowski, A. (2004) Bouquet for the smoking ban. Letter to the Editor. *The Irish Times*, 18 August.

When health means illness: analysing mental health discourses and practices in Ireland

Introduction

The last ten years have witnessed significant developments in mental health policy and practices in Ireland. As Foucault and other authors have noted, discourses constructing mental health have been strongly tied to biomedical understandings of mental *illness* and the medical speciality of psychiatry (Foucault, 1965; Rogers and Pilgrim, 2005; Middleton, 2007). The recent questioning of these biomedical discourses in Ireland, as in other countries – by critical psychiatrists, survivors of the mental health system and others – has led to the emergence of different, and sometimes conflicting, ways of constructing 'truths' about mental health. In this chapter, I use ideas drawn from governmentality to explore the emergence, and sometimes uneasy co-existence, of these discourses in the mental health policy arena. In particular, I seek to expose a key tension in recent policy pronouncements between broad statements about the universal relevance of our mental health (the notion that *we all have mental health*) and narrow, deficit-based, medical conceptions of mental *illness* which lead to policies and practices being focused around a particular segment of the population who use mental health services. By exploring this tension, I argue that we can expose not just the different ways in which the self-identities and subjectivities associated with mental health are constructed, but also the mismatches between rationalities of governing and the technical aspects of putting particular visions and mentalities into practice – practices which, in turn, have very real consequences for the way in which we 'do' mental health in Ireland.

My analysis in this chapter is based primarily on a number of mental health policy documents published in the past ten years. The most significant of these is *A Vision for Change: Report of the Expert Group on Mental Health Policy* (AVFC) (Government of Ireland, 2006) which is recognised as Ireland's core policy document setting out the direction, and plan for the delivery of, mental health services in the state from 2006 until 2015. At the time of its publication, *AVFC* was described as having 'widespread support across the political spectrum and among people who use mental health services, their family supporters and professionals delivering services' (Mental Health Reform, 2015: 1). While providing a blueprint for the delivery of mental health services in Ireland, *AVFC* also established an apparently more comprehensive understanding of mental health than previous biomedical definitions, with the document acknowledging 'that there is a range of factors which can influence mental health, including physical, psychological, social, cultural and economic' and that 'mental health is broader than an absence of mental disorders' (Government of Ireland, 2006: 15–16). However, as I seek to show in this chapter, these assertions have not been matched by the document's recommendations, which remain resolutely oriented towards mental health service users, mental health service provision, and the interaction between mental health services and other specialist services. This apparent mismatch is also evident in other documents, such as *Healthy Ireland: A Framework for Improved Health and Well-Being 2013–2025*, a broader public health strategy which references mental health (Government of Ireland, 2013), and in policy in the area of children and youth affairs such as *Brighter Outcomes, Better Futures* (DCYA, 2014).

Exploring these documents through a governmentality framework provides an opportunity to examine how particular ideas emerge and are given meaning in the mental health policy arena in different contexts. As mental health policy develops, new concepts are emerging which are shifting our understandings of mental health. One such concept, that of *recovery*, for example, has been a central theme in the discourse related to the implementation of *AVFC*. The deployment of the concept of recovery offers an interesting insight into the tensions between clinical and social understandings of mental health as both clinical and social models of this concept are used interchangeably in discourse. Notions of mental health literacy, similarly, have gained attention internationally, and have recently been incorporated into Irish policy in the area of children and youth affairs (DCYA, 2014). The chapter, therefore, seeks to trace the emergence of some of these discourses, and asks how they might build into, or develop, more holistic understandings of mental health and mental health practices.

Overall, then, my aim in this chapter is to expose the tensions between broad public mental health statements and the narrow, deficit-based approaches taken in practice as a way of articulating a holistic understanding of mental health that goes beyond illness. In exploring this tension, broad-based messages about *our* mental health in current policy documents can be interpreted as invitations to develop discourses in this area and establish new possibilities for collective understanding that can make a real and positive difference to the everyday ways in which we, as a society, practice mental health. The significance of these possibilities lies in the very real impact our understanding of mental health has on our lives, individually

and collectively. For example, the ways in which we understand and interpret mental health and mental health difficulty have a significant bearing
on our willingness to ask for support. In turn, the likelihood of personal
difficulties escalating into crises can be increased if our cultural framing of
mental health is narrow. As I suggest, then, new possibilities for collective
understanding will involve a widening of our gaze in mental health beyond
the medical ontology which has historically underpinned, and arguably still
dominates, mental health policy and practice(s) in the state.

Exploring mental health through governmentality

The theoretical framework of governmentality can be helpful in exploring
tensions between the mentalities and practices of governing, and discourses
as they have developed around mental health policy and practice in Ireland.
Governmentality, as an analytical tool, can be used to open up understandings of the ways in which social institutions such as the education system,
the health system or the penal system function, and can help to explain
the philosophies that guide the day-to-day functioning of those institutions. Foucault began to develop his thinking around governmentality in
the 1970s as an 'activity that undertakes to conduct individuals throughout their lives by placing them under the authority of a guide responsible
for what they do and for what happens to them'; as he later described it,
governmentality can be 'understood in the broad sense of techniques and
procedures for directing human behaviour' (Foucault, in Rose, O'Malley
and Valverde, 2006: 83). Governmentality allows us to analyse dominant
regimes of practices and *regimes of truth* in relation to various aspects
of human life. Dean (2010: 40) describes regimes of practices as 'historically constituted assemblages through which we do such things as cure,
care, relieve poverty, punish, educate, train and counsel'. A governmental analysis allows us to explore the logic underpinning practices so that
we can ask questions such as, How do we do mental health? or How
do we do economic policy?, and therefore 'takes as its central concern
how we govern and are governed within different regimes, and the conditions under which such regimes emerge, continue to operate, and are
transformed' (*ibid.*: 33).

In the context of mental health, governmentality approaches have been
used to explore identity formation and mental health within a professional
setting (Ball, 2010) and to critically analyse emerging policy and discourse
as bound to advanced neoliberal modes of governing (Teghtsoonian, 2009).
Ball's (2010) work on strategies designed to tackle depression within the
legal profession, for example, illustrates how a range of prescriptive texts
concerned with the problem of depression works to create a range of identities among law students which can be summarised as 'responsibilising'.

Analysing texts such as handbooks for lawyers and law students in Australia, his work identifies the different identities which coalesce around 'psychological subjects', 'neurochemical selves' and 'virtuous persons'; in all cases, these texts seek to govern depression in a way which makes the individual responsible for his or her mental health. Ball (2010: 9) concludes in his analysis that 'while some attention is still paid to the environment within which students must study or will be employed, the focus is on the individual and not on changing broader social factors that may contribute to depression'.

Katherine Teghtsoonian similarly notes the individualising focus of mental health policy in her governmentality-inspired analysis of mental health policy in the Canadian province of British Columbia (Teghtsoonian, 2009). Teghtsoonian highlights the emphasis placed on the individual's role in fighting depression, something which she connects to the individualising and responsibilising agenda associated with neoliberal modes of governance. Rather than address issues related to the provision of state mental health services, policy in British Columbia identifies the individual and his or her community as the key resource in responding to mental distress. Among the concepts gaining popularity in mental health discourse in Canada – and indeed Ireland – is the concept of mental health literacy, described by Jorm and colleagues (1997) as 'knowledge and beliefs about mental disorders which aid their recognition, management or prevention'. Yet as Teghtsoonian (2009: 31) notes, focusing on mental health literacy may mean that 'public policies and systematic inequities are ... kept out of view in this analysis, displaced by arguments about the need to ensure that individuals have access to information that will support them in making better decisions regarding their mental health and wellbeing'.

Like Ball (2010), Teghtsoonian examines the text of specific documents which have clear agendas and themes in keeping with a neoliberal policy orientation. These documents emphasise the importance of active citizens self-managing their mental health in order to be able to lead meaningful and fulfilling lives, and as she argues, put forward calculated recommendations supported by selectively chosen evidence, based on approaches to treatment that will minimise economic costs for the state. As an example, Teghtsoonian (2009: 33–34) notes that one document, the *Depression Strategy*, 'advocates for a number of strategies for ensuring that practitioners adhere to standardized, evidence-based treatment protocols and presents as self-evident an interpretation of current evidence that points to a treatment approach that minimizes costs, group-based CBT [cognitive behavioural therapy]'. In so doing, Teghtsoonian clearly argues that British Columbian mental health policy is purposefully aligned with overall provincial economic policy. These studies provide helpful analyses of the ways in which mental health is constituted in discourse, and how particular policies construct subjectivities which are amenable to 'intervention' in different types of ways.

My own analysis of the Irish mental health policy domain builds on Dean's (2010) ideas about valued knowledges and identity formation in the context of governmentality. For Dean, any given regime of practices is underpinned by different dimensions, which include *fields of visibility*, *techniques*, *knowledge* and *identity formation*. In brief, fields of visibility refers to the ways in which particular 'things' or 'people' that are to be governed are framed or illuminated within particular spaces, and the ways in which they are envisaged. Techniques encompass the specific mechanisms or procedures through which governing is enacted and achieved. Knowledge refers to the ways in which particular forms of expertise or know-how are deployed in the process of governing – expertise which becomes bound up in the rationalities and mentalities of rule. Finally, identity formation draws attention to the ways in which programmes of government hinge around the creation of identities of both those who are to be governed, and those who are deemed to be in authority, and who are responsible for implementing processes of governing. Thus as Dean (2010: 43) outlines, governmentality studies ask, 'what forms of person, self and identity are presupposed by different practices of government and what sorts of transformation do these practices seek?' In the remainder of the chapter, I utilise Dean's framework as a way of interrogating regimes of practices shaping the governance of the Irish mental health policy arena. As the chapter argues, a governmental analysis of policy and practice allows us to unpack *how* we are governed in relation to mental health, by making visible dominant discourses, but also illuminating those 'counter-conducts', or ways of articulating mental health which sit outside mainstream *fields of visibility*. This, in turn, may open up new possibilities and alternative approaches to the everyday ways in which mental health is constructed and practised in Ireland.

Mental health policy in Ireland: the context

The history of mental health and mental health policy in Ireland can broadly be said to have emerged out of a nineteenth-century legacy of the management of what was perceived as 'madness'. As in many other Western nations, the asylums of nineteenth-century Ireland housed two different classes of person, categorised as either lunatics or idiots to broadly correspond with the mentally ill, or, in contemporary language, the intellectually disabled (Walsh and Daly, 2004). In this context, the medical speciality of psychiatry has historically played a defining role in mental health policy and practices, albeit with recognisable shifts in thinking and practices. Thus, dominant practices in psychiatry informed by accepted, contemporary knowledge have moved from incarceration in the asylum, to the psychoanalyst's couch through to the pharmacological treatment of the mentally ill. Such shifts are reflected in Rose's (2007: 188) observation that 'human beings, characteristically try to reform and improve themselves. Inescapably, at any historical moment, they do so in terms of knowledges and beliefs about the kind of creatures they are.'

The historical deficits of Ireland's mental health system – evidenced in the over-reliance on institutionalisation, the lack of rights of those detained in such institutions and the liberal use of psychotropic medications – have been highlighted by survivor groups such as Mind Freedom and organisations like the Critical Voices Network Ireland who have been instrumental in challenging biomedical discourses of psychiatry in Ireland. From 1984, with the publication of *The Psychiatric Services – Planning for the Future* (Government of Ireland, 1984), the government indicated a shift from 'treating' mental health in large-scale psychiatric institutions to community-based facilities, and this is a shift which has continued through the publication of *AVFC*. As Considine and Dukelow (2009: 397) describe it, however, mental health has frequently been seen as the 'Cinderella' of the health services, with developments such as the *Mental Health Act 2001*, the establishment of the Mental Health Commission and, more recently, the publication of a strategic vision for mental health services, as set out in *AVFC*, only happening in the past ten years. Developments have therefore been slow and poorly resourced, arguably impeding the potential for change aspired to, and set down in, documents such as *Planning for the Future* and *AVFC*.

Within this system, biomedical psychiatry remains a dominant form of expertise. Mental health services in Ireland are led by medically trained health professionals while key roles in the management of state agencies such as the Mental Health Commission are also taken up by medical experts. As an indication, the Mental Health Commission (which was established under the terms of the *Mental Health Act 2001* to protect the interests of people who are detained in mental health services involuntarily) comprises as its members a lawyer; three registered medical practitioners of whom two are consultant psychiatrists; a social worker; a psychologist; an employee of the Health Service Executive (HSE) nominated by the Executive; two registered nurses; a representative of the general public; and three representatives of voluntary bodies (at least two of whom must have or have had a diagnosed mental illness). The make-up of the Commission membership is indicative of the relatively narrow range of interests represented on public sector mental health institutions.

That said, there are today an increasing number of alternative voices and discourses evident in the mental health policy arena. The emergence of critical psychiatry, of which West Cork-based psychiatrist Pat Bracken is a leading member, is providing a challenge to biomedical understandings of mental illness and health from within the profession of psychiatry, and raises particular questions about the overuse use of psychotropic medication as a basis for treatment (Bracken, 2012). Moreover, movements such as the Critical Voices Network Ireland, a network of people comprising those with self-experience of mental distress and critical thinking health professionals, are increasingly articulating the need for a mental health system which does not work from a biomedical tradition. At another level, a vast number of small voluntary organisations also play a role in providing support services for people experiencing mental health difficulties and mental distress.

Situated within this complex network of actors, current Irish mental health policy increasingly uses the language of recovery and references the expertise of service users. The key document providing the focus for this chapter, *AVFC*, is the framework which has guided mental health practice in Ireland for the past ten years, and at the time of publication was viewed as something of a sea-change in setting out a more coherent understanding of, and vision for, mental health in the state. Informed by an Expert Group whose members included 'all the mental health professions, from voluntary groups and from service users, in order to reflect all the stakeholders in mental health' (Government of Ireland, 2006: 7), the document provided a roadmap for the delivery of mental health services in Ireland, but also acknowledged apparently broader understandings of mental health than those rooted in biomedical knowledge. For example, under the heading 'What do we mean by mental health?', it is stated that 'different cultures have different definitions of mental health, or can place varying degrees of importance on different aspects of mental health' (*ibid.*: 16). Elsewhere, whether consciously or not, the notion of mental illness as 'problems in living' which was developed by Szasz (1961) is invoked in the document's statement of 'the need to recognise that service users are primarily held back from recovery by practical problems of living rather than by their symptoms' (Government of Ireland, 2006: 13).

Since the publication of *AVFC*, mental health has also appeared in other health policy arenas and documents in Ireland, and I refer to these in my analysis. The publication of *Healthy Ireland: A Framework for Improved Health and Well-Being 2013–2025* (Government of Ireland, 2013), described as a 'new government framework for action to improve the health and wellbeing of people living in Ireland over the coming generation' (DoHC, 2014), places an emphasis on cross-departmental work and getting the most out of existing resources to improve the population's health and well-being, and includes mental health as one of its key areas of interest. Mental health issues are also visible in policies targeting young people (e.g. *Brighter Outcomes, Better Futures*, DCYA, 2014) and in the area of suicide prevention, which has become a discrete area of policymaking in its own right. In particular, two key suicide prevention policies have been published in recent years: *ReachOut: National Strategy for Action on Suicide Prevention*

2005–2014 (HSE and DoHC, 2005) and *Connecting for Life: Ireland's National Strategy to Reduce Suicide 2015–2020* (DoH, 2015). These strategies have led to the development of the *Your Mental Health* and the *#littlethings* public mental health campaigns, which have provided a relatively broad framework through which understandings and knowledge about mental health have become visible. In the three sections that follow, then, I seek to explore how these various documents constitute mental health as a regime of practice in Ireland.

What does mental health look like? Exploring fields of visibility

Taken-for-granted systems of acceptability in the context of mental health policy and practice should not necessarily be seen as the deficient starting points for critical analysis 'but rather the effects of historical practices' (Lemke, 2011: 31). Whether the object of critique is our understanding of madness, the penal system or our education system, it is possible to view current practice as but one possible approach. With reference to the penal system, for example, imprisonment is not the only form of response to law-breaking but is an outcome of just one possible approach associated with time-specific social practices motivated towards shifting outcomes from punishment to contemporary notions of rehabilitation. This rejection of the use of deficit in social analysis opens up the possibility and awareness of multiple historical and contemporary rationalities and allows investigation not of social problems per se but of *systems of acceptability*. The difference between what we understand as a social problem and what we come to see as systems of acceptability lies in the nature of reality as a socially constructed, rather than an a priori, social reality.

As outlined in the previous section, the *system of acceptability* surrounding mental health in Ireland emerged out of the historical practices and management of what was perceived as madness, of illness and deficit. On the surface, *AVFC* can be seen as initiating an approach which moves away from such a deficit-based approach, by recognising mental health as something which is of relevance to the whole population, and not just those experiencing illness. For example, the policy was launched with a message from the then Minister of State, Tim O'Malley, who asserted that 'good mental health is an integral component of general health and well-being, allowing a person to realize his or her abilities' (Government of Ireland, 2006: 4). The Chairperson of the Expert Group formed to oversee the writing of *AVFC*, Professor Joyce O'Connor, echoed the Minister's message, stating that

> we can attain it [mental health] through the attachments and the supportive relationships we form at each stage of our personal development, through learning to cope with challenging and difficult aspects of life, and finding ways

to belong and to contribute to others in line with our core values and aspirations. (Government of Ireland, 2006: 5)

Throughout the document, there are further statements and observations
reflective of broader, indeed critical, perspectives on mental health. The
report observes the social and demographic context of mental health in
Ireland and describes 'a society that is now more rushed, less caring and
more materialistic', and which has changed to a point 'where the oddities
and "eccentricities" of some individuals would in the past have been toler-
ated or incorporated into the community, such individuals are now viewed
with indifference or even fear' (Government of Ireland, 2006: 53). In
responding to the question as to 'what do we mean by mental health?' the
policy document states, 'mental health and mental well-being are therefore
part of everyday life, in that mental well-being is influenced, both positively
and negatively, in every area of life; in families, schools, the workplace and
in social interactions' (*ibid.*: 16).

AVFC communicates aspirational visions of a mentally flourishing population based on a more holistic vision of mental health as 'everyone's business', and these ways of viewing mental health have become increasingly
commonplace in other policy documents: for example, the high-level vision
of *Healthy Ireland* is one 'where everyone can enjoy physical and mental
health and wellbeing to their full potential, where wellbeing is valued and
supported at every level of society and is everyone's responsibility' (Government of Ireland, 2013: 5). Meanwhile, in the context of young people, Irish
Government policy puts an emphasis in its objectives on youth mental
health, identifying as one of five objectives that children and young people
'are active and healthy, with positive physical and mental wellbeing' (DCYA,
2014: xiv). Such discourses appear to build on the popularity of 'positive
psychology', which is motivated towards establishing ideas about mental
health that focus on enhancing well-being and indeed happiness (Seligman
et al., 2005).

Yet, I would suggest that the overall orientation of *AVFC* – and indeed
these other documents – highlights a tension between statements regarding
the mental health needs of the whole population and narrative discussion
and recommendations which emphasise an otherness in how mental health
should be viewed. Arguably reflecting the legacy of the historical sequester-
ing of those groups deemed to be mentally 'unfit', *AVFC* makes references
to mental health in terms of the language of disability, stating for example
that, 'if this policy is to fulfil its vision, the proportion of funds allocated
to mental health must reflect the level of disability in the population' (Government of Ireland, 2006: 58). Moreover, while *AVFC* claims to describe
a 'framework for building and fostering positive mental health across the
community', it also 'proposes a holistic view of mental illness' (not health)
(*ibid.*: 8), and states that its vision is 'to create a mental health system that

addresses the needs of the population through a focus on the requirements of the individual' (*ibid.*: 14).

Indeed, the object of direction in *AVFC* is not public mental health in Ireland but the provision of services for mental illness. The policy framework proposed in *AVFC* describes three levels of intervention including the community, primary care and mental health services. However, the ultimate focus within the policy document is very much on the latter and this is justified in the report by the argument that 'mental health services are more complex in their organisation than the services or interventions that feature in the other elements of the population model' (Government of Ireland, 2006: 23). There are ten chapters in all comprising the 'plan' section of *AVFC* which has a clear focus on mental health service delivery and emphasises the orientation shift towards the resourcing of community mental health teams with health professionals from a range of disciplines. As noted above, *AVFC* was preceded by the policy document *The Psychiatric Services – Planning for the Future* (Government of Ireland, 1984). The orientation shift in *AVFC* towards community mental health is in keeping with *Planning for the Future* which proposed that the site of service delivery would move from the old Victorian psychiatric institutions to the community. However, in *AVFC* it is noted that this process of de-institutionalisation which began in the 1980s often meant that while structures changed, users of services found that 'the treatment they received and their daily lives often did not change substantially' and that 'many of these people, though now outside the institutions that might formerly have housed them, remained "institutionalised" and isolated from the general community' (Government of Ireland, 2006: 56). Similar criticisms of the de-institutionalisation process have been noted elsewhere, with Grob (2008: 98) pointing out that, based on the experience of de-institutionalisation in the United States, 'the ideology of community mental health and the facile assumption that residence in the community would promote adjustment and integration was illusory'.

Thus, areas of action which constitute 'the plan' in *AVFC* concentrate on mental health service delivery, reflecting a somewhat narrow conceptualisation of mental health. The two exceptional areas within 'the plan' which sit outside of mental health services are primary care and suicide prevention which are included under 'special categories'. The fact that primary care warrants only minor consideration in *AVFC* is of relevance in its own right as the vast majority of health service responses to mental health need in Ireland are through primary care services, and the standard advice dispensed to the general population is that if you have a mental health problem you should visit your GP. 'Suicide prevention' is referenced within mental health policy because it has become a discrete area of policy and service provision in its own right. Wide-ranging and somewhat nebulous in nature, the suicide prevention strategy *Connecting for Life: Ireland's National Strategy* to *Reduce Suicide 2015–2020* states that 'implementation of Connecting for Life will be a complex process because it is a cross-cutting, whole-of-society strategy, which requires consistent co-operation and communication between relevant stakeholders' (DoH, 2015: xvi). Suicide prevention policy is of considerable significance here because specific actions arising out of suicide prevention policy documents have had an important influence on the visibility of mental health in Ireland. In particular, respective suicide prevention policy documents, *Reach Out* (HSE and DoHC, 2005) and *Connecting for Life*, led to the implementation of the *Your Mental Health* and the *#littlethings* public mental health campaigns.

These campaigns, directed by suicide prevention policy, have attempted to change what mental health looks like in Ireland. Following on soon after the launch of *AVFC* (though unconnected to it), the conception of mental health portrayed in the 2007 *Your Mental Health* campaign was broader than the deficit-based understanding of mental health reflected in the national mental health policy report. The *Your Mental Health* public awareness campaign targeted the general adult population and clearly framed mental health as an everyday issue relevant to all of us. The television advertisement which fronted the campaign included the following references to mental health; 'it's about how we see ourselves and those around us' and, 'it helps us get the best out of everyday life'. The advertisement also included references to stress and isolation – everyday terms that can be widely understood and are more relatable than clinical terminology. While the *Your Mental Health* campaign was a direct action arising out of the 2005 national suicide prevention strategy, the *#littlethings* campaign has been developed by the HSE's National Office for Suicide Prevention following the launch of *Connecting for Life* in 2015. Focused on communicating the impact and value of minor lifestyle changes and informal social support on individual mental health, the *#littlethings* campaign addresses the area of informal support, which was highlighted within *AVFC* but which was never the subject of concrete actions. *AVFC*, for example, stated that 'informal care and support offered by family and friends – and perhaps having a confidant – can be a great help. A person can take simple steps, such as getting more sleep and making similar minor lifestyle changes' (Government of Ireland, 2006: 21). This extract from *AVFC* can be read as an instructive brief for a campaign ultimately developed nearly ten years later arising out of a suicide prevention, rather than mental health, policy document. The *#littlethings* campaign is a highly visible public health campaign utilising television advertisements, online media and outdoor advertising to promote 'the little things that make a big difference to how we feel' (HSE, 2016, www.yourmentalhealth.ie). The campaign is based on the promotion of minor lifestyle changes to improve mental health and includes messages such as '8 hours sleep make the other 16 easier', 'the more you move, the better your mood' and 'do things with others – there's strength in numbers'. The messages of this campaign clearly have the potential to broaden our gaze in mental health and illuminate wider determinants beyond the biological and psychological factors that remain dominant in public discourse and professional practice.

Valued knowledge and techniques in mental health

Analysis of health and social policy in any given jurisdiction has the potential to shine a light on the types of knowledge and techniques that are most highly valued and indicates the disciplines from where experts and key advisors are recruited. Furthermore, analysis of policy can highlight broader orientations of the political system as Teghtsoonian (2009) has demonstrated in her exploration of mental health policy in British Columbia. Teghtsoonian identified an association between mental health policy and neoliberal modes of governing whereby a discourse which responsibilises individuals to take care of their own mental health has emerged. Her analysis also highlights the orientation of policy which can be seen as saving provincial finances and cutting costs in the delivery of services, for example through the promotion of relatively inexpensive interventions such as group-based cognitive behavioural therapy. While not the main focus of my analysis here, similarities can be seen in Irish mental health policy discourses, through statements in *AVFC* such as 'mental health problems have a high prevalence, have a wide-ranging impact on the individual and others, and are costly to the economy' (Government of Ireland, 2006: 17), and a policy direction which responsibilises service users by exhorting them to build on the resources within themselves as a way of achieving 'meaningful integration and participation in community life' (*ibid.*: 8).

In terms of valued knowledges and techniques, *AVFC* would seem to acknowledge a broad range of actors and different ways of understanding mental health. For example, the document discusses the 'spectrum of mental health' and acknowledges that 'individuals live and function in an environment made up of family, friends, community and society. Their mental health is influenced by this environment: how supportive or unsupportive it is, the richness of experience it facilitates, and many other features' (Government of Ireland, 2006: 20). Cultural influences on mental health are recognised and it is suggested that 'culturally sensitive mental health services will be aware of the different understanding of such things as mental health, mental health services, healing, family structure, sexuality and spirituality that exist in other cultures' (*ibid.*: 40). Recommended actions following on from such broad perspectives, however, remain confined to efforts within standard mental health service delivery encapsulated by Recommendation 4.8 that 'Mental health services should be delivered in a culturally sensitive manner. Training should be made available for mental health professionals in this regard, and mental health services should be resourced to provide services to other ethnic groups, including provision for interpreters' (*ibid.*: 41).

As outlined above, the vast majority of recommendations contained in *AVFC* pertain to the organisation and development of health services. In the current absence of a fundamental alternative to the way mental health is viewed within mainstream practice, the narrow gaze in mental health is consistent with the value placed on medical expertise and techniques directed by medical practitioners. Even within the more progressive and potentially transformative principles and recommendations of *AVFC*, the policy reverts to a traditional medical framing, as with the principle of 'recovery'. A contested concept, commentators such as Middleton (2007) and Pilgrim (2008) have highlighted how a distinction can be drawn between clinical models of recovery, focused on symptom reduction, for example, and social models in which personally meaningful indicators of recovery, related to subjective well-being, are central. Within the policy document, *AVFC* stresses

> The need to adopt a *recovery* perspective at all levels of service delivery. While recovery does not necessarily imply a cure, it does suggest that the individual can live a productive and meaningful life despite vulnerabilities that may persist, equipped with the necessary self-understanding and resources to minimize relapse. Service users also wanted services to treat them with *dignity and respect*. (Government of Ireland, 2006: 13; original emphasis)

The approach to recovery implied by this section of the document is, I would argue, a clinical one based on symptomatology, rather than a social understanding of recovery. In this sense, then, *AVFC* negates the more holistic descriptions of mental health and its determinants set out elsewhere in the report, by focusing on recovery only in the context of service delivery. Middleton (2007: 41), in acknowledging the tension between different understandings, advocates for a holistic concept of recovery 'rather than the relief of symptoms' so that it is possible to move beyond a view that 'an individual's mental health difficulties can be somehow wholly understood in terms of a diagnosis'. In *AVFC*, references to recovery remain bound to service delivery settings and a clinical framework whereby, for example, an operational principle of the Community Mental Health Team set out in *AVFC* is that 'contact with primary care services should be maintained to inform GPs, or other referral agencies, of the user's progress in recovery and their discharge from secondary or tertiary services back to the community' (Government of Ireland, 2006: 82).

Meanwhile, practices of mental health, and mental health advice, remain strongly rooted in biomedical practitioners and services. The standard advice dispensed by the HSE and other mental health agencies is that, in responding to a mental health problem, you should visit a GP. This is despite the fact that many GPs have received no formal training in the area of mental health. According to a 2004 report by the South Western Area Health Board (abolished when the HSE was launched in 2005) and the Irish College of General Practitioners, 68% of GPs indicated that they had no specific training in mental health (South Western Area Health Board and the Irish College of General Practitioners, 2004). A more recent study (Agyapong, Jabbat and Conway, 2012) of randomly selected Irish GPs indicates that as many as three out of four GPs (76.6%) are assigned to psychiatric rotation as part of their training. Nevertheless, it remains the case that formal mental health training is not a prerequisite for GPs despite their role as the first point of contact for patients experiencing mental health difficulty. Where training does take place, the focus is on a medically informed curriculum and generally takes place in settings that are inappropriate to future practice at primary care level. As acknowledged within *AVFC*,

> much of this training occurs in specialist mental health services; in psychiatric in-patient units and community based mental health services. This type of psychiatric placement means that GPs often do not experience the type of mental health and social problems they will experience in primary care settings. (Government of Ireland, 2006: 67 – with reference to the *Progress Report of the Primary Care Steering Group*)

Furthermore, given the relative shortage of alternative therapies such as counselling psychotherapy as referral routes for GPs, especially within the public healthcare system, and the significant demands on GP services in terms of patient numbers, there is a concern that some GPs may prescribe medication for mental health difficulties before exploring other, more time- and resource-intensive, support options.

While public messaging encourages a GP visit for mental health difficulties and the vast majority of mental health support is at the very least channelled through primary care, psychiatrists retain their status as the specialist doctors in the field of mental health, drawing on biomedical, technical expertise to govern the prescription of medication and the administration of treatment such as electro-convulsive therapy (ECT). Notwithstanding a recent amendment to the Mental Health Act, 2001, whereby the clause related to a patient being 'unable or unwilling' to consent to ECT was modified by removing 'or unwilling' (Mental Health (Amendment) Act, 2015), in the case of people who are involuntarily admitted to mental health services 'once a patient is detained all power is put into the hands of the consultant psychiatrist' (Bracken, 2012: 55).

However, within psychiatry, there is increasing debate with regard to the 'technical' dimensions of the work with some psychiatrists drawn to neuroscience and brain function with others arguing for a fundamental shift in the role of psychiatry. A 2012 article in the *British Journal of Psychiatry* authored by twenty-seven psychiatrists, mostly practising in clinical settings in Ireland and the UK, contextualises a call for change in psychiatry by acknowledging that 'All forms of suffering involve layers of personal history, embedded in a nexus of meaningful relationships that are, in turn, embedded in cultural and political systems' (Bracken *et al.*, 2012: 433). Bracken and his colleagues argue that if psychiatry orients further towards biomedical and neuroscientific approaches, the discipline 'will not only sell our patients short, but risks leading the profession down a single narrow alley, when what is needed is openness to alternative routes' (*ibid.*: 433).

The views of the *Critical Psychiatry Network*, a largely UK-based network of psychiatrists and mental health professionals, of which Bracken is a member, suggest that there is a potential for *counter-conducts* to emerge within psychiatry in relation to the ways in which we do mental health. The concept of *counter-conduct* was developed by Foucault to encapsulate elements of resistance or refusal with respect to the dominant ways of governing people. According to Davidson (2011: 28), Foucault chose the term *counter-conduct* 'after rejecting the notions of "revolt", "disobedience", "insubordination", "dissidence" and "misconduct", for reasons ranging from their being notions that are either too strong, too weak, too localized, too passive, or too substance-like'. Counter-conducts in relation to the governing of mental health in Ireland are represented by knowledge and techniques that are currently outside mainstream practices but possess a political and ethical quality worthy of exploration and may ultimately expand the field of visibility in mental health.

In the context of Irish mental health policy, it is interesting to note that the principles of critical psychiatry, which developed in response to concern with proposed legislation to increase the coercive nature of psychiatric care in the UK, echo some of the statements within *AVFC*. Thus, critical psychiatry's emphasis on 'the critically appraised value of neurobiological, psychological, social, economic, political and spiritual determinants of well-being', and its critique of 'the influences of a dominant biomedical hegemony and abuses of power' (Middleton, 2007: 41), can be witnessed in *AVFC*'s reference to environmental determinants of mental health. However, *AVFC*'s broad policy statements, as has been discussed, do not necessarily translate into actions. Similarly, the question remains as to whether the discourse of critical psychiatry can be impactful in terms of shifting practices, particularly in a context where it appears marginal within Irish psychiatry, which retains an emphasis on biomedical knowledge and practices of mental health.

Identity and mental health

A key contribution of governmentality studies has been to explore the subjectivities and identities that are produced through processes of governing, or which act as a means of promoting and activating governmental ends and visions. My analysis of *AVFC* demonstrates that the processes of identity construction at work in the policy reinforce ideas of otherness in mental health. While Rose refers to subjectivities such as 'neurochemical selves' and the 'biological citizen' (Rose, 2003), *AVFC* identifies the 'service user' and bestows upon him or her epistemic privilege by virtue of expertise gained through experience. Nevertheless, while a number of concrete recommendations are made in *AVFC* regarding the value of experts by experience, service users are consistently referred to in ways which reinforce otherness. It is acknowledged that 'service users have a unique insight into the experience of mental ill health and a greater awareness of the public perception of mental health and the provision of services. Their expertise is very different to the expertise of other stakeholders in mental health' (Government of Ireland, 2006: 24). The discussion continues with the recommendation that 'service users should be involved in implementing and evaluating the new mental health policy. This means involving them at all management levels and functions' (*ibid.*: 26). However, the notion of deficit in relation to human subjectivity, and in particular, the human experience of mental health problems, remains insofar as *AVFC* suggests the need to 'value the expertise of service users and assist *them* to develop new skills and confidence' (*ibid.*: 28; emphasis added). The abiding theme throughout in relation to identity and mental health is the sense of 'them and us' characterised by whether one has experience of using the Irish mental health services or not. This is further evidenced by the suggested requirement for potential 'advocates' who would play a supportive role for service users when it is noted that 'the advocate should be a person who has had occasion to use the mental health services themselves' (*ibid.*: 26).The sense of otherness is also evidenced in *AVFC*'s discussion of 'children of service users' where it is observed that

> the experience of having a service user in the family can negatively impact on the development, health and education of children in the household. Children may be undertaking a range of caring responsibilities, including household and financial management; care of other siblings and family members and administering medication. (*Ibid.*: 29)

If the human identity related to mental health inspired by national policy is negative, narrow, and deficit-based, most independent, not-for-profit mental health organisations could also be said to reinforce the otherness of the mental health subject. This is evidenced by the close working relationships, built on funding arrangements under Section 39 of the Health Act (2004), between mental health organisations and both the HSE and the Department of Health and Children (DoHC). *AVFC* highlights the importance of the non-statutory sector in Ireland and observes that such formally organised, non-profit organisations are 'ideally placed to seek improvements in the way mental health services are delivered' (Government of Ireland, 2006: 53). The role identified by national policy, therefore, is limited to operating within existing approaches to practice and is explicitly relevant to 'mental health services'. The human rights-based approach to mental health campaigns underlines this focus, and Amnesty International's 2003 Irish campaign provides one example of this. Developing from 2003, the focus of Amnesty International Ireland's mental health campaign across three distinct phases was the improvement of the lives of people experiencing mental illness. A highly visible public awareness campaign was rolled out featuring people who had experienced mental health difficulties with personal messages about their circumstances in an effort to 'end mental health prejudice and discrimination' (Amnesty Ireland, 2016). Amnesty combined media advertising with strong lobbying for the implementation of *AVFC*, and sought to establish mental health as a political priority. Other national organisations have rallied to the call surrounding *AVFC* thereby strengthening the current *system of acceptability* in the area of mental health which is to focus on improving the lives of people experiencing mental health difficulties through increasing and improving the level of current mental health service provision.

Apart from campaign work, the day-to-day focus of most mental health organisations in Ireland is to work within existing frameworks and the existing system, to improve the experience of those who are experiencing difficulty and need help. Aware offers to be 'your supporting light through depression', Shine is 'dedicated to upholding the rights and addressing the needs of all those affected by mental ill health' and Mental Health Reform 'promotes improved and prioritised mental health services in Ireland' (Aware, 2016; Shine, 2016; and, Mental Health Reform, 2016). The public-facing work of most not-for-profit organisations reinforces that current system of focus on mental illness or a deficit-based approach to mental health within a medical framework. While this work is undoubtedly valuable and makes untold positive differences to the lives of many people, it is not reflective of the holistic vision of mental health and the Irish population alluded to, but, I would argue, not delivered on, by *AVFC*.

A major challenge to a reimagining of our identity as humans with mental health at the core of our being lies in the popular appeal of stigma reduction campaigns, messaging and organisations. An interesting development in this area since 2010 has been the establishment of *See Change*, a national mental health partnership campaigning to reduce the stigma associated with mental health problems. While *See Change* has adopted an engaging approach by employing everyday language to encourage public conversations about mental health, it does not do anything to extend the gaze of mental health. *See Change* reinforces a narrow ontological foundation with respect to the concept of mental health, given that the focus of the campaign is the stigma of mental ill-health. As it becomes more and more acceptable that we talk about mental health in Ireland, there has been less reflection on *how* we talk about mental health. Public discourse remains framed by medical understandings of mental health which manifest in statements such as 'my mental health is just as important as my physical health'. However, the subjective and complex nature of the 'symptoms' of mental health problems are not easily measured, nor is there a widely shared understanding of the aetiology of mental health problems. In this context, the 'illness like any other' approach merely serves to maintain the current regimes of practices in mental health within a medical framework. A genuinely transformative 'sea change' in relation to cultural attitudes to mental health could involve a framing of mental health as neither good nor bad, but as a quality of human existence, without constructions of deficit. Such an approach might encourage closer personal identification with mental health among a greater number of the population thereby shifting subjectivity towards a sense of shared humanity with respect to mental health rather than reinforcing the characteristic of otherness.

Concluding remarks

An analysis of Ireland's national mental health policy (*AVFC*) and other documents reveals a tension between statements regarding the importance of mental health for the whole population and the practical recommendations intended to improve service delivery for people experiencing mental health difficulties. Using a governmental analysis based on the key dimensions of dominant practices outlined by Dean (2010), I suggest that it is possible to uncover the influence of *AVFC* on how mental health is envisioned, the relative value placed on different forms of knowledge and techniques in mental health, and the type of human subjectivities imagined in mental health policies.

AVFC simultaneously advocates the role of policy in supporting the mental health and well-being of the population while insisting that funds which are allocated to mental health must reflect the level of 'disability' in the population (Government of Ireland, 2006). Psychiatric medical expertise is placed at the centre of the knowledge base and education and training recommendations within *AVFC*, while it is equally acknowledged that there are other cultural interpretations of mental health and other approaches to the alleviation of human distress. With regard to human identity, *AVFC* reinforces the mental health subject in the context of otherness based on expertise gained by experience of using mental health services. The operational elements of *AVFC* betray the claims to whole-population relevance of mental health and reinforce a narrow conception of mental health as a euphemism for mental illness. Nevertheless, *AVFC* contributes in significant ways to the broader, public discourse on mental health, and those elements of mental health policy that relate to a more holistic sense of mental health have been incorporated into policy in the related arena of suicide prevention. The coming years will determine whether the public mental health messaging directed by suicide prevention policy will have sufficient impact to change the ways in which we see mental health in Ireland. The extension of our gaze beyond a model which privileges medical knowledge offers the potential to shift understandings of mental health difficulties and distress, and foster a sense of shared humanity in the ways in which we conceptualise our mental health, for better or worse, as human beings.

References

Agyapong, V., Jabbat, F. and Conway, C. (2012) Shared care between specialised psychiatric services and primary care: the experiences and expectations of General Practitioners in Ireland. *International Journal of Psychiatry in Clinical Practice*, 16(4): 293–299.

Amnesty International Ireland (2016) Available from: www.amnesty.ie/reports/evaluation-end-mental-health-prejudice-and-discrimination-campaign. Accessed 8 March 2016.

Aware (2016) Available from: www.aware.ie. Accessed 8 March 2016.

Ball, M.J. (2010) Governing depression in law students and the shaping of legal personae. IN: *Proceedings of TASA conference 2010: Social Causes, Private Lives*. The Australian Sociological Association Annual Conference, December 2010, Macquarie University, Sydney, Australia.

Bracken, P. (2012) Psychiatric power: a personal view. *Irish Journal of Psychological Medicine*, 29(1): 55–58.

Bracken, P. *et al.* (2012) Psychiatry beyond the current paradigm. *British Journal of Psychiatry*, 201(6): 430–434.

Considine, M. and Dukelow, F. (2009) *Irish Social Policy: A Critical Introduction*. Dublin, Gill and Macmillan.

Davidson, A. (2011) In praise of counter-conduct. *History of the Human Sciences*, 24(4): 25–41.

DCYA (2014) *Better Outcomes, Brighter Futures. The National Policy Framework for Children and Young People 2014–2020*. Dublin, Government Publications.

Dean, M. (2010) *Governmentality: Power and Rule in Modern Society*. London, Sage.

DoH (2015) *Connecting for Life: Ireland's National Strategy to Reduce Suicide 2015–2020*. Dublin, Ireland.

DoHC (2014) Available from: www.dohc.ie. Accessed 11 April 2014.

Foucault, M. (1965) *Madness and Civilisation*. New York, Random House.

Government of Ireland (1984) *The Psychiatric Services: Planning for the Future*. Dublin: Stationery Office.

Government of Ireland (2006) *A Vision for Change: Report of the Expert Group on Mental Health Policy*. Dublin, Stationery Office.

Government of Ireland (2013) *Healthy Ireland: A Framework for Improved Health and Wellbeing 2013–2015*. Dublin, Stationery Office.

Grob, G. (2008) Mental health policy in the liberal state: the example of the United States. *International Journal of Law and Psychiatry*, 31: 89–100.

HSE (2016) Your Mental Health. Available from: www.yourmentalhealth.ie/Get-involved/LittleThings-campaign/. Accessed 6 January 2016.

HSE and DoHC (2005) *Reach Out: National Strategy for Action on Suicide Prevention, 2005–2014*. Dublin, HSE/DoHC.

Jorm, A. (2012) Mental health literacy: empowering the community to take action for better health. *American Psychologist*, 67: 3.

Jorm, A., Korten, A., Jacomb, P., Christensen, H., Rodgers, B. and Pollitt, P. (1997) 'Mental health literacy': a survey of the public's ability to recognise mental disorders and their beliefs about the effectiveness of treatment. *Medical Journal of Australia*, 166: 182–186.

Lemke, T. (2011) Critique and experience in Foucault. *Theory, Culture and Society*, 28 (4): 26–48.

Mental Health Reform (2015) *A Vision for Change Nine Years On: A Coalition Analysis of Change*. Dublin, Mental Health Reform.

Mental Health Reform (2016) Submission for Budget 2015. www.mentalhealthreform.ie. Accessed 8 March 2016.

Middleton, H. (2007) Critical psychiatry. *Mental Health Review Journal*, 12(2): 40–43.

Pilgrim, D. (2008) 'Recovery' and current mental health policy. *Chronic Illness*, 4: 295–304.

Rogers, A. and Pilgrim, D. (2005) *A Sociology of Mental Health and Illness*. Maidenhead, Open University Press.

Rose, N. (2003). Neurochemical selves. *Society*: 46–59.

Rose, N. (2007) *The Politics of Life Itself: Biopolitics, Power and Subjectivity in the 21st Century*. Princeton, Princeton University Press.

Rose N., O'Malley P. and Valverde, M. (2006) Governmentality. *Annual Review of Law and Social Science*, 2: 83–104.

Seligman, M., Steen, T., Park, N. and Peterson, C. (2005) Positive psychology progress: empirical validation of interventions. *American Psychologist*, 60(5): 410–421.

Shine (2016) About Us. Available from: www.shineonline.ie. Accessed 8 March 2016.

South Western Area Health Board and Irish College of General Practitioners (2004) *Mental Health in Primary Care*. Kildare, Irish College of General Practitioners.

Szasz, T. (1961) *The Myth of Mental Illness: Foundations of a Theory of Personal Conduct*. New York, Harper and Row.

Teghtsoonian, K. (2009) Depression and mental health in neoliberal times: a critical analysis of policy and discourse. *Social Science & Medicine*, 69: 28–35.

Walsh, D and Daly, A. (2004) *Mental illness in Ireland 1750–2002. Reflections on the Rise and Fall of Institutional Care*. Dublin, Health Research Board.

Governing organ donation: the dead body, the individual and the limits of medicine

Introduction

In the twenty-first-century biomedical imaginary where the diseased body can be restored to health through surgical and therapeutic intervention, the procedure of organ transplantation is for the most part unproblematic, except in respect of the availability of organs. Imagined as spare parts (Shildrick, 2014), enlisting the public to novel moral and bodily imperatives to make their organs available for transplantation after their death has become the focus of many policy initiatives internationally, including Ireland. A list of commitments under the heading 'Bioethics' in the *Fine Gael / Labour Programme for Government 2011–16* (2011: 38) included a pledge to legislate for 'an opt-out system for organ transplantation ... so as to improve the availability of organs for patients in desperate need'. In policy deliberations, such as those conducted by the Joint Committee on Health and Children in 2013, a repeated concern is how an 'opt-out' or 'presumed consent' system can be made the new norm. For example, in a statement to the Joint Committee by a Principal Officer in the Cancer, Blood and Organs Unit of the Department of Health (DoH) she stated,

> We must change the cultural attitude towards organ donation and make organ donation the norm in Ireland. The present system of consent will change to one of 'presumed' or 'deemed' consent, which means that the consent of an individual to organ donation is deemed or presumed to have been given unless they objected during their lifetime. (Houses of the Oireachtas, 2013: 37)

As explained in a DoH public consultation document, in Ireland in 2012 there was a total of 78 deceased donors, which resulted in 244 organs being transplanted. This equated to a donor rate of 17.03 per million of the population, a rate considerably lower than the Spanish rate of 35.3, a country with an organ donation system based on presumed consent. The public consultation document went on to report that there were 650 people on the organ transplant waiting list and emphasised that given 'the scarcity of organs available in Ireland for transplantation, it is important that as a society we do all that we can to increase the number of organs available for transplantation' (DoH, 2013: 1).

This commitment in the *Programme for Government* was at odds with the findings of a public consultation process conducted in 2009 regarding the (still long-delayed) Human Tissue Bill. This legislation was a response to the organ retention scandal, which revealed a paediatric post-mortem practice whereby parents were not told about the retention of their dead children's organs. The aim of the Bill is to ensure that such practices cannot happen again without parents' knowledge and consent. Addressing how consent to organ donation should best be secured, that consultation process outlined the three options of 'presumed consent' (opt-out), 'explicit consent' (opt-in) and 'mandated choice' which requires people by law to specify if they do or do not consent to the donation of their organs after death. Of the 30 submissions received from organisations, only one favoured presumed consent. However, by 2013, a number of organisations (e.g. Cystic Fibrosis Ireland, the Irish Heart and Lung Transplant Association, and the Irish Lung Fibrosis Association) that had previously opposed the presumed consent option had changed their position in favour of it. Crucial to this change was the proposal to introduce a *soft* opt-out system of organ donation, one that requires the consent of the family of the deceased.

This policy objective of transforming the prevailing cultural attitude towards organ donation can be seen as an instance in which the state seeks not to act *on* us by forcing us to do something, but *through* us, shaping our dispositions, preferences and behaviour. To employ the now widely cited explanation of the French philosopher and historian Michel Foucault's concept 'governmentality', it can be seen as a policy objective to 'conduct the conduct' of people in regard to organ donation. In this era of neoliberal austerity when the Irish state is withdrawing responsibility for the provision of health services, evident in 'cost-shifting by government back onto households' (Thomas, Burke and Barry, 2014: 1546), this is a new form of intervention it has taken on. Foucault's fusion of 'government' with 'mentality' to form the term 'governmentality' signified a radical rethinking of the notion of government in the social sciences and of how the exercise of power can be understood (Dean, 1999). Breaking with the habit of thinking of government as pertaining only to the exercise of power by the state, here government is understood as any form of activity that deliberately attempts, more or less subtly, to shape human behaviour. From this perspective, to analyse government 'is to analyse those practices that try to shape, sculpt, mobilise and work through the choices, desires, aspirations, needs, wants and lifestyles of individuals and groups' (Dean, 1999: 12). Through mundane and everyday reiteration of procedures of intervention into the body, these practices reinforce particular modes of power. To analyse power is to consider *how* the effects of power are produced, based on a recognition that 'nothing is more material, physical, corporeal, than the exercise of power' (Foucault, 1980: 58). Viewing the recent organ donation policy initiative through the lens of governmentality studies helps us to see how diverse 'governmental technologies' are being used (by the state together with a network of other actors) to shape the body and its dispositions, and more specifically, to alter people's thinking and habitual behaviour with regard to organ donation. This consideration of how a novel bodily imperative to consent to making one's cadaveric body available to others includes attention to how 'technologies of subjectification' are used to mould the subjectivities of the governed, and the identities presupposed and promoted by the practices of governing organ donation. Additionally, a governmentality approach encourages us to critically scrutinise the institutional forms and power relations established by these efforts to increase the availability of organs (Wehling, 2011).

In this chapter I explore how these efforts to increase the availability of human organs by moving to an institutional arrangement based on presumed consent necessarily extend beyond shaping people's cultural attitude towards organ donation. Transforming the prevailing cultural attitude and habitual behaviour in respect of organ donation also requires subtle but significant shifts in how people imagine the dead body, the individual and her or his responsibilities to others, and the limits of medicine. Presumed consent has been a focus of many recent debates about organ donation for transplant medicine. Some commentators, such as Peter Wehling (2011), argue that these institutional arrangements can potentially instigate new ways of governing human bodies that restrict individuals' autonomy, create new moral duties and bolster unrestricted claims to access to transplant medicine. More positively, others, such as Anne Phillips (2013), contend such arrangements can counter the constitution of the human body as private property, thereby tapering the destructive and pervasive individualism that is a feature of contemporary Western societies. I consider these debates in light of the ideas of Foucault about the construction and government of the modern individual. Central to Foucault's conceptualisation of governmentality is that the modern sovereign state and the modern autonomous individual, *homo economicus*, co-determined each other's emergence. Using the Joint Committee on Health and Children's public consultation process and 2013 report, I have drawn on these debates and concepts to critically scrutinise the government of organ donation in Ireland.

Governmentality and *homo economicus*

As noted above, adopting a very broad meaning of government as a continuum that extends beyond regulation by the state to regulation of the family, self and even soul, governmentality refers to a distinctive form of governing whereby the exercise of power is combined with its rationalisation. In Thomas Lemke's (2001) appraisal of the potential of the concept of governmentality, he emphasises that study of the operation of 'technologies of power' must be combined with study of the political rationalities underpinning them. These rationalities are the ways of thinking that make the exercise of power possible. He explains the two sides to the governmentality coin: the term refers to the representations, arguments, justifications and definitions that enable a problem to be recognised and addressed, but also the structuring of the forms of intervention deemed necessary and appropriate.

Lemke reminds us that Foucault used the concept to highlight the articulation of power relations and processes of subjectification, the production of particular conceptions of what it is to be human. His history of governmentality was concerned with revealing the co-determination of the modern state and the modern autonomous individual. Many theorists have considered what they regard as this fiction of the modern autonomous individual, perhaps most forcefully theorists of the commons. 'Commoners' such as Gustavo Esteva (O'Donovan, 2015: 749) call on us to recognise that 'we are constructed as individuals, we see and experience the world as individuals but we cannot *be* individuals'. For them, the individual as we know it is a destructive, historically specific but very strong social construction. In modern capitalist society, the individual and the commodity are the basic cells of society. For those in the commons movement, the commons is the new basic unit. Foucault explored diverse governmentalities, both liberal and neoliberal, acknowledging they are shaped by context-specific possibilities and constraints. A key feature of neoliberal governmentalities that he addressed is the eclipsing of the social by the economic whereby an economic rationality or mentality pervades the ways of thinking and criteria for decision-making in all spheres of life. In some versions, this goes even further, as the social sphere becomes redefined as a form of the economic domain. As explained by Lemke (2001: 197), 'the economy is no longer one social domain among others with its own intrinsic rationality, laws and instruments. Instead, the area covered by the economy embraces the entirety of human action to the extent that this is characterized by the allocation of scant resources for competing goals.' A neoliberal governmentality thus encourages us to understand all human action and relations in economic terms. It is premised on a particular conception of human nature, *homo economicus*, and encourages us to regard ourselves and *be* autonomous consumers and entrepreneurs with full responsibility for how we choose to invest our life.

For Lemke, one of the ways in which the concept of governmentality is theoretically innovative is that it encourages us to make the dividing lines between the state and society, and between the public and private spheres, objects of study. In the context of studies of neoliberal forms of government, rather than just focusing on the withdrawal of the state from society (associated with the demise of the welfare state), a governmentality approach directs our attention to the new tasks, functions and forms of intervention it takes on. These include the

> indirect techniques for leading and controlling individuals without at the same time being responsible for them. The strategy of rendering individual subjects 'responsible' ... entails shifting the responsibility for social risks such as illness ... and for life in society into the domain for which the individual is responsible and transforming it into a problem of 'self-care'. (Lemke, 2001: 201)

Similar to this assessment of neoliberal governmentalities, according to Ivan Illich (2010: 104), crucial to the project of development, central to which are putative advances in medicine, have been efforts to get people to recognise their newly *invented* needs, but once conscious of these needs people have to 'fend for themselves in satisfying them'.

Neoliberalism, therefore, refers not just to a way of governing economies, but is intimately tied to the governing and self-governing of the individual, and her or his needs and responsibilities. This approach attunes us to how neoliberal rationality constructs moral and responsible actors as those who are economically rational, where their 'moral quality is based on the fact that they rationally assess the costs and benefits of a certain act as opposed to other alternative acts' (Lemke, 2001: 201). From this perspective, neoliberalism is a political rationality and project that endeavours 'to render the social domain economic' and render the individual body and collective bodies (such as the state) '"lean", "fit", "flexible" and "autonomous"' (*ibid.*: 203). The invention of the rational autonomous individual by neoliberal forms of governing became a focus of much of Foucault's work in which he took his analysis of the 'genealogy of the modern state' further by developing a 'genealogy of the modern subject'. Indeed, as argued by Jason Read (2009: 3), 'the nexus between the production of a particular conception of human nature, a particular formation of subjectivity, and a particular political ideology, a particular way of thinking about politics', was at the heart of Foucault's research.

Presumed consent, ownership of the body and biological citizenship

Concerns about the implications of thinking about the body as private property motivate Anne Phillips's (2013) contribution to debates about organ donation. For her, when we think about the body as our property 'we minimise the significance of our bodies to our sense of self and encourage a mind/body dualism that makes it easier to think of bodies as marketable resources' (2013: 104). According to this rationality, to be human is to own, rather than to be, one's body. Even in the context of an almost worldwide ban on the trade in human organs, the mentality of *homo economicus* is evident in the permeation of the language of commerce in discussions of organ donation. As she points out, organs are frequently spoken about as being *extracted*, *harvested* and *procured* in a new kind of *gold rush* where the territory is the body. Additionally, she reminds us that speaking about organs as *resources* is by implication the language of property. The defining of the sphere of organ donation as a form of the economic domain is further evident in talk about the *supply* and *demand* of organs.

Phillips's consideration of different organ donation systems does not so much explore those that do and do not encourage us to think about the body as property, but rather the different property regimes they can presuppose and promote. For example, organ donation based on the idea of gifting is not inconsistent with thinking about the body as property. However, in keeping with Richard Titmuss's classic text *The Gift Relationship*, Phillips argues it promotes different attitudes towards others and their bodies, and different power relations, to those that would be promoted should a trade in organs be legalised. She is an advocate of organ donation based on presumed consent as a policy response to the shortage in organs for transplantation, so long as it applies to everyone and that opting out can be easily done. She points out that one reason why presumed consent is controversial is that it weakens the dominant economic understanding of the body as the individual's private property. For her, one of the problems with understanding the body as private property is that in policy deliberations it focuses our attention too narrowly at the micro-level, on the individual and her or his rights. In discussions addressing the dilemmas generated by new developments in medicine, it reinforces individualism and makes it more difficult to address broader societal concerns. Thinking about the body as private property governs 'the kinds of arguments that become available when societies are considering policies on body matters. Property claims make the individual property owners the centre of attention and establish their preferences and choices as the predominant concerns' (Phillips, 2013: 142). Some bioethicists, such as Daniel Callahan (2012: 51), have long bemoaned 'the almost complete triumph of liberal individualism in bioethics' and have sought ways to promote a more communitarian approach. For Phillips, by emphasising communal bonds and interdependency, the governmental rationality underpinning a system of presumed consent can encourage such a different understanding of the dead body and responsibility to others, and disrupt neoliberal conceptions of human nature. Under such a system Phillips (2013: 121) says,

> I think of my body as a resource that becomes available for others when it is no longer of use to me ... My relationship to my body then becomes closer to the relationship to the land under systems of communal land tenure: the body is very much mine so long as I use it, but is not mine to sell. I owe it, in some sense, to others when I can no longer use it.

Organ donation based on presumed consent, she argues, encourages us to think of the dead body as a 'commons', an understanding that is more conducive to policy deliberations about macro-level concerns that extend beyond the claims and preferences of individuals or specific groups.

Phillips concludes her analysis by turning to the macro-level question of the limits of medicine. Developments in transplant medicine, she notes, are likely to intensify the scarcity of organs. However, referencing the arguments of Ivan Illich, she accepts that the very idea of an organ scarcity rests upon what he referred to as an 'artificially created need'. As explained by Nancy Scheper-Hughes, this is a need 'invented by transplant technicians, doctors and their brokers, and dangled before the eyes of an ever expanding sick, aging, desperate and dying population' (cited in Phillips, 2013: 153). According to this argument it is only since medical technology offered a way of circumventing organ disease through transplantation that we can talk meaningfully of a *desperate need* and *scarcity* of organs. Phillips acknowledges that this is a scarcity that can never be met:

> if we consider all those the world over who could benefit from an organ transplant, and then add in the unknown millions who would be able to benefit from the new kinds of transplant that are no doubt being worked on, it becomes apparent there cannot be enough donors ... to go around. (*Ibid.*)

No system of organ donation therefore is likely to result in the availability of organs for all those in *need*.

The emergence of the 'biological citizen' as a particular form of the modern individual provides the focus for Peter Wehling's (2011) discussion of organ donation policy. What distinguishes this new form of citizenship is that the individual is construed as somatic; it entails the linking of citizenship claims to biology, or an articulation of 'claims to participation in social and political life and to recognition of certain individuals' or groups' identities, expertise and specific needs based on their (supposedly) biological or genetic conditions' (Wehling, 2011: 226). These are *supposed* conditions in the sense that they are constructed as such by medicine and its particular ways of thinking. Wehling points to the significant contribution being made by biological citizens and the patients' organisations they mobilise in generating demands, optimism and hope for improved medical therapies. The proliferation of patients' organisations is occurring in a context in which twenty-first-century medicine is increasingly being used to 'enhance' and 'optimise' the human body and extend its capacities beyond what was previously thought of as natural. Wehling (2011) is ambivalent about the emergence of active biological citizenship, which he regards as a new and significant element in contemporary governmental regimes of medicine. Using organ donation policy as an example he considers some potentially undesirable consequences of biological citizenship. Biological identities, he argues, might be ascribed to individuals and groups, new forms of inequality and discrimination might develop, and 'freedom of choice might subtly be transformed into an obligation to act as an active, responsible and prudent biological citizen' (2011: 227). These new obligations could include bodily imperatives to donate organs, but also to avail of transplant medicine. Furthermore, organ donation policy based on presumed consent potentially promotes a way of thinking about the body where 'every human body contains valuable biological materials that might help to save the life of others or to improve their quality of life' (*ibid.*: 237). This reductionist way of thinking about the body as a container of future spare parts or resources for biomedical intervention can in turn potentially result in a moral duty to help others by making our 'healthy' cadaveric body available to them. In such a system, he argues, the principle of informed consent is weakened and the autonomy of the individual is restricted. Wehling's concern, therefore, is with the new responsibilities and moral duties promoted by an organ donation system based on presumed consent, and the potential erosion of individual autonomy. A further concern is that in a system based on presumed consent, unrestricted claims to access to transplant medicine from biological citizens could be further bolstered, and 'the right to treatment' converted into a moral obligation to undergo treatment. For him, this gives rise to the question of the limits of medicine that demands consideration of the political question 'of whether and to what ends we should believe in and comply with powerful and seductive promises of a "better life" brought about by medical and pharmaceutical interventions' (*ibid.*: 238). He fears the political rationalities underpinning organ donation based on presumed consent may preclude a 'politics of enough'.

Irish organ donation policy discourses

What are the political rationalities underpinning current Irish organ donation policy discourses and what ways of thinking and behaving do they cultivate? To explore these questions, I examine the Joint Committee on Health and Children's 2013 report on organ donation. This is a 149-page report on the Irish government's public consultation process regarding the proposal to change the system of organ donation to one based on presumed consent. The largest section of the report (73 pages) is a transcript of three public hearings held in April 2013. The first of the public hearings included contributions from people with personal experience of donation and advocacy groups, organisations of biological citizens such as the Irish Kidney Association, Cystic Fibrosis Ireland and the Irish Donor Network. The perspectives of medical, legal and bioethical professionals were heard on the second day, and those of officials from the DoH and elsewhere on the third. Another section of the report is a 20-page Briefing Paper, prepared by the Oireachtas Library and Research

Service. Other contents of the report include details of the membership and terms of reference of the Joint Committee, and copies of submissions it received.

The Briefing Paper provides little by way of support for the proposed change in policy. Overwhelmingly, it mobilises evidence in support of maintaining the existing opt-in system, albeit with some adjustments. Its executive summary includes a reminder that in the 2009 DoH consultation process, most advocacy organisations favoured retention of the opt-in system. Furthermore, its review of other countries' organ donation policies describes the rejection of systems based on presumed consent in four countries (Britain, the USA, Canada and Australia). Reasons for the rejection of presumed-consent models that are noted include economic ones (insufficient evidence that the required financial investment is worthwhile) but also the view that it could constitute a violation of civil rights by converting everyone into an organ donor and weakening the commitment to the principle of informed consent. Even though most European countries have institutionalised presumed consent, the only country with this institutional arrangement profiled in the Briefing Paper is Spain, the country with the highest donation rate in the world. However, the country's high donation rate is attributed largely to the success of its programme of 'professionalisation' of organ donation, and the establishment of transplant coordinating teams. Criticisms of the Spanish model of presumed consent are noted, including that it allows for subtle coercion of family members to consent. Notwithstanding the Briefing Paper's status as a governmental device that encourages ways of thinking contrary to the policy objective (possibly reflecting the internally fractured nature of the state or a change in the prevailing governmental rationality), in the foreword to the report the chairperson states that the public hearings 'greatly enhanced the Joint Committee's understanding of the position pertaining to organ donation in Ireland and reaffirmed our view that the transition to a *soft opt-out* system is a necessary one' (Houses of the Oireachtas, 2013: 6). From a governmentality perspective, the recommendations of the Joint Committee reflect successful government as its members were enlisted to what had been rendered a thinkable, practicable and imperative policy change.

Organ donation policy – problems and solutions

Let us now turn to the ways of thinking about organ donation policy promoted by these policy deliberations. What were the political rationalities or arguments, justifications and definitions that enabled organ donation to be recognised as a problem that needs to be addressed by Irish policymakers? What were the ways of thinking that structured the forms of intervention that were deemed necessary and appropriate to address the organ donation problem?

One of the key ideas promoted during the public hearings was that there is an organ donation 'crisis' due to the scarcity of organs for transplantation, a crisis that urgently needs to be addressed. Economic rationalities featured prominently in the urgency narratives about this crisis. These included assertions that without more organs for transplantation, the growing need for medical treatments, specifically dialysis, will bankrupt the health services. The potential for the commodification of organs, objectified as spare parts exchangeable between bodies (Shildrick, 2014), was emphasised. A forceful example of this way of thinking can be found in the scenario envisaged by the Director of the National Kidney and Pancreas Programme. He asserted,

> There is a global shortage of organs for transplantation, particularly kidneys, as renal failure is increasing at an alarming rate, it is accepted that it will bankrupt most health services in the next 20 years if not addressed in a radical fashion now. Without a significant increase in both deceased organ and living donors, we are going to be at a situation in the very near future where dialysis is going to be rationed i.e. Nobody over 55 being dialysed leading to as already happens in the developing world, reliance on commercial illegal (backstreet) transplantation. (Houses of the Oireachtas, 2013: 22)

Another contributor to the discussions, a senator and also a medical professional, warned that this 'apocalyptic scenario involving the rationing of dialysis should not be dismissed as a Cormac McCarthy-like future fiction' (*ibid.*: 99). The crisis situation, at a national level, was described by the Joint Committee's chairperson in his foreword to the report. Identifying the policy problem as the low rate of organ donation, he stated,

> In June 2012, more than 1,700 Irish adults were receiving haemodialysis, yet throughout all of 2012, just 163 renal transplants were carried out in the Republic of Ireland. To meet the needs of those receiving haemodialysis our health system should be performing in the region of 300 kidney transplants each year. This low rate of organ donation is reflected in Ireland ranking 23rd in European league tables for organ donation. (*Ibid.*: 4)

League tables such as this were a key governmental technology used to establish the organ crisis as one that is particularly acute in Ireland and warranting the intervention of policy makers. The Director of the National Kidney and Pancreas Transplant Programme similarly bemoaned that Ireland has been 'stuck at 21 donors pmp [per million population] for the past 20 years, and whilst this was in the top 5 in Europe for a long time, we have now fallen significantly in the league table' (*ibid.*: 23). With dialysis ranked as the most costly procedure for hospital day patients, the threat to the health service of the growing need for this service was noted repeatedly. This growth in need was attributed to advances in medicine and the greater survival rates of people with kidney disease, but also because of growing rates of obesity and diabetes. Assertions of how the demand for dialysis could bankrupt the health service were accompanied by calculations of the potential savings of each kidney transplant, calculations that ranged from €680,000 to €830,000. Calculations of the costs in terms of the numbers of lives lost were also made; the CEO of the Irish Kidney Association stated that 'as many as 10 people a day now die because of the lack of donated organs' (*ibid.*: 13).

The role of new medical technologies in the creation of the need for organ donation was acknowledged by the CEO of the Irish Kidney Association in his presentation to the Joint Committee. Noting that the first kidney transplant took place in Ireland in 1964, he highlighted how the development of the drug Cyclosporine which helps prevent the body's rejection of a new organ contributed to not only making transplantation possible but also to it becoming 'normal surgery and expected by society' (Houses of the Oireachtas, 2013: 12). The growing 'demand' for organs overtime together with the 'explosion in the number of patients coming onto the [kidney] transplant waiting list' (*ibid.*: 22) was described by many participants in the public hearings. One of these who emphasised the urgency of growing numbers of people waiting for a transplant was a biological citizen who concluded his address to the Joint Committee saying,

> Finally, I will give one last statistic which for me, as a long-term renal patient, is the most concerning of all. In 2000, there were only 150 patients awaiting kidney transplants. Today, that figure is closer to 650, a 413% rise. People are living longer. Type 2 diabetes sufferers are on the increase and the current waiting list will not dissipate any time soon unless we make this very subtle change. (*Ibid.*: 53)

The official definition of the organ donation problem as primarily the low donation rate was, however, repeatedly challenged during the public hearings. For many of the participants, the lack of public investment and/ or the poor management of organ donation services in Ireland was the foremost problem. Highlighting the need for 'massive public investment', the Director of the National Kidney and Pancreas Transplant Programme rejected the definition of the problem as primarily a shortage of donors stating, 'More donors mean more transplants and we currently cannot deal with what we have' (Houses of the Oireachtas, 2013: 23). A representative of the Intensive Care Society of Ireland also argued that the key problem is inadequate public expenditure on organ donation services. Challenging the governmental rationality underpinning the presumed consent policy initiative, he said that because in practice intensive care personnel always secure the consent of family members to organ donation, the debate about presumed consent was much ado about nothing; it 'is not the big issue. It is not the big ticket and I do not think changing this will make any difference' (*ibid.*: 89). Similarly, a senator acknowledged that 'the organ crisis' contributes to the problem, but for him the main problem, which is a 'microcosm of the health service in general', is that 'we have a system which is under-resourced, grotesquely understaffed and mismanaged by people who should not be managing it' (*ibid.*: 98). It is not that the service is underfunded, he claimed, but 'severely malfunded' and in need of reform. The Norwegian organ transplant service was repeatedly held up as a model to be emulated. As argued by one clinician, even though the two countries have similar population sizes, in Ireland an average of 150 kidney transplants are performed every year whereas in Norway it is as many as 300 (*ibid.*: 40). For him, with 'appropriate investment within a few years [Ireland could] be achieving transplantation results similar to Norway with enormous benefit to patients with kidney failure' (*ibid.*: 40). These alternative governmental rationalities constituted not only a redefining of the primary problem, but also a challenge to the mentality that rendered individuals who failed in their obligations to donate their organs responsible for the problem. They also rendered appropriate forms of intervention that extend beyond changing the system of consent to organ donation that emphasise broader social responsibility for the problem.

These arguments about the lack of public investment in the health services that were expressed repeatedly during the public hearings were made in the macroeconomic environment of neoliberal austerity policies enforced by the International Monetary Fund and European Central Bank, though no reference was made to this broader context. For the Irish health services, austerity resulted in 'radical resource cuts', such as a reduction of public financing for the Health Service Executive (HSE) of 22% or €3.3 billion between 2009 and 2013, and significant 'cost-shifting' onto patients (Thomas, Burke and Barry, 2014: 1545). There is widespread acknowledgement that the International Monitory Fund and European Central Bank were 'pushing an open door' in insisting on these austerity measures that weakened poverty alleviation and intensified emigration (Dukelow, 2015). Nonetheless, a recurring theme in contributions to the public hearings were celebrations of the generosity of the Irish people, who if facilitated properly would willingly 'gift' their organs. Replete with a rhetoric of altruism, Ireland was variously imagined as a 'neighbourly' (Houses of the Oireachtas, 2013: 72) and 'altruistic' (*ibid.*: 60) society, and 'a giving country full of compassionate people' (*ibid.*: 53).

Many of those who rejected the definition of the policy problem as primarily the low donation rate nonetheless saw a necessity for, and favoured the introduction of, a donation system based on soft presumed consent. In contrast to the ways of thinking about the 'international perspective' presented in the Briefing Paper, which overwhelmingly pointed to controversial aspects of presumed consent, accounts of experiences of systems based on presumed consent in other countries were crucial to establishing its appropriateness as a policy response. Some of these accounts were represented as highly authoritative, such as a review published in the *BMJ* cited by the

Director of the National Organ Donation and Transplant Office that concluded 'it is associated with a 25% increase in organ donation rates', a
conclusion supported by a 'UK health technology assessment report' (Houses
of the Oireachtas, 2013: 115). League tables were mobilised in this context
too, as in 'European league tables of organ donation rates are consistently
dominated by those countries which have presumed consent in partnership
with form organ donation infrastructures, including Spain, Portugal and
Croatia' (*ibid.*: 115).

A prominent organ donation campaigner and a live kidney donor represented the proposed presumed consent policy as entirely unproblematic:
it is 'a no brainer' and he reported that when he discusses it with people
the response is, 'Why have we not done this already?' (Houses of the
Oireachtas, 2013: 52). He identified people's failure to register their willingness to donate their organs as a weakness of the existing system and argued
that presumed consent 'will more properly accord with the overwhelming
view in society that organ donation is good. Who does not want to save
seven lives after he or she is dead?' (*ibid.*). Supporting this argument, a
fellow campaigner and renal patient reported that in a survey of 1000
people, and without any education on the issue, 71% agreed with presumed
consent to organ donation. For this biological citizen, there is no option
but to introduce presumed consent: 'I see no plan B' (*ibid.*: 53).

The appropriateness of organ donation based on presumed consent was
nonetheless contested during the public hearings. Key arguments made
against it include that it is coercive, and undermines individuals' autonomy.
In this context too, images of Ireland and the Irish were evoked, such as
'The Irish people like to be asked, not told, to do something' (Houses of
the Oireachtas, 2013: 14), an image which critics of Ireland's willingness
to comply with International Monetary Fund and European Central Bank
austerity measures are likely to dispute. Another criticism was that it could
potentially undermine the 'gifting' of organs and thus result in resistant
counter-conducts, as happened in Brazil where the introduction of a system
based on presumed consent was followed by a decrease in organ donation.
A further argument made against the soft opt-out system is that it may be
impracticable as what constitutes 'family consent' is not always clear and
may not always be achievable.

The dead body

Historically, the contribution of transplant medicine to redefining the
boundaries between the dead and living body, and to the emergence in
the 1960s of the idea of 'brain death', is widely recognised (Miller, 2009).
Articles in bioethics journals such as 'Are DCD donors dead?' (Marquis,
2010) and publications such as the US President's Council on Bioethics'
2008 paper 'Controversies in the Determination of Death' indicate that

the definition of death in the context of transplant medicine continues to be contentious. Multiple ways in which death is medically defined and determined were discussed in the course of the public hearings, particularly in the contributions from representatives of the Intensive Care Society of Ireland. However, the discussions steered away from consideration of the changing, complex and contentious issue of defining death, and for the most part encouraged acceptance of what it is to be dead as something straightforward.

The specialist interest of one of these representatives of the Intensive Care Society of Ireland was 'donation after determination of death by cardiovascular criteria ... cardiac death, DCD, or non-heart beating donation' (Houses of the Oireachtas, 2013: 90). This he explained is distinct from donation after brainstem death, DBD. In the written submission from the Society it is noted that one of its concerns was whether presumed consent would apply to donors after cardiac death. His colleague pointed out that many people struggle with the idea of brain death, and described the difficulties faced in explaining it to the families of potential donors. Highlighting how the idea of brain death entails a governing of people's understanding of what it is to be dead, he explained, 'Their relative is warm and has a pulse, the screen monitor looks normal and yet he or she is dead' (ibid.: 103). The instability of what constitutes a dead body was also evident in the contribution of the Chief Bioethics Officer in the DoH. She noted that as the need for organs for transplant medicine increases, transplantation systems have explored a number of innovative strategies to increase their availability, many of which are ethically challenging. Amongst these strategies are 'expanding the criteria for declaring death' (ibid.: 44). The dead body, therefore, was constructed as something historically specific and determined by changing medical criteria. However, it was not this but the issue of ownership of the dead body (even though in common law the body cannot be owned), or who should have decision-making authority in the donation of organs, that emerged as a predominant concern in the public hearings.

In keeping with the saturation of transplant medicine with the altruistic rhetoric of gift-giving (Scheper-Hughes, 2007), the 'most precious gift' is how one contributor to the hearings encouraged us to think about the donated dead body. For her, and many others, concerns about presumed consent centred on its potential to undermine gifting. In order to retain its status as a gift, she said the dead body must be 'given unconditionally and wholeheartedly with such goodwill to the organ recipient' (Houses of the Oireachtas, 2013: 21). An organ recipient spoke about the body part that she received, a lung, as 'the ultimate gift' that had given her 'a second shot at life' (ibid.: 54). Opposing the proposed change, a clinician noted his commitment to the idea of 'the gift of life', and that 'nothing can ever be presumed in a gift and nothing should be taken for granted' (ibid.: 90).

Outlining arguments made by bioethicists defending presumed consent, the DoH's Chief Bioethics Officer noted that their arguments hinge on an understanding of the dead body as something that cannot be harmed, and consequently 'any curtailment of individual freedom is legitimate in the interest of the common good, that is the survival of other citizens' (*ibid.*: 46). However, given the emphasis on the necessity for *soft* presumed consent throughout the public hearings, it was not the choice and autonomy of the deceased but their family members that was often regarded as being in question. The dead body was widely constructed as the property of 'the family', not a commons as envisaged by Anne Phillips (2013). The family, rather than the common good, was the centre of attention of most of the deliberations, and their preferences and choices emerged as the principal concerns.

Without a doubt, for many, the distinction between *hard* and *soft* presumed consent, and the different ways of thinking about ownership of the dead body structured by these two forms of intervention, was crucial to presumed consent being rendered an appropriate institutional arrangement. By shifting from a proposal to introduce a hard opt-out system to a soft one, the representative of the Irish Donor Network explained that there had been a 'major change' in the government's proposal and this change led to his coalition of organisations altering its position in respect of presumed consent. He declared that: 'Under no circumstances would the groups we represent ... support a hard opt-out approach whereby next of kin would not be consulted. Next of kin should always be consulted in respect of organ donation' (Houses of the Oireachtas, 2013: 61). Hard presumed consent, which implicitly constructs the dead body as public property or a commons, was characterised as allowing organs to be 'taken', whereas the soft version, which retains provision for choice on the part of the family, was deemed to facilitate organs being 'given'. The difference between these property regimes and their varying provisions for choice on the part of the family were critical to the policy deliberations.

The advocates of presumed consent all encouraged an understanding of death as something that should always be linked with organ donation, and where people have a moral duty to be organ donors. The dead body was constituted as a means to saving lives and saving money. One of the high-profile organ donation campaigners explained that with presumed consent 'everybody is a donor [as] in Belgium and it is merely a normal part of the dying process' (Houses of the Oireachtas, 2013: 52). As noted earlier, for him, a donated dead body is the means to saving seven lives. For some others, the dead body was spoken about as a container of materials for medical intervention and a means to saving the health services money. Articulating the mentality of *homo economicus*, one clinician said 'one could consider a kidney donor to be a pot of gold' (*ibid.*: 104), given the savings on dialysis therapies that can accrue over time from transplantation.

This kind of economic mentality was also evident in depictions of the bodies of organ donors as a 'scarce resource' (*ibid.*: 40).

The individual

Three key constructions of the individual are apparent in the policy deliberations about organ donation, namely, a citizen with rights, a member of a family, and a potential organ donor. In many of the contributions death was assumed to entail the transformation of the autonomous citizen into a family member, where the wishes of the former can be overruled by those of their family members.

What was deemed by many to be the foremost controversial aspect of organ donation based on presumed consent was its potential to violate individuals' rights. For example, a legal expert explained to the Joint Committee that even though in the 30 years in which presumed consent has been introduced in European countries it has not been legally challenged, he outlined a number of rights 'relevant in this territory' (Houses of the Oireachtas, 2013: 95). These included provisions in the European Convention on Human Rights, such as the right to a private and family life, and the right to freedom of conscience and religion. He also mentioned Irish citizens' constitutional rights to bodily integrity, freedom of conscience and religion, and the constitution's recognition of the family as a fundamental unit. In a similar vein, the DoH's Chief Bioethics Officer noted that the principal ethical objection to presumed consent models of organ donation is 'the loss of autonomy and right to self-determination of potential donors ... [and that it] violates the principle of respect for autonomy that underlies the concept of informed consent'. She pointed out that some ethicists have rejected the very term presumed consent as a misnomer because consent is an active process involving the individual and cannot be given passively. In the Briefing Paper these objections were noted to have been crucial to the decisions not to introduce presumed consent in Canada.

This construction of the human as an autonomous individual with citizen rights is, however, in tension with the almost universal acceptance during the public hearings that the family should have authority to give final approval for the donation of their relative's dead body for organ transplantation. In this instance, to be human is first and foremost to be a member of a family. Here, it is worthwhile noting the familism inherent in the Irish constitution of 1937 that privileges the family over the individual (Yeates, 1999). It defined the marital family as 'the natural primary and fundamental unit group of Society' that the state 'guarantees to protect ... in its constitution and authority, as the necessary basis of social order and as indispensable to the welfare of the Nation and the State'. Consistent with the property regime implicit in the provisions of soft presumed consent in which the family is understood as 'owning' the dead body, a repeated refrain during the public hearings was that 'the ultimate choice must rest with the Family', as declared in the submission by the representative of the Organ Procurement Office (Houses of the Oireachtas, 2013: 20). The alteration of the policy proposal to introduce a *hard* opt-out system to a *soft* opt-out system in which the consent of the family is required was after all crucial to many of the advocacy organisations changing their position in regard to presumed consent. A rare exception to this way of thinking was evident in the contribution of one of the Joint Committee members who argued the preferences of family members should not take precedence over the preferences of the deceased. He said, 'I would be strongly of the view that my family has no right to object' (*ibid.*: 106). In this instance, the construction of the individual as first and foremost an autonomous actor trumped its construction as a family member.

The question of who is the donor is raised by much of the discussion of family consent. In many instances, it can be seen that it is not the deceased but the family who are constituted as the donors. This can be seen in the contribution of a TD who spoke at the public hearings about his experiences of being from a 'donor family'. Referring to the two people who received organs from his deceased sister he said, 'We gave them a whole new life' (Houses of the Oireachtas, 2013: 69). Similarly, one of the organ donor campaigners referred to organ donation as a 'family gift' (*ibid.*: 73). Concerns about the potential for presumed consent to undermine gifting hinged not so much on fears that it would undermine the rights of the individual but rather those of the family. 'We must bear in mind ... that it is within the right of the family' not to donate, was a reminder offered by a representative of the Irish Intensive Care Society (*ibid.*: 104).

The third construction of the individual is as an organ donor. Asserting this bodily imperative, one of the organ donor campaigners stated that all 'people must become donors', that 'everybody is a donor' (Houses of the Oireachtas, 2013: 51/52). As explained by the Chief Bioethics Officer, for some, this construction of everyone as a donor can be consistent with the construction of the human as an autonomous individual. She said, 'it has been argued that an opt-out system enhances autonomy as public surveys have shown a high willingness on the part of the public to donate their organs and by failing to remove people's organs, one is thus acting contrary to their (unexpressed) wishes' (*ibid.*: 45). Within the discussions, however, there are indications that not everyone is deemed to be a potential donor. This was most evident in the statement by one of the Joint Committee members that 'gay people are not allowed to be organ donors' (*ibid.*: 67). More subtly, however, references to the 'quality' of organs and to the importance of asking family members about the 'lifestyle' of the deceased suggest that there are good and bad organ donors, useful and not so useful dead bodies.

The construction of the individual as someone who inevitably becomes an organ donor after death rests squarely on the idea that we have a responsibility to each other to do so. For one of the most vociferous advocates of this position, this new moral duty is not burdensome, as 'Who does not want to save seven lives after he or she is dead?' (Houses of the Oireachtas, 2013: 52). As a live donor, this campaigner's experience of euphoria having donated a kidney to a friend was described by one of the medical professionals who addressed the Joint Committee, in a way that further underlined the positive features of giving the 'gift of life'. Others too spoke about the benefits of donation to families, emphasising, 'it is a key element to support families in their grieving process' (*ibid.*: 21). This kind of argument potentially extends responsibility beyond responsibilities to organ recipients to the families of the deceased, where a decision not to donate could become a way of depriving the grieving family of 'comfort and consolation' (*ibid.*: 20).

Presentations of emotional personal stories from the biological citizens who were organ recipients had strong responsibilising dynamics. These presentations were replete with references to the virtues of donors, such as the 'selfless generosity' of donor families and how they had given the chance of a 'second shot a life'; they were accompanied with assertions that advances in medicine that allow such second chances at life 'should encourage more people to be organ donors' (Houses of the Oireachtas, 2013: 54). But the responsibilisation of organ recipients themselves was also evident, as in the comments of one woman who noted that while the average life of a kidney transplant is 15 years, 'I am certainly aiming for many more' and hence 'the saving of €830,000 ... could possibly be greater' (*ibid.*: 56). Furthermore, recognition of the potential new responsibilities and retributions that the proposed new measure might entail are evident in the Chief Bioethics Officer's statement that the introduction of organ donation based on presumed consent would also produce a new responsibility for the state 'to prevent social stigmatisation of individuals who opt out and might thus be regarded as "lacking in solidarity"' (*ibid.*: 46).

Limits to medicine?

The policy deliberations about the proposal to introduce a system of organ donation based on presumed consent were devoid of a 'politics of enough' (Wehling, 2011) in respect of medicine. At no point was the 'organ crisis' called into question, nor was the inevitability of an increasing need and demand for organs. These were taken-for-granted aspects of the political rationality underpinning the policy initiative. Repeatedly, the imperative to 'maximise the number of patients who benefit' from transplant medicine was asserted (Houses of the Oireachtas, 2013: 27). As stated by a representative of the Cancer, Blood and Organs Unit in the DoH, we must 'maximise the number of organs available for transplantation' (*ibid.*: 39). This objective of maximising the availability of organs so as to maximise the number of people who can benefit from transplants was not disputed, only the means of achieving it. As stated by one TD, 'everybody is sincerely working towards the objective of improved donor availability and the consequent access for those in need. It is a matter of trying to find the appropriate response' (*ibid.*: 97).

As seen earlier, rationing access to medicine was depicted as apocalyptic and in the realm of the horrors of science fiction. At no point was the informal rationing of medicine that takes place acknowledged. Austerity, as noted by Thomas, Burke and Barry (2014: 1546), 'has yielded increased rationing' in forms such as growing waiting lists due to a 10% reduction in the number of public hospital beds between 2008 and 2012. But neither was there any acknowledgement that healthcare rationing can be just, as argued by bioethicists such as Leonard Fleck, who encourages a kind of questioning of the limits of medicine that Peter Wehling (2011) fears active biological citizenship and claims to the right to treatment can discourage. The kind of questioning Fleck (2009: vii) encourages was absent from the policy deliberations, questioning such as 'what does it mean to be a "just" and "caring" society when we have only limited resources to meet virtually unlimited health care needs?'

Greater access to organs and transplantation was represented as a means to avoiding the possible necessity for rationing in the future. As explained by one renal physician, 'we have revenue locked within the programme for treatment of end-stage kidney disease … If a proportion of those patients received a transplant, that revenue would no longer be required' (Houses of the Oireachtas, 2013: 102). This kind of argument was made in respect of kidney transplantation only, an argument that may not have the same force in respect of other organs, such as hearts and lungs. Despite these constructions of the rationing of medicine, which are in sync with the assertion of one biological citizen that 'One cannot put a cost on a human life' (*ibid.*: 53), one participant did acknowledge that on a global scale this happens by default. The Clinical Director of Transplantation Urology and Nephrology at Beaumont Hospital said, 'It is true to say that most patients in the world with kidney failure die without any significant treatment, as the treatment, although effective, is extremely expensive and requires a very sophisticated medical system to deliver it' (*ibid.*: 83). The limits placed on some people's access to medicine, therefore, was recognised, but the seeming limitlessness of people's need for medical treatments was beyond the range of consideration of the public hearings. Ever-expanding needs for transplantation arising from the growing number of people who are obese and have diabetes were taken for granted. Perhaps because of the emphasis on soft presumed consent, which established the preferences and choices of the family of the deceased as central concerns, there was little evidence that the property regime implicit in the proposed system of organ donation based on presumed consent encouraged consideration of broader macro-level concerns, as predicted by Anne Phillips. Her analysis, however, which imagines the dead body as a commons, presumes a hard model of presumed consent, whereas in the Irish policy deliberations the soft model in which the dead body is presumed to be property of the family was deemed imperative.

Conclusion

This chapter has explored how the Irish state has endeavoured to act *through* its citizens to transform the prevailing cultural attitude to organ donation whereby consent is presumed and (almost) everybody's cadaveric organs become available for transplantation. It has highlighted that efforts to shape people's organ donation behaviour and sensibilities have entailed government of how other matters are thought about too, namely the dead body, what it is to be an individual and the limits of medicine. Focusing on the public hearings about organ donation conducted by the Joint Committee on Health and Children 2013, the analysis offered here points to the messiness of public policymaking and the exercise of power, evident for example in the different governmental rationalities underpinning the Briefing Paper that forms part of the Joint Committee's report and the Committee's recommendations. However, even though the Briefing Paper mobilised arguments in favour of retaining the existing opt-in system of organ donation, albeit with modifications, and the Joint Committee's conclusions encouraged ways of thinking that regard the proposed opt-out system as necessary and practicable, both are founded on a recognition of the scarcity of human organs for transplantation as a policy problem that warrants intervention. Counter-conducts on the part of many of the participants are also apparent in their eschewing of the representation of Ireland's relatively low rate of organ donation as the primary organ donation policy problem, and their proffering of an alternative governmental rationality that defined poor healthcare resourcing and organisation as the main problems. But many of these nonetheless subscribed to the idea that, combined with infrastructural improvements, the introduction of institutional arrangements for organ donation based on presumed consent is imperative.

While Anne Phillips (2013) has suggested that presumed consent weakens the dominant understanding of the dead body as the individual's private property and thus can weaken the neoliberal individualism that can pervade policy deliberations on body matters, what we see in the policy deliberations considered here is that they were governed by commitments to familism. Instead of steering the policy debate to broader communal concerns, the new bodily imperative of *soft* presumed consent contributed to establishing the family of the deceased as the centre of attention and making their choices the predominant concern. The overriding conception of what it is to be human produced by the technologies of subjectification at play in this policy domain was not an autonomous individual, but a member of a family. Consideration of the dilemmas generated by seemingly limitless increases in the numbers of people in *desperate need* of organ transplantation, and biological citizens' claims that a cost cannot be put on a human life, were subtly rendered beyond the scope of the policy deliberations about Ireland's organ donation policy. So too were other complex and contentious issues, such as the controversy surrounding new ways of thinking about the passage from life to death that have been promoted since the advent of transplant medicine. The origins of bioethics have been traced to the terrible task faced by US hospital committees in the 1960s of deciding which patients would be given access to the then new but in short supply dialysis machines, decisions that would result in the death of those not selected (Callahan, 2012: xii). The terrible task of deciding what limits should be placed on people's access to transplant medicine remains unaddressed in Irish organ transplant policy deliberations, and reliance on unacknowledged rationing continues.

References

Callahan, D. (2012) *The Roots of Bioethics. Health, Progress, Technology, Death.* Oxford, Oxford University Press.

Dean, M. (1999) *Governmentality: Power and Rule in Modern Society.* London, Sage.

DoH (2013) *Public Consultation. Introduction of an Opt-Out System of Consent for Organ Donation.* Dublin, DoH.

Dukelow, F. (2015) Pushing against an open door: reinforcing the neo-liberal policy paradigm in Ireland and the impact of EU intrusion. *Comparative European Politics*, 13(1): 93–111.

Fine Gael / Labour (2011) *Towards Recovery: Programme for a National Government 2011–2016.* Dublin, Fine Gael, Labour Party.

Fleck, L. (2009) *Just Caring: Health Care Rationing and Democratic Deliberation.* Oxford, Oxford University Press.

Foucault, M. (1980) *Power/Knowledge.* Brighton, Harvester.

Houses of the Oireachtas (2013) *Joint Committee on Health and Children Report on Organ Donation.* Dublin, Houses of the Oireachtas.

Illich, I. (2010) Needs. IN: Sachs, W. (ed.) *The Development Dictionary: A Guide to Knowledge as Power.* London, Zed Books: pp. 88–101.

Lemke, T. (2001) 'The birth of bio-politics': Michel Foucault's lecture at the College de France on neo-liberal governmentality. *Economy and Society*, 30(2): 190–207.

Marquis, D. (2010) Are DCD donors dead? *Hastings Center Report*, 40(3): 24–31.

Miller, F. (2009) Muddling through? A commentary on controversies in the determination of death. *Hastings Center Bioethics Forum.*

O'Donovan, O. (2015) Conversing on the commons: an interview with Gustavo Esteva – part 2. *Community Development Journal*, 50(4): 742–753.

Phillips, A. (2013) *Our Bodies, Whose Property?* Princeton, Princeton University Press.

Read, J. (2009) A genealogy of homo-economicus: neoliberalism and the production of subjectivity. IN: Binkley, S. and Capetillo-Ponce, J. (eds) *A Foucault for the 21st Century: Governmentality, Biopolitics and Discipline in the New Millennium*. Newcastle upon Tyne, Cambridge Scholars: pp. 2–15.

Scheper-Hughes, N. (2007) The tyranny of the gift: Sacrificial violence in living donor transplants. *American Journal of Transplantation*, 7: 507–511.

Shildrick, M. (2014) Visceral phenomenology: organ transplantation, identity and sexual difference. IN: Zeiler, K. and Kall, L. (eds) *Feminist Phenomenology and Medicine*. New York, SUNY Press.

Thomas, S., Burke, S. and Barry, S. (2014) The Irish health-care system and austerity: sharing the pain. *The Lancet*, 383: 1545–1546.

Wehling, P. (2011) Biology, citizenship and the government of biomedine. IN: Brockling, U., Gasmann, S. and Lemke, T. (eds) *Governmentality: Current Issues, Future Challenges*. New York, Routledge: pp. 225–246.

Yeates, N. (1999) Gender, familism and housing: Matrimonial property rights in Ireland. *Women's Studies International Forum*, 22(6): 607–618.

PART II

Governing neoliberal healthcare agendas: politics, strategies and practices

Neoliberal governmentality and public health policy in Ireland

Introduction

Since 1994 the Irish government has developed policies that set out its vision, priorities and direction for improving and sustaining the health of its people. This chapter critically appraises how these strategies have been configured to structure responsibility for health. Informed by the work of Rose and colleagues (Rose, 1999, 2000; Rose and Miller, 2010; Rose, O'Malley and Valverde, 2006), our analysis exposes a number of key characteristics of neoliberal governmentality, including the shift towards a market-based model of health; the distribution of power across a range of agents and agencies of health ('governing at a distance'); and the increasing individualisation of health, which places responsibility upon each citizen to look after his or her own health by behaving in appropriate and recommended ways. We conclude that while the decision to devolve responsibility to others may avoid claims of paternalism, an increasing focus on the individual prioritises individual agency as the means to advancing health at the expense of wider, macro social structures and processes.

Background

Strategic health policies are heavily politicised blueprints (or grand narratives) of health and its need for governance (Roe, 1994). Health policy strategies provide a snapshot of the state of the nation's health at a particular point in time, framing it as a problem to be solved (see Bacchi, 2012). They also provide solutions in the form of recommendations that reflect the complexity of health and recognise the need for intersectoral collaboration and action, as well as the need to provide opportunities for individuals to improve, manage and protect their own health (Newman and Vidler, 2006).

Over past decades policy recommendations to improve population health have increasingly targeted individuals and individual risk factors (see, for example, DoH, 2004; HM Government 2010; Jennings, 2014; Lalonde, 1974; Michailakis and Schirmer, 2010; WHO, 1981, 1985, 1986). This is largely the result of describing and explaining health behaviours in terms of 'lifestyle' and choice (see DoH, 2004; WHO, 1981, 1986, 2013; WHO Regional Office for Europe, 1985; Voigt, 2013). There is a wealth of evidence that links lifestyle choices, such as smoking, binge drinking and lack of physical activity, to the development and progression of chronic diseases, including obesity, Type 2 diabetes, cardiovascular disease and even cancer (Alwan *et al.*, 2010; Lee *et al.*, 2012). Resnik (2007), for example, suggests that six of the top ten causes of death and disability are related to lifestyle choices. In the UK, the *Global Health Strategy 2014 to 2019* recognises that non-communicable diseases (cancers, cardiovascular diseases, chronic respiratory diseases and diabetes), which cause 'more than 36 million deaths annually', are caused by lifestyle factors 'such as tobacco use, alcohol use, unhealthy diet and sedentary lifestyles' (Public Health England, 2014: 14). Similarly, in Ireland, lifestyle factors are said to contribute to 'almost 35% of cancer deaths and cases of cancer, and almost 65% of cardiovascular disease deaths and cases' (Jennings, 2014: 13). Furthermore, the economic costs of treating and managing such chronic diseases, which are constructed as largely preventable, place undue burden on healthcare services. For example, the cost of obesity alone in Ireland was estimated to be €1.13 billion (Jennings, 2014).

Consistent with other countries, targeting the risk factors of ill-health and the associated costs not only requires the Irish government to take action, but also necessitates action by industry, other government agencies and public agencies (HM Government, 2010; Newman, 2006; WHO, 2013; Wilson, 2014). Individuals are also required to bear responsibility for the lifestyle choices that they make. This has led to the development of health policies that promote self-management, patients as experts, and making individuals responsible and accountable for their behaviours. Using the rhetoric of engagement, empowerment and participation, such strategies endeavour to mobilise all – people, communities, industry – to share responsibility for health and reduce the overall social and economic burden of disease. In Ireland, for example, this notion abounds in health promotion strategies and is suggestive of a new mode of governmentality (see Foucault, 2009; Newman, 2003; Rose and Miller, 2010). In the words of the EU White Paper, *Together for Health*, 'healthcare is becoming increasingly patient-centred and individualised, with the patient becoming an active subject rather than a mere object of healthcare' (Commission of the European Unions, 2007: 4).

Focusing on poor lifestyle choices as a cause of mortality and morbidity is in keeping with a market-driven, neoliberal model of healthcare policy. As explained in Chapter 1, neoliberalism is a style of governmentality (that is, the art of governing) that is characterised by a liberal attitude to social behaviour and a willingness to apply free-market principles as readily to matters of welfare and education as to matters of business and economics, and increasingly, to matters of health. Within this context, it refers to a range of measures used by the government to reduce healthcare expenditure, while simultaneously maximising users' choices as consumers (Prince, Kearns and Craig, 2006; Peedell, 2009; Gallagher 2012). As such, the process normally involves the deregulation and privatisation of health services in order to ensure sustained economic growth, competition and innovation; the reframing of patients as 'clients' and 'consumers'; and the deployment of market-driven techniques to measure and monitor the performance of staff and service providers. What is usually ignored is that health has social determinants, as well as individual and behavioural determinants.

In an organisational framework, the neoliberal state aims to function as a contractual commissioner of healthcare rather than as a provider of care. As a result, most Western societies now encourage the development of a mixed economy of provision ('any willing provider') with the implicit understanding that by privatising public services the state can reduce costs and render services more affordable and efficient via the operation of market forces. However, the introduction of market forces is only one aspect of change in the organisation of healthcare. In successive sections, we use the concept of neoliberal governmentality to understand how health policy strategies in Ireland have structured responsibility for health. In doing so, the chapter adds to the many research papers exploring neoliberal forms of governance (for example, Prince, Kearns and Craig, 2006; Peedell, 2009; Gallagher, 2012; Barcelos, 2013; Van Houdt and Schinkel, 2013).

Methodological framework

The concept of governmentality refers to systematic and regulated ways – discursive as well as concrete (usually bureaucratic) practices – in which the state/government exercises and justifies its power (or form of political technology), according to a particular form of rationality (mode of thought or reasoning), so as to control and manage its populace (Lemke, 2002, 2007; Gallagher, 2012). Different political rationalities provide a means for the state to define, imagine and identify solutions to any given 'problem' or risk set and are commonly identifiable in policy documents. Such problems are subsequently addressed through various 'technologies of government' (that is, techniques) that the state has at its disposal to achieve governance. Given that 'health' is an example of an imagined governable space – what Rose (1999: 32) terms the 'irreal' (neither quite real nor imagined) – it is not surprising that the neoliberal state uses discursive resources to imagine, construct, justify and legitimise health policies within its jurisdiction (Lemke, 2002, 2007). It is partly through such policies (or rationalities) that health becomes an intelligible and knowable realm, with specific problems, urgencies and strategies.

In successive sections, we apply a governmentality lens to analyse how Irish strategic health policies promote a neoliberal agenda when structuring responsibility for health. Health policies often present a narrative (story) of a particular problem to be solved (Bacchi, 2012). By analysing these narratives, we explore the process by which a neoliberal rationality for health responsibility is promoted. Examining narratives is a part of the 'argumentative turn' in policy analysis, which places considerable importance on the content and structure of the text in producing and maintaining policy, including health policy. Understanding how responsibility for health is constructed in policy discourse requires understanding the 'discourse coalition'; that is 'the ensemble of a set of story lines, the actors that utter these story lines, and the practices that conform to these story lines, all organised around a discourse' (Hajer, 1993: 47). Scrutinising the argumentative turn not only gleans insight into the particular narrative surrounding arrangements for governance, including how we govern and are governed, but extends the informational space to include those counter-positions that helped to construct the argument in the first instance (*ibid.*: 45).

To this end we searched the website of the Department(s) of Health/and Children for all health policy strategies published between 1994 and 2013. We chose 1994 as the cut-off point as this is when the first strategic public health policy was published. We identified three strategies: *Shaping a Healthier Future* (DoH, 1994), *Quality and Fairness: A Health System for You* (hereafter *Quality and Fairness*; DoHC, 2001), and *Healthy Ireland: A Framework for Improved Health and Wellbeing* (hereafter *Healthy Ireland*; DoH, 2013). We scrutinised and identified the main claims or arguments of each document according to the dimensions of analysis discussed above, which we subsequently placed within a grid to facilitate their comparison. Our results illustrate three evolving rationalities in strategic public health policies in Ireland: (1) a market-based model of healthcare (2) devolution of responsibility: governing at a distance, which depicts the ever-expanding hand of the state while responsibility for health is shared between public, private and voluntary spheres, and (3) capabilities and techniques to manage the self and ensure individual behaviour aligns with political objectives.

A market-based model of healthcare

The need to reduce healthcare expenditure appeared in the first national, strategic public health policy – *Shaping a Healthier Future* (DoH, 1994). At the time of publication, life expectancy in Ireland had increased by 11 years for women (from 67.1 to 77.5 years of age) and 8 years for men (from 64.5 to 72 years of age) between 1950 and 1990. In addition, the country was beginning to feel the effects of an economic boom that was set to last until 2008 (McDaid *et al.*, 2009). Yet, despite this positive outlook, the language of the document was mostly subdued and cautious. This is not surprising; previous years (1980 to 1987) had been marred by a prolonged economic recession, which saw living standards plummet, unemployment escalate (employment decreased by nearly 6% and 25% in manufacturing), and mass emigration rise (O'Donnell, 1998).

Fearful of national insolvency and of a declining tax base, the document authors deployed an apparently objective and technical narrative of 'efficiency' to justify and legitimise real cuts in healthcare expenditure. They argued that the state was spending too much, given that more affluent countries were spending less and apparently getting more: 'In Ireland, however, we are already committing as high a proportion of our national wealth to healthcare as some countries which are significantly wealthier' (DoH, 1994: 8). Yet, at the time of publication, the amount of money spent on health in Ireland was lower than anywhere else in the EU: 8.4% of GDP (Gross Domestic Product); 6.5% expenditure on public health and 1.9% expenditure on private health (Cowman, 1996). The document also spoke of a desire to free up resources to tackle other areas of governance, thus: 'In addition to the human costs of ... premature illnesses, disabilities and deaths, there are, of course, very heavy financial costs to the health services which, if they could be reduced, would make more resources available to meet the many other priority needs' (DoH, 1994: 20). Part of the problem was that while life expectancy had improved, it remained below the EU average (72.8 years for men and for 79.4 years of age for women). There were also concerns in relation to premature mortality in those under 65 years of age from chronic diseases, notably cancer, cardiovascular disease, as well as other causes such as accidents.

To this end, and as the prevailing rhetoric of this document demonstrates, the authors of *Shaping a Healthier Future* turned towards a market-based model of health; the language bears the hallmark of an efficiency savings approach with frequent references to notions of 'greater savings', 'value for money' and being 'cost-effective'. Patients featured strongly as purchasers as well as users of services, and from the outset there were references to 'clients', 'consumers', 'users', 'user satisfaction and participation' and 'consumer-oriented' provision. Throughout the document the need for austerity was clear as efforts were geared towards trying to 'extract maximum efficiency so that the volume and quality of patient services could be maintained at the greatest level possible at a time of very tight financial constraint' (DoH, 1994: 8). By means of these concepts, the Department of Health (DoH) had developed and mobilised a narrative based on efficiency, performance management and other market principles that legitimised the proposed actions and interventions suggested at that time (Bourdieu, 2003; Raco, 2009).

Given that reforms couched within a narrative of austerity were likely to be poorly received by voters, the authors of the document placed a heavy emphasis on 'quality', especially a desire to provide 'high quality' services, and quality assessment and the need to improve the patient's 'experiences' of healthcare. The document thus explained that the best-quality outcomes must be achieved in return for the level of investment undertaken, and that customer satisfaction will function to reflect the quality of the service offered and received. Health staff employees were not only to be accountable to the state but also to the patients – in accordance with the call for health services to be 'consumer-orientated' (DoH, 1994: 39). In an attempt to gauge customer satisfaction, the state aimed to gather 'comprehensible and good quality information' on a range of issues, including 'information on needs, information on activity, information on detailed costs and information on outcomes' (ibid.: 17). These features of the actuarial state were to be operationalised via an array of tools: 'clinical audit mechanisms', contracts, 'appropriate complaints procedures', 'annual reports', as well as the collection of 'baseline data' and preference data from 'consumer surveys'.

The language of measurement and assessment enabled the operations of governance to be executed at a distance and more easily subjected to political as well as administrative scrutiny. Standards of care and provision were also to be developed and set out in specific charters (for example, 'The Charter of Rights for Hospital Patients', DoH, 1994: 39). Once again, market-influenced performance management and monitoring tools were to be used to assess the success of placing 'greater emphasis on the importance of the patients and clients who receive the services and the staff who provide them' (DoH, 1994: 44). Such quantification of activity and the deployment of an increasing array of actuarial tools and performance indicators are, of course, characteristic of governance in all neoliberal regimes. They allow the disciplinary state to count, evaluate and distribute goods, information and services across the population in an apparently neutral and 'objective' manner beyond the bounds of 'ideology' (Gallagher, 2012; Prince, Kearns and Craig, 2006). In adopting such practices – increased emphasis on transparency, accountability and managerial programmes – the government sought to improve productivity, increase efficiency and make a profit. However, as we come to see in Quality and Fairness (DoHC, 2001), these gains would come at a cost: greater inequality.

The publication of Quality and Fairness (DoHC, 2001) bore witness to a more robust and persuasive narrative of 'efficiency savings'. Consistent with its predecessor, Quality and Fairness was also underpinned by market techniques. At the time of publication, Ireland had experienced unprecedented economic growth. Yet, although life expectancy had increased (75.1

years for men and 80.3 years for women, compared to 1995 to 1997 when it was 73 years for men and 78.5 years for women), it had not increased as quickly as other parts of the EU and the gap between nations was widening. Similarly, life expectancy was lower for men than for women. Such variations gave rise to a new, mutated narrative for health focused not on addressing chronic health problems, but the imbalance in the distribution of health across specific pockets of the population and the population as a whole. Subsequently, there was an increased emphasis on inequalities as evidenced by references to 'inequalities in health', 'disparities in health status', 'occupational class gradients in mortality' given the document's intention to make 'Ireland a healthier nation and making sure that good health is enjoyed more equally across society' (DoHC, 2001: 39). *Shaping a Healthier Future* had not mentioned the word 'inequality' but instead made reference to 'equity', and then only tangentially with regard to 'achieving equity in the healthcare system' and to 'reducing waiting-times' (DoH, 1994: 10).

The Department of Health and Children (DoHC) – authors of *Quality and Fairness* – argued that, by privatising public services, the state could increase competition and make healthcare services more affordable and efficient thereby deflecting some of the expenses involved. And so, we find clear references to 'quality of the service', 'maximising efficiency' and 'accountability'. Indeed, the language of value echoes loudly in this document with references to 'a value on quality of life', 'the value of investment in health', 'direct economic benefits' and 'value for money' (DoHC, 2001: 16). In other words, the state could reduce the provision of social services and relieve some of the financial costs that had increased in recent years from the decline of the birth rate; increase in life span due to improved healthcare; the associated increase in degenerative diseases at older ages such as dementia; changes in unemployment; and the development of new technologies to expand the range of treatments available.

Quality and Fairness also referred to the importance of adopting 'an evidence-based approach' to healthcare (DoHC, 2001: 88). The evidence-based approach naturally lends itself to technocratic decision-making and the apparent exclusion of ideology from healthcare. In line with this policy, the authors argued that 'Improving quality in the health system requires implementation of internally-recognised evidence-based guidelines and protocols, and on-going education and commitment from health-care institutions and professionals' (*ibid.*: 19). Consequently, it stated that '[d]ecisions in all areas must be supported by reference to this kind of evidence or to agreed standards, protocols or models of best practice' (*ibid.*: 88). In keeping with the dominant rationality, the collection and analysis of comprehensive data would facilitate 'the planning and delivery of services' according to need as well as alternative technologies and approaches to service delivery (*ibid.*: 24). As it stands, the document suggests that there is a lack of evidence to make informative healthcare decisions: 'There are considerable gaps in information related to morbidity'; 'Information from out-patient and primary care services is limited. Data on mental health and chronic disease are also incomplete' (*ibid.*: 34). And so there is a need for evidence to inform policy. In that spirit, the document drew its own evidence from a variety of national and international sources, including 'The European Home and Leisure Accidents Surveillance System (EHLASS) Report for Ireland (1998)', 'The National Health and Lifestyle Survey (Slán)' and the 'Health Behaviour in School-Aged Children (HBSC)' (DoHC, 2001: 28–29). It also sought to conduct 'clinical audits' and develop 'improved customer care procedures', 'easily accessible complaints and appeals procedures', and 'mechanisms that capture customer feedback'. Under a neoliberal regime these techniques not only enabled a detailed monitoring of activity on the ground, but also displaced responsibility for any adverse outcomes on to 'street level' (rather than central) bureaucracy.

In 2013, following eight consecutive austerity budgets, the DoH published its new strategy: *Healthy Ireland*. In the wake of the collapse of the Irish banking system in 2008 the unemployment rate had soared from 4.9% in January 2008 to 15% in January 2012 (Central Statistics Office, 2012). Unsurprisingly, this was matched with a fall in per capita annual health expenditure of 6.6% between 2009 and 2011. This fall reflected the substantial reforms taken at this time coupled with the price cuts paid for healthcare in the form of wages and pharmaceuticals. In 2010, the country agreed to international financial assistance and subsequently accepted an €85 billion bailout package for the period 2010 to 2013 (European Commission, 2014). At that time life expectancy at birth in Ireland was 81 years, one year higher than the OECD average of 80 years (83 years for women and 78 years for men) (OECD, 2016).

Consistent with its predecessors, the authors of *Healthy Ireland* continued to develop and mobilise a more nuanced and selective narrative concerned with efficiency savings. This narrative, like its ancestors, was socially constructed by the state to describe an imagined social reality that prescribed and legitimised those types of actions and intervention that the state endorsed (Bourdieu, 2003; Raco, 2009). Once again, the basic premise of this business approach to healthcare was that it was beyond both the capacity and the remit of the state to manage individual health. Consequently, the government should fund essential care only and outsource responsibility for health to other government departments and organisations, as well as empowering communities and individuals, providing them with the freedom and knowledge to behave as informed consumers of healthcare. The government was to be a commissioner of healthcare rather than a provider of healthcare. Underpinning the redistribution of responsibility and workload is, of course, a form of technocratic expertise based on the use of 'evidence'. Thus,

> Accelerating the take-up of new knowledge and innovating through advances
> in scientific knowledge is a key aspect of how we will achieve [our] goals.
> The consistent application of evidence of what works and what interventions
> positively impact on health behaviours, in a cost-effective way, is critical to
> setting policy and investing in prevention programmes. (DoH, 2013: 28)

As one might expect under neoliberal forms of governing, '[t]his will require
an audit of resources, skills and infrastructure to inform actions to consoli-
date, co-ordinate and improve the efficiency of our research, evaluation,
and implementation activities' (*ibid.*: 28). In addition, '[e]xcellent data-
monitoring capacity and systems to track progress in achieving targets will
be required to evaluate the success of Healthy Ireland' (*ibid.*: 30). The
problem is that what counts as evidence and how evidence is itself assessed
are never beyond contention, as studies in the sociology of science have
persistently shown (Collins and Pinch, 1993).

Devolution of responsibility: governing at a distance

For all documents the technology of governance devised by the state as a
means to streamline services to deal with the identified problems (increasing
inequalities in health, spiralling costs) involved the devolution of responsibility. The basic premise was that it was beyond both the capacity and the
remit of the state to manage the health status of individuals. Consequently,
the state sought to empower individuals, communities and organisations
(via the provision of information and 'choice') to manage health risks.
   Shaping a Healthier Future presaged the beginning of an era that would
see the expansion and roll-out of the health service as it strived for solidarity
and equity in health, and the participation and accountability of individuals,
groups, institutions and communities for continued health development
(DoH, 1994). This was to be achieved by delegating power and responsibility for population health to those further down the bureaucratic ladder both
within the health sector and also across the public sector. For example, the
remit of the GP was to change: GPs were to become integrated into the
health system and given greater responsibility for health (Cowman, 1996).
At face value, this approach suggests a reduced role for the state and seemingly provides evidence of its retreat. However, such a move should not be
interpreted as the relinquishing of the state's interest in health. Indeed, the
document highlights that the 'Minister for Health will ... continue to have
ultimate responsibility to the Oireachtas [Government] for all health services' (DoH, 1994: 31). Rather, then, it reflects the delegation of work roles
and responsibility such that 'his Department will no longer be involved in
the detailed management of individual services' (*ibid.*: 31). In other words,
the state was to retain a supervisory and commissioning role – ultimately
essential to its legitimation – but would delegate care tasks to those with

the relevant 'expertise' and local knowledge – highlighting the increasing role for technocrats in public health governance whereby 'operational decisions are best taken locally, with local knowledge' (*ibid.*: 31).

Quality and Fairness built on this line of reasoning by delegating responsibility for health not only to organisational structures but also to individual citizens (DoHC, 2001). The off-loading of risk necessitated a greater appreciation that 'many other factors, and therefore, many other individuals, groups, institutions and public and private bodies have a part to play in the effort to improve health status and achieve the health potential of the nation' (*ibid.*: 16). There was a nod to cooperation and partnership as the mechanism by which this would be achieved, as well as the need to develop 'high quality, integrated health-care at local, regional and national level' (*ibid.*: 19), given that 'co-operation between statutory and voluntary providers allows for a more responsive and dynamic approach to meeting needs' (*ibid.*: 47). This 'integration' sought to expand not only 'the role of the other sectors in keeping people healthy' (*ibid.*: 23) but to lead to 'integrated information systems' and 'improved inter-disciplinary team-working' too (*ibid.*: 49). In this way, the document made suggestions as to how others might work *with* the state to co-produce health (McDaid *et al.*, 2009), which is completely in keeping with the broader aim of the neoliberal state to download the management of risk.

Once again, at first sight, the invisible hand approach suggests a reduced role for the state. Yet, as we have argued, in place of retreat, what we see is the early beginnings of the advancement and extension of the state as contractor and regulator into a vast network of organisations and activities. In many ways the mutation of state responsibility for health actually reflects the redistribution of workload as opposed to the redistribution of power. This is akin to 'governing at a distance'. In the words of Gallagher (2012: 466), 'while a neoliberal ideology may suggest less government, it does not signify less governance'. Indeed, despite the intent to devolve responsibility for health, there was consensus that overall accountability rests with the government and, in particular, the Minister for Health and Children and the DoHC (McDaid *et al.*, 2009). Thus, it is more in keeping with an attempt to outsource responsibility as opposed to retract responsibility. Indeed it is recognised that 'The Department has a leadership role in areas such as equity, quality, accountability and value for money' (DoHC, 2001: 39).

Healthy Ireland continued to expand on the 'efficiency' theme but now the rationality of cooperation alluded to in previous documents came to the fore (DoH, 2013). The document argued that the 'old ways' of working were no longer valid and that a new 'cooperative' approach was needed. Terms such as 'clients', 'consumers' and 'users', which abounded in previous documents, had languished and were replaced with a new rhetoric on collaboration and teamwork. The impact of this on the welfare state, and on the health services in particular, is a constant sharing of 'responsibility'; a constant call for 'partnership'; and a constant claim that matters of health are matters for 'all', matters for 'us', and matters for 'every one' – together. Indeed the text is imbued with words and phrases such as 'partners', 'partnerships', 'cross-sectoral work', 'joined-up', 'working together', 'cooperation', 'shared vision' and 'shared responsibility'. The document stipulated a need to pull together towards a 'common purpose' (*ibid.*: 21), 'common agendas', and to draw on 'individual and collective strengths' (*ibid.*: 24). This cooperative rationality builds on the previous market-based efficiency strategy and seemingly stems from an understanding that the government needs assistance to meet its core objective: reducing expenditure by sharing the burden of ill-health.

Consistent with previous strategies, within *Healthy Ireland*, devolving responsibility for health was gradually promoted, not so much as a means of relinquishing power but rather by securing buy-in to government ideas. This is particularly evident in statements such as the following: 'Building partnerships wins support for action at grassroots level and contributes to community development' (DoH, 2013: 14), and,

> It is beyond the capability of any one Government Department or organisation to promote society wide health and wellbeing. This can only be done through society-wide involvement in and engagement with health and wellbeing promotion and improvement activities – from individuals making positive lifestyle choices and projects run by community and local groups, to policy and legislative changes at the highest level of government. (*Ibid.*: 7)

This latter quote illustrates how the neoliberal state intends to reinvent itself as a key agent in a network of agents. There is emphasis on decentralising functions, including roles and responsibilities from the state to local government, organisations and the community and voluntary sectors as well as individual citizens. The state, it would seem, is establishing itself as a regulatory state (as opposed to a providing state), providing guidance and support, and downloading 'risk' and the management of risk to others. Furthermore, it intends to support this cooperative form of governance by establishing new working relationships with a wide range of stakeholders from each and every sector of society: 'from business, enterprise, academia, media, professional bodies, philanthropic organisations, community and voluntary bodies to representative bodies, organised societies, associations, foundations, community fora and individuals' (*ibid.*: 21).

The government expresses its decision to devolve responsibility and expand its control over other sectors via a narrative of cooperative and collaborative action: 'A core aspect of solidarity is that populations share the benefits, risks and burdens of public health policy' (DoH, 2013: 51). The justification for the dispersal is couched in a rhetoric of mutual gain, thus, 'Identifying partners at every level of society, from government to business, to community and family will contribute to the implementation of mutually beneficial health and wellbeing programmes' (*ibid.*: 14). Growth remains important but there is an understanding that it cannot be achieved alone or by working against one another. Responsibility for health is to be shared and 'balanced between the State, private sector and employers, communities, families and individuals' (*ibid.*: 21).

Indeed, the document makes it clear that it still retains the power to 'review and update public health laws and instruments', 'review regulation, enforcement, licensing, accreditation and quality control' (*ibid.*: 27) and that 'A balance will need to be struck between clear national leadership and accountability mechanisms and autonomy at the local level for innovation and advancement' (*ibid.*: 26). And so, the traditional role of the state as a 'heavy handed' provider of care has been dissolved and a new mode of governance has emerged in its place; a mode in which the state has expanded its range of influence and concern by developing ever-more complex, networked relations across different terrains. In one respect, this broad-stroke approach creates subjectivities by leaving room for other partners to decide how to intervene in promoting and improving health at the population level. However, there is no recognition that the interests of these various stakeholders might ever be in conflict.

Capabilities and techniques to manage the self

In contemporary Western neoliberal societies, the individual is valued and prized as autonomous, capable, self-serving and in control of his or her life. This stance constructs health problems and solutions as lying within the individual's control, thereby aligning personal and political objectives, and has appeared with increasing regularity in public health policies across the industrialised world, including Ireland.

Within *Shaping a Healthier Future* population health gains were to be achieved by delegating power and responsibility to those further down the bureaucratic ladder both within the health sector and also across the public sector: 'Hospitals, general practitioners and other community services should operate as elements of an integrated system within which patients can move freely as their needs dictate' (DoH, 1994: 26). Individual citizens were also to be encouraged 'to take responsibility for their own health' and given information to improve their 'skills relating to making healthy choices in lifestyle' in six key areas: smoking, alcohol, nutrition and diet, cholesterol and blood pressure, exercise and causes of accidents (DoHC, 2001: 48). Together, these priorities marked the beginning of an era that would see the expansion of the health service as 'it strives for solidarity and equity in health, and the participation and accountability of individuals, groups, institutions, and communities for continued health development' (DoH, 1994: 8). The emphasis on greater primary care and preventive health services, as well as individual responsibility for health, reflected a trend to account for the 'themes and targets' of the WHO 'Health for all' programme. At that time, governments the world over were actively pursuing the objective that all people of the world would attain a level of health that would allow them to lead economically and socially productive lives by the year 2000 (WHO, 1981). A core objective of this strategy was the promotion of healthy lifestyles, which was operationalised in targets 13 to 17 (see *Targets for Health for All*; WHO Regional Office for Europe, 1985).

Individual responsibility for health encapsulates Foucault's concept of self-governing ethics (or technology of self-governance). The implication is that coercion, intimidation and punishment are not necessary as individuals are rational beings and, with the right support, every individual can be an Adam Smith in the making, capable of self-governing their own health to the point of maximum benefit for one and for all (Newman, 2003, 2006). In this regard, the neoliberal agent is free to make decisions about his or her health, although this only stands true insofar as being able to use the correct actions for self-improvement, or what Foucault calls 'technologies of the self'. Thus, it is technologies of the self that come to define and differentiate the healthy subject from the unhealthy subject. In a disciplinary world, a healthy self requires intensified notions of self-awareness and of conceptualisations as to one's identity (that is, one's 'sense of self'). Healthy subjects are able to demonstrate the agency, care, discipline and responsibility needed to look after their own health, and also have the capacity to govern other individuals in line with governmental expectations or rationalities. And, in the contemporary world, a perpetual focus on the care of the body, of mind and above all of 'self', have become de rigueur with ideas of personal identity and health dominating over notions of social welfare (HM Government, 2010; Michailakis and Schirmer, 2010; Wilson, 2014). The implication is that individuals should be responsible for their own health. This conceptualisation of responsibility dovetails neatly with other emerging market-driven ideas of health behaviour such as those encompassed in ideas about 'nudging' – influencing another's behaviour in subtle ways that do not affect his or her freedom of choice (Thaler and Sustein, 2009). However, this new governance requires much work as people can contest the rationality; indeed, quite often, it fails to produce the aspired subject, as exemplified by the rising obesity epidemic.

In *Quality and Fairness*, the dominant 'regime of truth' extended this political rationality by outwardly constructing health and concomitant ill-health as a consequence of lifestyles choices (DoHC, 2001). As a result, there is an understanding that if health is to improve, individuals must learn to look after themselves better, since their behaviour (particularly that of men) puts them at increased risk of premature mortality, which is

largely 'preventable' (DoHC, 2001: 154). The document sells the need for
individuals to become accountable for their health in two ways: first by
suggesting that individuals have a responsibility to look after themselves,
through the statement, 'Personal and community health is the responsibility not only of government and other providers of healthcare but also of
individuals and communities' (ibid.: 67); and second by stating 'that the
system does not have the capacity to meet the current demands being placed
on it' (ibid.: 79). In such ways, 'risk' is transferred from the state onto its
subjects (Beck, 2000).

In the context of public health a basic premise of this neoliberal approach
is that it is beyond both the capacity and the remit of the state to manage
the health status of individuals. Consequently, the state seeks to empower
individuals (via the provision of information and 'choice') to take control
of their health and manage their own health risks: 'A health system that
supports and empowers you, your family and community to achieve your
full health potential' (DoHC, 2001: 8). This increasing representation of
the citizen as a rational, utility-maximising being prescribes a cogent argument that only the self-governing agent has the power, freedom and skills
to procure health (see Rose, 1999, 2000; Rose and Miller, 2010; Rose,
O'Malley and Valverde, 2006).

To improve individual responsibility, there are efforts to provide the
correct information to individuals: '[t]he health system must focus on providing individuals with the information and support they need to make
informed health choices' (DoHC, 2001: 16). There is an assumption that
the provision of information will help individuals behave rationally: 'consumers need access to high quality information on health to fully benefit
from health and social systems and to participate in decisions relating to
their health; readily available information is seen as underpinning self-help
and informed choice' (ibid.: 18). The use and dissemination of information
under the guise of 'knowledge' is, as we have already suggested, a hallmark
of a neoliberal form of governance. It informs people of how they ought to
live – what is normal, acceptable and appropriate behaviour – without fear
of reprisal. Its intention is to produce and reproduce individuals as engaged,
responsible citizens with the agency and capabilities to behave as expected,
to realise their obligations and to take proactive action that benefits their
health.

The increased role for individuals thus reflects an extension of the hand
of the state who views the individual as an autonomous subcontractor, and
seeks his or her approval and help in attaining its prescribed recipe for
health. On the one hand, this suggests that individuals, as active participants in regulation, have the power to improve their health and the health
of those around them. It also recognises that individuals have agency to
pursue valuable goals and implies that people ought to have the freedom
to behave in ways they see fit. Thus, not only does this stance blame

individuals for the status of their health, poor or otherwise, but it saddles them with 'greater control' and 'greater responsibility' for taking action to improve and manage their 'own health' (DoHC, 2001: 18). However, as we have demonstrated earlier in the chapter, the government retains power to intervene when these choices are deemed counterproductive. In other words, the government is able to exploit agency to ensure deference to economically and politically defined objectives, rather than advancing true collective freedoms that enable individuals to pursue the ambitions they have reason to value. Furthermore, such technologies of 'managing the self' assume that everyone has access to the same resources and so fail to consider the material and social contexts that influence the choices available to people and the decisions they in turn come to make. It also assumes that individuals want to make these changes and have the skills, opportunities and resources to do so, which may not be the case. In short, by emphasising the individual and ensuring that responsibility for improving health rests with the person, wider macro social structures and processes are ignored (see Rose, O'Malley and Valverde, 2006; Thaler and Sustein, 2009).

This dominant political rationality of responsibility continues to underpin *Healthy Ireland* where there continues to be a heavy emphasis on personal risk and responsibility: '[m]any health and wellbeing indicators are affected by individuals' personal lifestyle choices' (DoH, 2013). A central plank of neoliberal healthcare reform supports the idea that 'health' (and therefore ill-health) is primarily a matter of personal responsibility, of, say, needless tobacco consumption more than of air pollution; of self-indulgence rather than reckless marketing of industrialised food and alcohol products; of personal indolence rather than poorly planned and designed transport systems and urban spaces.

As argued, this approach reflects an intention to expand power, governmentality and governance beyond a focus on the plight of specific population groups (such as those with chronic diseases), to a focus on the health of the whole person and whole populations. The implication of this approach is that individuals are perceived to be deficient in health (a person's actual health is falling short of its potential), and until this is remedied, they cannot fully partake as a valued member of civilised society. It is thus crucial that individuals take affirmative action and realign health with that of the imagined mainstream (Raco, 2009), particularly given that '[t]he effects of these risk factors can be minimised if individuals can be motivated and supported to make healthier choices' (DoH, 2013: 14).

As with its predecessor, part of the solution will involve 'informing people and communities about how to improve their health and wellbeing and empowering and motivating them to do so, whilst working to remove or at least minimise any legislative or practical barriers that impede their ability to make healthy choices' (DoH, 2013: 14). Consistent with a technocratic approach to health, individuals are to become 'experts' of their own health. In this regard, ill-health is no longer viewed as the government's responsibility as they have provided individuals with the information and knowledge that they need to remedy their situation. In this view, the role of the state, as with the market, is to serve only as an invisible hand supporting and guiding free and aspirational agents (Raco, 2009). Thus, while there is ample rhetoric in the document about the social determinants of health, actions to improve health target the individual and his or her lifestyle choices.

What we see in *Healthy Ireland* then is the conflation of globalised neoliberal economic forces as well as social forces. Economic crises and declining state revenues require stringency, whilst the style of governance demands a downloading of risk and responsibility onto various agents, and most importantly, the 'individual'. Given information, evidence and choice, the individual can adapt his or her behaviour to ensure health for all. So unlike sovereign power which is observable, direct and open to resistance, the disciplinary society exerts its power indirectly through knowledge, surveillance and an invisible gaze (Foucault, 2009).

Conclusion

Using multiple examples from three strategic public health policy documents – *Shaping a Healthier Future* (DoH, 1994), *Quality and Fairness – A Health Service for You* (DoHC, 2001) and *Healthy Ireland* (DoH, 2013) – we have used the concept of neoliberal governmentality to understand how different strategic health policies configure responsibility for health and render its subjects governable in the neoliberal era.

In undertaking our brief review we have shown that all three of our chosen policy documents developed and expressed a form of political rationality wherein individual subjectivities are aligned to neoliberal values via the use of ideas such as accountability, autonomy, choice, ownership and responsibility. It was also evident that market values and actuarial tools have been fully integrated into public health policy so that the 'field' is regarded very much like a business with clients, consumers, league tables, performance management systems and quality control mechanisms. In this respect, health, firmly entrenched in a neoliberal model, is yet just another 'good' or service, available in the marketplace to those who have the money and the capability to choose one service from another. Yet, it is also clear that this approach to strategic health policy has downsides given that each document reports evidence of ever-widening health inequalities. Indeed, according to recent figures, Ireland has the third highest infant mortality rate and Irish people have one of the lowest life expectancies compared to other EU member states (McDaid *et al.*, 2009).

Broadly speaking, Ireland is indeed moving closer to Boston than Berlin (see Schäffer, 2009), and it is principles of efficiency and effectiveness that guide public health policy rather than overt political values. What we see is the emergence of a technocratic approach to health in which 'experts' can apparently solve all problems (except growing inequality). These efforts to depoliticise policy underpin an ethic of simply supporting whatever 'works' (Parsons, 2002; Pawson, 2006). Yet assessments of what 'works' are never entirely objective (Head, 2008), and therefore never apolitical; what 'works' for whom, for how long, under what conditions, at what cost and with what unintended consequences?

Over the years, successive Irish governments have endeavoured to stream-line and improve the 'effectiveness' and 'efficiency' of healthcare services while simultaneously reducing the cost of public health spending. As the tax-base of the modern state increasingly moves beyond its control (to international outposts) it is also increasingly forced to do 'more' with 'less'. One strategy for achieving this is to off-load duty and responsibility on to its subjects. In a neoliberal age this means that care of the self increasingly comes to be seen as a matter for 'us' rather than 'them', with all that that implies for personal behaviour and political action.

We have shown how the neoliberal state is reinventing itself as a key agent in a network of agents. It is establishing itself as a regulatory state rather than a providing state, downloading 'risk' and the management of risk to others (Newman, 2006). The impact of this on the welfare state, and on the health services in particular, is a constant sharing of 'responsibility'; a constant call for 'partnership'; and a constant claim that matters of health are matters for 'all', matters for 'us', and matters for 'everyone', together. These calls manifest themselves in a number of ways. First, there is a dispersal of centres of governance – institutes, 'agencies' and commissioned providers multiply in place of a monolithic centre (such as a 'Ministry'). Second, there is a dispersal of duty such that individuals in particular are re-created as rational, utility maximising actors who, given the correct information and evidence, can be motivated or even nudged towards being 'healthy'. Third, there is an emphasis on regulation and monitoring and a consequent focus on service 'outcomes' rather than inputs (especially financial inputs).

The argument that the role of the state is to be 'hollowed out' rests on the belief that people are self-interested and motivated to behave in their own best interests (Newman, 2006; Wilson, 2014). In particular, we have highlighted how the traditional role of the state as a 'heavy handed' provider of care has slowly dissolved and a new mode of governance has emerged in its place; a mode in which the state has expanded its range of influence and concern by developing ever-more complex, networked relations across different terrains through which it outsources some of its responsibilities to other organisations beyond the health sector (including

NGOs) and individual citizens. Thus, contrary to popular belief, these changes are not indicative of an attempt or intention to reduce power and government.

As demonstrated, Irish health policy has reflected most if not all of these characteristics, although in the context of a system that has evolved through a unique blend of public, private and charitable financing and provision. In many ways this is unsurprising given that health policy these days is globalised via agencies, such as the WHO, and the modern state tends merely to adapt global health policy templates and guidelines to local conditions. Thus, the WHO Alma Ata Declaration of 1978, presaging the emphasis on primary rather than secondary healthcare, and the Ottawa Declaration of 1986, with its emphasis on enabling, informing and promoting, as well as the related and repeated calls for 'health in all' and 'health for all', have left clear and easily recognisable traces in Irish health policy documentation (and the 'for all' tag has been explicitly used to entitle a number of health policies in Northern Ireland). In like manner, many national guidelines on diet, exercise, mental health and so forth are usually little more than adaptations of global WHO recommendations. The contents of *Healthy Ireland: A Framework for Improved Health and Wellbeing* stands as a testament to these claims (DoH, 2013). Perhaps most interestingly, in this mixed economy, provision of public health is seen neither as the sole responsibility of government nor of the individual, but rather as a matter for 'all' and 'everyone'. In such ways it is not only responsibility for healthcare that is dispersed across a range of agents, but also the task of identifying health risk and devising strategies for managing such risk, as we have demonstrated.

References

Alwan, A., MacLean, D.R., Riley, L.M., D'Espaignet, E., Mathers, C.D., Steven. A.G. and Bettcher, D. (2010) Monitoring and surveillance of chronic non-communicable diseases: progress and capacity in high-burden countries. *The Lancet*, 376(9755): 1861–1868.

Bacchi, C. (2012) Introducing the 'What's the problem represented to be?' approach. IN: Bletsas, A. and Beasley, C. (eds) *Engaging with Carol Bacchi. Strategic Interventions and Exchanges*. Adelaide, University of Adelaide Press: pp. 21–24.

Barcelos, C.A. (2013) Producing (potentially) pregnant teen bodies: biopower and adolescent pregnancy in the USA. *Critical Public Health*, 24(4): 476–488.

Beck, U. (2000) *Risk Society: Towards a New Modernity*. London, Sage.

Bourdieu, P. (2003) *Language and Symbolic Power*. Cambridge, MA, Havard University Press.

Central Statistics Office (2012) Seasonally adjusted standardised unemployment rates (SUR). Available from: cso.ie/en/statistics/labourmarket/principalstatistics/seasonallyadjustedstandardisedunemploymentratessur/. Accessed 23 February 2016.

Central Statistics Office (2013) Measuring Ireland's progress. Available from: cso.ie/en/releasesandpublications/ep/p-mip/measuringirelandsprogress2012/introduction/#.UwRwDGJ_vTo. Accessed 23 February 2016.

Collins, H. and Pinch, T. (1993). *The Golem. What Everyone Should Know about Science*. Cambridge, Cambridge University Press.

Commission of the European Communities (2007) White paper. Together for health: a stategic approach for the EU 2008–2013. Available from: ec.europa.eu/health/ph_overview/Documents/strategy_wp_en.pdf. Accessed 23 February 2016.

Cowman, S. (1996) View from Ireland. *Quality in Health Care*, 5: 6062.

DoH (1994) *Shaping a Healthier Future. A Strategy for Effective Healthcare in the 1990s*. Dublin, The Stationery Office.

DoH (2004) *Choosing Health: Making Healthy Choices Easier*. London, The Stationery Office.

DoH (2013) *Healthy Ireland: A Framework for Improved Health and Well-being 2013–2025*. DoH, Dublin. Available from: dohc.ie/publications/pdf/HealthyIrelandBrochureWA2.pdf?direct=1. Accessed 23 February 2016.

DoHC (2001) *Quality and Fairness: A Health System for You. Health Strategy*. Dublin, DoHC. Available from: dohc.ie/publications/pdf/strategy.pdf?direct=1. Accessed 23 February 2016.

DoHC (2008) *The Minister's Foreword to, Tackling Chronic Disease. A Policy Framework for Managing Chronic Disease*. Available from: dohc.ie/publications/tackling_chronic_diease.html. Accessed 23 February 2016.

European Commission (2014) *Economic Adjustment Programme for Ireland*. Available from: ec.europa.eu/economy_finance/assistance_eu_ms/ireland/index_en.htm. Accessed 23 February 2016.

Foucault, M. (2009) *Security, Territory, Population: Lectures at the Collège de France, 1977–78*. Ed. M. Senellart. Trans. G. Burchell. Basingstoke, Palgrave Macmillan.

Gallagher, A. (2012) Neoliberal governmentality and respatialisation of childcare in Ireland. *Geoforum*, 43: 464–471.

Hajer, M.A. (1993) Discourse coalitions and the institutionalization of practice: the case of acid rain in Britain. IN: Fischer, F. and Forester, J. (eds) *The Argumentative Turn in Policy Analysis and Planning*. London, Duke University Press: pp. 43–76.

Head, B.W. (2008) Three lenses of evidence-based policy. *Australian Journal of Public Administration*, 67(1): 1–11.

HM Government (2010) *Healthy Lives, Healthy People: Our Strategy for Public Health in England*. London, The Stationery Office.

Jennings, S. (2014) *Preventing Chronic Disease: Defining the Problem. Report from the Prevention of Chronic Disease Programme*. Dublin, HSE.

Lalonde M. (1974) *A New Perspective on the Health of Canadians: A Working Document*. Ottawa, Government of Canada. Available from: phac-aspc.gc.ca/ph-sp/pdf/perspect-eng.pdf. Accessed 23 February 2016.

Lee, I.-M., Shiroma, E.J., Lobelo, F., Puska, P., Blair, S.N. and Katzmarzyk, P.T. (2012) Impact of physical inactivity on the world's major non-communicable diseases. *The Lancet*, 380 (9838): 219–229.

Lemke, T. (2002). Foucault, governmentality, and critique. *Rethinking Marxism: A Journal of Economics, Culture & Society*, 14(3): 49–64.

Lemke, T. (2007) An indigestible meal? Foucault, governmentality, and state theory. *Distinktion: Scandinavian Journal of Social Theory*, 8(2): 43–64.

Marmot, M. and Wilkinson, R. (eds) (2005) *Social Determinants of Health* (second edition). Oxford, Oxford University Press.

McDaid, D., Wiley, M., Maresso, A. and Mossialos, E. (2009) Ireland: health system review. *Health Systems in Transition*, 11(2): 1–268.

Michailakis, D. and Schirmer, W. (2010) Agents of their health? How the Swedish welfare state introduces expectations of individual responsibility. *Sociology of Health & Illness*, 32(6): 930–947.

Newman, J. (2003) *Modernising Governance: New Labour, Policy and Society*. London, Sage.

Newman, J. (2006) Modernisation and dynamics of welfare governance. *Zeitschrift für Sozialreform*, 52(2): 165–179. Available from: oro.open.ac.uk/17473/2/Newman_06_zeitschrift.pdf. Accessed 23 February 2016.

Newman. J. and Vidler. E. (2006) Discriminating customers, responsible patients, empowered users: consumerism and the modernisation of health care. *Journal of Social Policy*, 35(2): 193–210.

O'Donnell, R. (1998) Ireland's economic transformation: industrial policy, European integration and social partnership. Working paper no. 2. University of Pittsburgh, Center for West European Studies European Union Center. Available from: aei.pitt.edu/27/1/Odonnell.pdf. Accessed 23 February 2016.

OECD (2016) *Better Life Index*. www.oecdbetterlifeindex.org/countries/ireland/. Accessed 1 September 2015.

Parsons, W. (2002) From muddling through to muddling up – evidence based policy making and the modernisation of British government. *Public Policy and Administration*, 17(3): 43–60.

Pawson, R. (2006) *Evidence-based Policy: A Realist Perspective*. London, Sage.

Peedell, C. (2009) Global neoliberalism and the consequences for healthcare policy in the English NHS. IN: Lister, J. (ed.) *Europe's Health for Sale. The Heavy Cost of Privatisation*. Faringdon, Libri: pp. 107–118.

Powell, D. (2014) Childhood obesity, corporate philanthropy and the creeping privatisation of health education. *Critical Public Health*, 24(2): 226–238.

Prince, R., Kearns, R. and Craig, D. (2006) Governmentality, discourse and space in the New Zealand health care system 1991–2003. *Health & Place*, 12: 253–266.

Public Health England (2014) *Global Health Strategy 2014 to 2019*. London, Public Health England.

Raco, M. (2009) From expectations to aspirations: State modernisation, urban policy, and the existential policies of welfare in the UK. *Political Geography*, 28: 436–454.

Resnik, D.B. (2007) Responsibility for health: personal, social and environmental. *Journal of Medical Ethics*, 33(8): 444–445.

Roe, E. (1994) *Narrative Policy Analysis, Theory and Practice*. Durham NC, Duke University Press.

Rose, N. (1999) *Powers of Freedom: Reframing Political Thought*. Cambridge, Cambridge University Press.

Rose, N. (2000) Government and control. *British Journal of Criminology*, 40(2): 321–339.

Rose, N. and Miller, P. (2010) Political power beyond the state: problematics of government. *British Journal of Sociology*, 61(S1): 271–303 (reprint of paper 1992).

Rose, N., O'Malley, P. and Valverde, M. (2006) Governmentality. *Annual Review of Law and Society*, 2: 83–104

Schäffer, M. (2009) The Irish welfare state: closer to Boston than Berlin? *Socheolas, Limerick Student Journal of Sociology*, 1(1): 106–123.

Thaler, R.H. and Sustein, C.R. (2009) *Nudge: Improving Decisions about Health and Happiness*. London, Penguin.

Van Houdt, F. and Schinkel, W. (2013) Crime, citizenship and community: neoliberal communitarian images of governmentality. *The Sociological Review*, 62(1): 47–67.

Voigt, K. (2013) Appeals to individual responsibility for health: reconsidering the luck egalitarian perspective. *Cambridge Quarterly of Healthcare Ethics*, 22(2): 146–158.

WHO (1981) *Global Strategy for Health for all by the Year 2000*. Geneva, WHO.

WHO (1986) *The Ottowa Charter for Health Promotion*. Available from: who.int/healthpromotion/conferences/previous/ottawa/en/. Accessed 23 February 2016.

WHO (2013) *Global Action Plan for the Prevention and Control of Non-communicable Diseases 2013–2020*. Geneva, WHO.

WHO Regional Office for Europe (1985) *Targets for Health for All. Targets in Support of the European Regional Strategy for Health for All*. Copenhagen, WHO Regional Office for Europe.

Wilson, J. (2014) *Understandings of Well-being in Public Health Policy*, PhD Thesis, The Queen's University of Belfast.

9 Cliona Loughnane

Governing healthcare: the case of Universal Health Insurance – by competition

Introduction

One of the defining features of the Irish health system, since the establishment of Voluntary Health Insurance (VHI) in the 1950s, has been a heavy reliance by those who can afford it on private health insurance. Thus the Irish health system, which is three quarters funded by taxation (Wren, Connolly and Cunningham, 2015), is a strange mix of a national health system with high levels of private insurance cover (with up to 50% of the population holding insurance). In 2011, the newly formed Fine Gael / Labour Government, signalled its intention to develop Universal Health Insurance, which would require everyone to hold health insurance:

> This Government is the first in the history of the State that is committed to developing a universal, single-tier health service, which guarantees access to medical care based on need, not income. By reforming our model of delivering healthcare, so that more care is delivered in the community, and by reforming how we pay for healthcare through Universal Health Insurance, we can reduce the cost of achieving the best health outcomes for our citizens, and end the unfair, unequal and inefficient two-tier health system. (Government of Ireland, 2011: 32)

This self-styled 'radical' (Fine Gael, 2011: 3) departure was anticipated to be 'the most comprehensive reform of Irish healthcare since the establishment of the State' (DoH, 2012: 6). The model proposed was Universal Health Insurance (UHI) provided by public and private insurers through managed competition (Government of Ireland, 2011). Universal Health Insurance by Competition (referred to as UHI-by Competition, or UHI-C here) was articulated in a number of policy documents (Fine Gael, 2011; Government of Ireland, 2011; DoH, 2012, 2013a, 2013b, 2014a, 2014b (the UHI-C documents)).

UHI-C represents a particular moment in Irish health policymaking. A number of delays, primarily the result of the costs of the system, means it is increasingly unlikely that UHI-C will ever be implemented. Without UHI-C implemented in practice, this chapter uses existing policy documents to critique the proposal as an example of the rationality and technology of advanced liberal government developed by Nikolas Rose and Peter Miller (Rose, 1996, 2000, 2001; and Rose and Miller 2010).

The 2011 Programme for Government had promised that UHI-C would begin to be rolled out in 2016 and be fully implemented by 2019. In July 2014, a cabinet reshuffle saw UHI-C's chief proponent, Minister of Health James Reilly, move to the Department of Children and Youth Affairs (DCYA). Almost immediately, his successor in the health portfolio, Minister Leo Varadkar, began to stretch the likely implementation timetable. By 2015, Minister Varadkar indicated that UHI-C could not be in place before a third term of government – a ten-year delay on the initial Programme for Government commitment (Varadkar, 2015). The reasons for the delay centred around emerging evidence on the likely cost of the UHI-C system, both to the state and to individuals (in the form of mandatory UHI-C premiums). While concerns had consistently been expressed about the cost of UHI-C from a number of quarters, it was the 2015 publication of a Department of Health (DoH)-commissioned report, 'An Examination of the Potential Costs of Universal Health Insurance in Ireland' (Wren, Connolly and Cunningham, 2015) which left the implementation of UHI-C in severe doubt. The economic analysis found that UHI-C would increase overall Irish healthcare expenditure by up to 11%, with the primary driver of the increase being the margins which would be earned by competing insurance companies. Until these government-commissioned figures emerged, exposing the cost to the state and citizens, and the monetary benefit to private health insurers, UHI-C had appeared to be a 'win-win' for Fine Gael, by enabling 'the party to promise what no government had done before – universal healthcare for all – as well as maintaining and increasing the profits of private health insurance companies' (Burke, 2015). The General Election in 2016, which removed the Fine Gael / Labour Government, signalled the final death knell for the policy. Whether UHI-C is ultimately implemented or not, the process around the articulation of a new model for the Irish health system is important as it exposes key rationalities of current government thinking about health policy, particularly an increasing reliance on private provision and individuals taking responsibility for their own health 'risks'.

UHI-C represents both an emerging discourse for governing healthcare and a governmental technology-in-development. Drawing on the concept of governmentality, this chapter seeks to attend to the patterns of thought (mentalities of rule and regimes of practice) which underlie how governing takes place (Bacchi, 2009). A reliance on individual autonomy through 'choice, personal responsibility, control over one's own fate, self-promotion and self-government' (Rose, 2000: 329) is characteristic of advanced liberal government. Advanced liberal governments seek to 'govern without governing *society*, to govern through regulated choices made by discrete and autonomous actors' (Rose, 1996: 328; emphasis original). The problems of advanced liberal government can be analysed in terms of their political rationalities – the discursive field to exercise power *and* their governmental technologies – their programmes and their techniques which give effect to governing (Rose and Miller, 2010). Dean (1999) outlines how regimes of practice can be identified in the fields of visibility of government – shedding light on certain governmental intentions and rationalities, whilst concealing others. With regard to UHI-C, the field of visibility of government shone a bright light on *health insurance* and darkened the spectre of *privatisation in healthcare*.

This discussion will bring attention to a specific policy in which the 'activity of governing is problematised' (McKee, 2009: 478). Problematisations in policies are 'central to governing process' (Bacchi, 2009: xii). Problem representations in policies simplify the problem, emphasising some aspects and silencing others. In this way, we can see that problematisations represented in policies are 'powerful yet contingent' (Bacchi, 2012: 7) ways in which to see the world. This analysis seeks to examine the 'problem' UHI-C was thought to solve, the policy problems which were silenced as a result and the likely effects of this policy approach. The shift to market principles in advanced liberal government has shifted the nature of government in social policy. The functions of health systems have been re-problematised through economic discourses which emphasise individual rights and responsibilities and the need to ration care in order to make the most of the healthcare system for all (Joyce, 2001). While once government may have sought to compensate for the operation of the market, now it seeks to redefine the social arena on market principles (Veitch, 2010). It will be argued that UHI-C emphasised the lack of health insurance amongst all the population and the lack of market efficiency in healthcare as the 'problem' of the Irish health system. In this way the policy obscured the lack of equal access to quality healthcare for all citizens and the health inequities between citizens.

This chapter continues with a discussion of how the trajectory of health policy in Ireland enabled the imagining of UHI-C. The UHI-C documents will then be examined in terms of four elements of governing in an advanced liberal state: seeking to govern at a distance; placing responsibility on individuals through choice; the management of risk; and the fragmentation of the social sphere into multiple communities. The analysis will suggest that the outcome of UHI-C was likely to mean increased responsibility for citizens for their own healthcare needs and a consolidation of private enterprise in the Irish health system.

Irish health policy and the development of UHI-C

The development of the Irish health system has followed an ad hoc, resources-allowing model (Considine and Dukelow, 2011), leading some to suggest that what was missing was 'a basic plan of what is to be created in the first place' (Murphy-Lawless and Quin, 2004: 139). The incrementalist nature of development enabled the state to operate 'its political ideologies silently by concealment of its true goals and purposes' (Lynch, 2010: 11), making it problematic to untangle the organising principles or the rationale behind health entitlements. The anomalous Irish health system has historically combined elements of a national health system, such as centrally funded basic hospital care since 1953, with high levels of private health insurance since the establishment of the VHI scheme in 1956 (Considine and Dukelow, 2009). Since the establishment of VHI, citizens have been encouraged by the state to take out private insurance through generous tax-breaks.

The hidden dimensions of welfare (who provides and who pays) are particularly salient in Irish healthcare policy where state-sponsored private health (through subsidies for health insurance and the use of public hospital beds by private patients) led to the provision of solidarity for the Private Health Insurance (PHI)-holding middle classes (see McDonnell and O'Donovan, 2009, and Wren, 2003). In 2014, almost 45% of the population held PHI; 40% were covered by a medical card and entitled to free GP care and free public hospital care; almost 3% to a GP visit card to free GP care; while the remainder had access to public hospital care (DoH, 2014a). McDonnell and O'Donovan (2009) have demonstrated how a myth of social solidarity was built around PHI by generations of Irish politicians. PHI – with its 'community rating' payment structure (Health Insurance Authority, 2016) – was constructed as a proxy form of social health insurance carried by responsible citizens. This PHI myth obscured the fact that all citizens were already entitled to hospital care and ignored those who could not afford to hold PHI. The valorisation of PHI in Irish health policy has concealed the fact that the vast majority of spending on healthcare comes from public sources – up to four fifths from taxation, with the remainder from a 50/50 split of out-of-pocket charges and health insurance. In total, PHI covers only 12% of health costs (DoH, 2014a).

The entrenchment of the public–private healthcare mix since the 1980s led to decades of patient complaints and care scandals based on the privileged access to care for private patients in public hospitals (Considine and Dukelow, 2009). Given the level of public ferment about healthcare provision, while languishing in political opposition for the best part of two decades, Fine Gael and Labour separately developed plans for universal access to healthcare. As early as 2000, Fine Gael, drawing on NHS market-style reform, proposed a UHI system to cover hospital care, followed in 2001 by a Labour Party election pledge of free GP care for all (Wren, 2003).

After long decades of waiting by patients, citizens and many healthcare commentators, in 2011 the newly formed Fine Gael / Labour Government finally committed to develop universal access to healthcare. While the UHI-C proposal was officially heralded as creating 'universality', 'solidarity' and 'fairness' in the Irish health system, many believed that the real impetus was to embed competition in the delivery of healthcare. In Ireland, where the health system is currently primarily funded through general taxation, UHI-C reform would lead to continued reliance on general taxation supported by UHI provided by mainly private companies (DoH, 2014a). Fine Gael (2011: 14) stated that the quality of healthcare would remain 'guaranteed by the State, which still pays for around three-quarters of healthcare costs through taxes'. This approach once again begs the question posed by Wren (2003: 322), speaking of earlier iterations of UHI-C by Fine Gael and Labour: 'But why go this route to equity and assured funding? Why not merely ban private practice in public hospitals and fund equitable public health care through taxation or social insurance, without the intermediary role of the insurance companies?'

The model of UHI-C, with its reliance on managed competition by multiple insurance companies, has been questioned by a number of players in the health sector, including the Adelaide Hospital Society (Thomas, Ryan and Normand, 2010), Amnesty International Ireland (2012) and the Irish Medical Organisation (2010 and 2012), who have all called on government to consider other options for the development of universal healthcare, such as a taxation-funded system, or a social health insurance administered by a single not-for-profit fund. As the Government's 2011–2016 term wore on, members of the public also began to question whether UHI-C was a daring departure or an additional tax for healthcare by another name. As one correspondent wrote to *The Irish Times*,

> It may come as a surprise to the Minister [for Health], but, the population already has a minimum mandatory health insurance policy in place. It's called 'the health service', and is paid for from general taxation. That includes his salary. I'm not sure I want to pay his any more. (Doran, 2014)

Managed competition in healthcare

The concept of 'managed competition' in healthcare was developed by the American economist Alain Enthoven, who declared that the 'problem' of health systems lay in the inefficiencies of their administration and 'the solution lay in reconceiving governmentality in terms of competition between comprehensive health care plans' (Light, 2001a: 1156). The idea behind managed competition, which involves citizens signing up for insurance from competing funds, is to take healthcare out of the political arena, with the invisible hand of the market instead setting priorities and allocating health services appropriately (Light, 2001b). Governments have often treated managed competition as amoral economic policy, without recognising that it is a constructed reality which will benefit some over others (Light, 2001a). Light (2001a: 1163) points to the 'economic myths and sociological realities' of managed competition:

First, 'managed competition' is not taken up in its full coherent version that enables beneficial competition to take place in health care. Rather, its rhetorical themes are taken up as an ideology to legitimate in varying degrees privatization, budget cuts, user fees, two-tier access, a commercial ethos, and the rationalization of services.

Over time, Enthoven's theory of managed competition based on strong regulation to control healthcare providers came to be applied to any cluster of the elements of the theory which suited a particular government and situation (Light, 2001b; Randall and Williams, 2006). In recent times, managed competition (in divergent forms) in Israel, the UK, New Zealand, Canada and the Netherlands has been criticised for creating less control of healthcare quality and more costs for individuals and the state (Gross and Harrison, 2001; Light, 2001a, 2001b; Fougere, 2001; Randall and Williams, 2006; Naderi and Meier, 2010; Rosenau and Lako, 2008; and Turquet, 2012). Despite these difficulties of implementation, managed competition has an 'enduring legacy' (Light, 2001b: 1177). The policy's resilience is likely due to three main attractions for governments: managed competition shows their capacity to introduce private markets into health; it can control costs for the state; and it enables government to shift citizens' dissatisfaction to insurers and providers (Randall and Williams, 2006). The effect of decades of managed competition in health systems across the world has been to reduce governments' healthcare role from provider to commissioners of care and to allow economic concepts of efficiency and costs to supplant the language of care and health in policy documents (Light, 2001b).

UHI-C for Ireland

> Insurance systems differ greatly. They can be a route to equity but how they are implemented is critical. (Wren, 2003: 323)

In Ireland, UHI-C developed from a long history of support for a public–private mix in the health system. In its 2011 *FairCare* document, Fine Gael outlined its vision of UHI as 'the Dutch system of mandatory health insurance, adapted to meet Irish circumstances' (2011: 12). Despite its claim to eliminate the 'unfair and inefficient public/private divide' (*ibid.*: 5), the proposal was based on neoliberal principles of cost savings and the creation of a more competitive insurance market. In keeping with the apparent neutrality of Irish health policy, Fine Gael (*ibid.*: 8) described the approach as 'essentially pragmatic' and 'not bound by ideology or dogma'. The value system behind *FairCare* remained relatively opaque, aside from the slippery concept of 'fairness', a concept which Lynch (2010: 14) has argued is 'built on dubious moral principles, is highly subjective and will be generally interpreted by those in power in their own interests'. Following electoral victory and the forming of a coalition government with Labour in 2011, the Fine Gael-led government published a reworked plan for UHI-C in the Programme for Government (Government of Ireland, 2011). As a government they had inherited an unprecedented economic crisis and a healthcare service reeling from cuts. The UHI-C proposal now promised both reduced costs and 'the best health outcomes for our citizens' (Government of Ireland, 2011: 32).

In its iteration in the Programme for Government (Government of Ireland, 2011: 32) UHI-C was described as 'designed according to the European principle of social solidarity'. Under UHI-C, insurance for a standardised level of care with a public or private insurer would be compulsory and related to ability to pay, with the state subsidising premiums for low- and middle-income earners. Insurers would not be allowed to sell higher-cost insurance, giving faster access to procedures covered by the UHI-C package, but would be able to provide comforting extras, such as single-occupancy rooms. A purchaser–provider split would be established between the insurers and hospitals. Public hospitals would be divided into groups, eventually becoming independent hospital trusts which would compete for care contracts from insurance companies. In seeking to achieve universal access to healthcare, UHI-C represented a new departure for Irish health policy; however, in seeking to provide such access through compulsory insurance in a managed competition process provided by private and not-for-profit companies, Ireland looked set to remain an outlier in European health policy.

UHI-C was being developed during a time of austerity and contraction of public spending. The reform programme made clear that Ireland could not have universal health insurance until 'responsible' health-cost cuts were made: 'by reforming how we pay for healthcare through Universal Health Insurance, we can reduce the cost of achieving the best health outcomes for our citizens' (Government of Ireland, 2011: 32). There was to be 'continued focus on the issue of costs through 2013 and beyond' (DoH, 2013b: 26). UHI-C appeared as a combination of lofty social democratic ideals underpinned by neoliberal efficiency; claims to 'fairness' were always coupled with requirements for 'cost reduction'. Once the health system could be cut into efficiency, the citizen would enjoy universal access fulfilled by at-arms-length insurance companies. As such, UHI-C enabled the ongoing 'framing of public, political and governmental choices through a universalising logic of cost calculation' and the continuation of 'what we can afford policies' (Clarke, 2004: 35).

The publication of the White Paper on UHI-C, which would clearly outline the specifics of the reform programme, was expected throughout 2013. By the start of 2014 it was clear that tensions had emerged between the two government parties and between the DoH and the Department of Public Expenditure and Reform. The tensions – as reported in the media – centred on the cost implications for the state. When the White Paper was finally published in April 2014 (DoH, 2014a) there was an obvious emphasis on cost control to limit the financial obligations of the state. For the first time in a White Paper, government indicated there would be no additional resources for the introduction of UHI-C and that the state would pay no more than it currently did for healthcare: 'total spending by the State on healthcare in Ireland under a single-tier UHI system should not exceed its total spending under the two-tier system which it replaces' (DoH, 2014a: 12). Despite the White Paper's heavy focus on economics and costs for the state, it failed to outline the ultimate price of UHI-C to individuals, and the contentious issue of what exact health services a person would receive as part of their UHI-C coverage.

Advanced liberal governing in UHI-C

In this section the UHI-C documents are considered in relation to the rationality and technology of advanced liberal government developed by Nikolas Rose and Peter Miller (Rose, 1996, 2000, 2001; and Rose and Miller, 2010). With policy documents as the primary source, this analysis examines the political rationalities of UHI-C and seeks to demonstrate the value of policy-questioning (Bacchi, 2009). UHI-C is examined here in relation to four specific rationalities and technologies of the advanced liberal state articulated by Rose (2000: 337):

> Central to these are the revised ambitions of political government, the aspiration to govern 'at a distance', the fragmentation of sociality and subjectivity into communities and identities, the emphasis upon creating active individuals who will take responsibility for their own fates through exercise of choice, and the organization of socio-political concerns around the management and minimization of risks to lifestyles of contentment and consumption. (Emphasis added)

Rose and Miller (2010) identify three elements of political rationalities. First, they have a moral form, naming the proper distribution of actions by different levels of society, familial and political. Second, they have an epistemological drive in articulating a particular concept of society, individuals and all the objects to be governed. Finally, political rationalities operate through an idiom to make the world understandable in a particular way to suit a certain form of governing.

Governing at a distance

In advanced liberal governing, the centre steers the system indirectly (Ferlie, McGivern and FitzGerald, 2012). The government may seem to cede power for implementation, but it strongly retains the framing of policy problems. Rose (2001: 6) identifies this as the 'enabling state, the facilitating state, the state as animator', which articulates the way in which the state seeks to free itself of some responsibilities which are instead pushed onto the citizen. In this way, the 'health-related aspirations and conduct of individuals is governed "at a distance", by shaping the ways they understand and enact their own freedom' (Rose, 2001: 6). Governing is thus concerned 'to structure the possible field of action of others' (Foucault, 1982: 790). Individuals seek to follow the established norms and engage in self-regulation, so that the 'arm of government can rest lightly' (Bacchi, 2009: 29).

Under UHI-C, the Irish state would move from having ultimate responsibility for the provision of healthcare to citizens, to focusing on the development of policy. The role of the state was reconceptualised from provider of healthcare, to be an overseer of quality and competition. Health policy – decided by the Minister – would be implemented by insurance companies and regulated by a number of new state agencies:

> The future model of UHI involves a sea-change in the role of the State. In essence, this change will see the State shift from direct financing and delivery of health services to regulation and oversight of a competitive system of purchasers and providers. Put more succinctly, it will involve a substantial shift from rowing to steering. (DoH, 2014a: 42)

The state would have an oversight role, in the 'highly regulated form of multi-payer UHI' (*ibid.*: 5) and would 'intervene sharply' (DoH, 2013a: 53) in cost overruns. Primarily, the state would be responsible for guaranteeing the UHI-C system through a statutory framework, controlling the costs 'for which central control is most effective' and determining the package of care to be covered by UHI-C (DoH, 2014a: 47). The cost of UHI-C insurance would be 'essentially determined by health insurers when actuarially forecasting claims costs' (*ibid.*: 82). Where once citizens had entitlements to the public healthcare system, disputes between citizens and their insurance companies about the care covered by the UHI-C package would 'ultimately be matters of private contract law' (*ibid.*: 62).

The state's circumscribed role primarily focused on those on low and middle incomes, rather than society as a whole. While in the earlier UHI-C documents the focus was on the state actively subsidising those on low and middle incomes, the 2014 White Paper stated that 'where a person is unable to afford UHI cover, *they may apply* for financial support' (DoH, 2014a: 40; emphasis added). The onus for the state to provide a safety net would shift to individuals seeking supplementation from the National Insurance Fund. For all other citizens, the state would operate at a basic level to monitor health insurers' provision of a 'standard package' of insurance and the operation of community rating.

Public hospitals would be reorganised into competing hospital groups. Hospitals would no longer be managed by state agencies or subject to central budget control, but be 'independent … accountable to their boards'

(Government of Ireland, 2011: 35). Their independence would be tempered by a plethora of new agencies and roles pushing government-led controls outwards into the heart of the health system. New bodies, such as the National Insurance Fund, Patient Safety Agency, Healthcare Commissioning Agency, Healthcare Pricing Office, Finance Reform Board and the Money Follows the Patient Oversight Group would lead the reform process and manage the future health system. Meanwhile, from the Special Delivery Unit, a 'small cadre of experienced managers, clinicians and health economists ... will ... ensure that targets are met, and to act as a source of expertise for healthcare professionals and managers' (Fine Gael, 2011: 20). By insulating the state from citizens' healthcare needs through the use of intermediaries, managed competition – and UHI-C – profoundly reconceptualised the role of the state and power relations in the health system (Light, 2001b). The state would retreat into a policymaking and dispute resolution role, ceding the provision of healthcare to competing insurers and healthcare providers. Less direct government intervention 'does not necessarily entail less governing' (McKee, 2009: 469). Foucault's analysis of neoliberal governmentality demonstrated that the seeming 'retreat of the state' actually represented a transformation of power relations (Lemke, 2002). In the UK, reforms of the NHS seeking to insert managed competition have demonstrated that the state does not 'divest itself of power', instead it uses managed competition to 'establish the market as a mode of organising' (Veitch, 2010: 326). Similarly, by devolving control out into the system, it was anticipated that UHI-C would bring 'increased independence and greater control at local level' (DoH, 2014a: 27).

Responsibility on individuals through choice

The proposal for UHI-C heralded a move from collective health needs to a limited consumer choice approach. Every activity of government presupposes an ideal person, organisation and society to be achieved through governing (Dean, 1999). The vision of UHI-C entailed the imagining of an ideal-type consumer who would identify their own risk, and plan and choose accordingly. This ideal type may conveniently overlap with the generally middle-class, PHI-holding, traditional Fine Gael voter. Choice and patient choice are central to consumerist approaches to healthcare (Nettleton, 2006; Veitch, 2010) which place demands on individuals, rather than endowing them with new rights. Patients are required to act as consumers, so that in making choices they can provide feedback for future patients and for policymakers. The notion of the 'consumer' embodies a different view of the citizen public (Clarke, 2004), with consumers marked out as individual active choice-makers engaged in individualised encounters and interactions.

Rose (2000: 328) identifies that in advanced liberal societies the 'politics of choice and lifestyle' through insurance helps us 'to be our own rock'.

Individuals must live their lives – and make their choices – with prudence and responsibility (Rose, 2001). It is in making these regulated choices that citizens enact their role in society. In UHI-C patient 'choice' was directly equated with a choice of insurance, embodied in the statement that 'The goal is not to take away their insurance, but to give everyone insurance and choice' (Fine Gael, 2011: 15). In advanced liberal societies, freedom is performed through the making of choices by entrepreneurial, independent individuals (Rose and Miller, 2010).

The reliance on the private market and price negotiation was seen as providing benefits to consumers, the state and to insurance companies to 'control costs and encourage innovation in the delivery of care' (Government of Ireland, 2011: 35). It was expected that the provision of healthcare through the private market would enable all citizens to have access to the level of care which was previously only available to those with PHI: 'UHI will provide guaranteed access to care for all in public and private hospitals on the same basis as the privately-insured have now' (Government of Ireland, 2011: 34). An economist's analysis was employed, highlighting a lack of 'appropriate incentives to achieve desired actions/behaviour' (DoH, 2012: 24). UHI-C rested on the perceived private-sector benefits of increased efficiency, innovation, transparency and competition for business. A managerial culture would ensure 'enhanced productivity and efficiency' (DoH, 2014a: 50). The development of a competition/managerial culture in advance of the establishment of UHI-C was expected to be effective in reducing bureaucracy and 'enormous duplication and waste' (Fine Gael, 2011: 7). Quasi-markets would be established in areas not deemed suitable for full privatisation. Public hospitals would no longer be centrally managed and would become 'independent, not-for-profit trusts with managers accountable to their boards' (Government of Ireland, 2011: 55). A purchaser–provider split would be established between the insurance companies and the hospitals. Hospitals would be paid according to the level of care they deliver and be incentivised to deliver more care through a Money Follows the Patient system. UHI-C thus signalled the 'injection of market forces in the name of consumer choice' (Lister, 2010: 49).

Where in the current system all citizens were entitled to centrally funded free hospital care, but many paid for primary-care services, under UHI-C citizens would 'be entitled to obtain healthcare cover from their choice of competing insurer and will be entitled to obtain treatment from their choice of healthcare provider in accordance with the terms of their UHI policy' (DoH, 2014a: 68). Citizen choice was constrained to a 'choice for the consumer in relation to who insures them' (DoH, 2014a: 5) when 'all individuals will enter into private contracts with their choice of multiple health insurers' (*ibid.*: 58). Health insurance was constructed as the socially responsible choice. Insurance would be 'universal and mandatory' (*ibid.*:

42) and 'everyone will have their choice between competing insurers' (*ibid.*: 39). Even this circumscribed 'choice' of insurance provider and treatment location was limited by budgetary concerns, as the state's ability to provide the access, choice and quality that people want 'at a price that they are prepared to pay is a growing challenge' (DoH, 2012: 3). The contract between the state and the citizen would be reduced to a 'health basket' which would determine what people would be entitled to under their UHI-C package. The decision on the composition of the health basket would be 'deeply value-laden' (DoH, 2014a: 8). It was proposed that the health basket and the values underlying it would be refined in consultation with the public and with experts. Participants would be asked a 'set of explicit questions' to 'force deliberation on difficult ethical issues and require hard choices to be made' (DoH, 2014a: 54): Thus, as was stated, 'This explicit approach will be vital to maintaining social solidarity and social protection under the future model of UHI whereby all individuals will enter into private contracts with their choice of multiple health insurers' (DoH, 2014a: 58).

The choice between a range of private and public health insurers in UHI-C is an example of a political responsibility 'transformed into commodified forms and regulated according to market principles' (Rose and Miller, 2010: 296). A reliance on individual choice obscures the fact that the healthcare system is ultimately the outcome of government's political choices (see Veitch, 2010). Further, it makes the limitations on people's choices opaque, implying that we all have equal choices open to us and ignores that in healthcare choices are primarily in the gift of providers, rather than users (O'Donovan and Casey, 1995). In UHI-C, choice represented a divesting of responsibility for care by government – people make their own care choices, the government cannot be blamed for the care which results from that choice. In this way, government could use regulated choices as 'indirect techniques for leading and controlling individuals without at the same time being responsible for them' (Lemke, 2001: 201). The question is whether Irish citizens would be rationally responsive to the market ideals to be imposed on them. 'Choice' is so limited in UHI-C to a choice between insurance products, that it inhibits our ability to question why patients must make choices, and these choices in particular. Why must they act like consumers, allowing their choices to feed the health system? Is choice created primarily as a means of limiting cost (Veitch, 2010)? Through UHI-C Irish citizens were reimagined as consumers and health insurance was contradictorily represented both as mandatory and the exemplar of a socially responsible 'choice'.

Management of risk

UHI-C embodied two forms of the management and minimisation of risk – individual risk which could be controlled through compulsory health insurance, and the risk of cost overruns in the health system which could be controlled by better management and regulation.

Insurance against individual risk

Through UHI-C the state would place a new obligation on citizens to have mandatory health insurance. The problematisation in the UHI-C documents was that people are not insured and the emphasis in the documents is a need for everyone to have access to what was previously the preserve of PHI-holders. The solution was not to ensure everyone has *access to health-care*, rather it was to ensure everyone has *access to insurance*:

> We believe it makes sense to construct a UHI system that acknowledges that 50% of the Irish people already have a relationship with a private insurance company. The goal is not to take away their insurance, but to give everyone insurance and choice. We want to level up the playing field, not level it down. (Fine Gael, 2011: 15)
>
> UHI will provide guaranteed access to care for all in public and private hospitals on the same basis as the privately-insured have now. (Government of Ireland, 2011: 34)

The 'pooling of resources' in the public and private health markets – through the pooling of tax resources in the first instance and through the risk equalisation of insurance rates for the young and old in the PHI market – were both construed as achieving 'a fundamental social solidarity objective, ensuring that the healthier cover the costs of those in need of care' (DoH, 2014a: 75). This understanding ignored the fact that many citizens, who cannot afford PHI, were excluded from sharing in the second 'pool' of resources for PHI-holders only. In the current PHI market collectivisation applies only to consumers who can purchase insurance. Yet, Irish health policy has eulogised PHI as a 'proxy form of social health insurance' (McDonnell and O'Donovan, 2009: 7). This construction of PHI empha-sises the 'caring nature of Irish *people* (solidarity as voluntary action)', while ignoring the role of the *'welfare state* (solidarity as state responsibility)', thereby consistently obscuring the precarious position of those without PHI (McDonnell and O'Donovan, 2009: 18; emphasis original).

The UHI-C documents demonstrated a consistent slippage between the terms 'health system' and 'health insurance system'. At one point, UHI-C was described as representing 'a fundamental change to our *current system of health insurance*' (DoH, 2014a: 41; emphasis added), rather than as a reordering of the *health system*. The decline in the rates of PHI, primarily amongst the younger, less claim-heavy holders, 'has made it even more important that a robust system of universal insurance is introduced as soon as possible' (DoH, 2014b: 6). In UHI-C, PHI anthropomorphised into a living being, or patient. Ireland must maintain a 'healthy and functioning voluntary private health market' (DoH, 2014a: 30). The task was to 'save'

PHI: 'The optimum long term solution is to establish a system where every-one has insurance, thereby ensuring that there are enough young people to help support the market as a whole' (DoH, 2014b: 6). This recourse to an 'insurance for all' solution failed to acknowledge that the reason most people hold PHI is because they don't believe they will receive access to adequate healthcare without it, rather than because of a desire to protect other citizens.

In addition to requiring individuals to insure themselves against risk, UHI-C also placed the responsibility for good health on each individual's shoulders, stating that 'health reform must lead to a healthy Ireland where health and wellbeing is valued by all individuals at every level of society, is embraced by every sector and is everyone's responsibility' (DoH, 2012: 14). Identifying health risks at an individual level is an example of Foucault's 'dividing practices' (Foucault, 1982) which separate individuals into active citizens who can manage their risks responsibly and those who cannot and require intervention (Bacchi, 2009). By minimising their health risks individuals can 'reduce the upward pressure on money' (DoH, 2012: 14). 'Patient empowerment and consumerism' would be 'a welcome develop-ment as it helps people to take more control over, and responsibility for, their health' (DoH, 2012: 2). Doing away with the collective provision of a social state, the advanced liberal rationality promotes a politics of risk and security through private insurance (Rose, 1996 and Rose and Miller, 2010).

Managing risks in the organs of the state through regulation and audit
Through UHI-C government would manage the risks of the health service (primarily constructed in terms of budget overruns) at a distance through the collection of data, new procedures for decision-making and new rela-tions between health-system actors. The reform would be achieved through 'strategic leadership, governance and development framework that ensures that services are delivered cost-effectively, are safe and of high quality and are managed in compliance with the highest standards of governance' (DoH, 2012: 47). The UHI-C model creaked with the burden of managers and experts ready to regulate, manage and audit the healthcare system. Even the Minister for Health would not be excluded from external oversight, with future additions to the 'health basket' (the combination of all of healthcare services, some of which would be funded in the standard UHI-C insurance package and others through taxation) 'subject to the approval of the Minister for Public Expenditure and Reform' (DoH, 2014a: 61).

A new governance system would be created that could give the 'benefits of increased independence and greater control of local clinical and manage-rial leaders to every hospital in Ireland' (DoH, 2012: 34). 'Upgrading the financial capability of managers' would be 'an immediate priority' (*ibid.*: 47). Data would be collected and used to 'reveal' quality (DoH, 2013a: 54).

The system would operate on the basis of a 'Governance Loop' (*ibid.*: 6) supported by 'regulatory building blocks' (DoH, 2014a: 28) to 'safeguard good governance and financial management of health services' (*ibid.*: 45). UHI-C imagined that risk in the health system could be mediated by transforming 'the terms of calculation from medical to financial' (Rose and Miller, 2010: 298). Financial reform would 'ensure that the financing system was based on incentives that are aligned to fairness and efficiency, while reducing costs, improving control and also improving quality' (DoH, 2012: iv). These incentives would be aligned to 'drive continuous performance improvement' (*ibid.*: 1). 'Priority-setting' would be used to distribute 'limited resources between competing demands in order to achieve the best health outcomes in an efficient and sustainable manner' (DoH, 2013b: 37). UHI-C therefore brought about two fundamental changes in the management of risk. The risk-averse state would relinquish its role for society's collective risk. To deal with the risks within – budget overruns and poor management – a maze of controls would be wrapped around the organs of the state. Health risks would be managed individually through private insurance contracts.

Fragmentation of the 'social' state into multiple communities

As discussed earlier, to date Ireland has not achieved universal healthcare provision. Instead of unifying healthcare provision in Ireland, UHI-C heralded a further fragmentation of the public healthcare system into communities of insurance. Rose (1996) tracks the 'mutation' of the state into communities – a limited and reduced version of the social state – in advanced liberal governing. Where the social state encompassed all citizens in an interconnected society built on collective obligations, communities must choose themselves, organise themselves, improve themselves, be responsible for themselves. In UHI-C, the purchasing of insurance would be a new security policy to be undertaken by individuals, mobilising a sense of community (Rose, 1996). Those who 'won't' hold insurance would be outside the newly constructed community of health, transformed from a citizen into a non-insured person.

In UHI-C, the differing and competing needs of the insured–uninsured–privately insured, the young–old and the healthy–less healthy strained against one another. The lines of what it is to be a 'competent citizen' (Rose, 1996: 337) were redrawn. UHI-C marked a changing of the relation of citizens to the health system from the collective to the consumer. The 'burden of health costs' must be 'shared' (DoH, 2013b: 23). Being ill is a drain on the system, to be limited and contained. In the new world of autonomous health insurance holders and competing independent hospital trusts, we could reach a utopia where 'patients will be a source of "income" rather than a "cost", just as they are in private hospitals today' (Fine Gael, 2011:

7). In the binaries of insured–uninsured, healthy–less healthy, the productive, insured, healthy subject who 'labors, in the analysis of wealth and of economics' (Foucault, 1982: 777) is divided from the irresponsible 'other'. The citizen-consumer enables the social space to be reconstructed as a series of individual interactions so that a veil can be drawn over collective need for and consumption of services (Clarke, 2004). The citizen as consumer is championed over the risk-taker who refuses to be morally enterprising and so is 'anti-community' (McDonnell and O'Donovan, 2009: 20). This positing of the poor or sick in terms of their status as 'uninsured persons' (DoH, 2014a: 42) marked out their deficiency as consumers, rather than the failure of the healthcare system (Malone, 1999).

Through UHI-C, the state would pull away from the governmental responsibilities implied in social government. Instead of providing for the healthcare needs of the population, the government instead would play *its part*. Multiple health insurers competing for healthcare business would be a further manifestation of a splintering political space. Government would develop a funding system which 'supports the health service to do its job in caring for our citizens' (DoH, 2013a: 9). The policy anticipated a need to step back from society's growing healthcare needs and proposed a 'shift towards service provision in the community, which includes natural supports (family, friends, etc.) as far as possible' (DoH, 2012: 38). The limited goal of the UHI-C system for society overall would be to 'provide financial protection against catastrophic out of pocket expenditure through universal coverage of the entire population' (DoH, 2014a: 17).

Solidarity was reduced to the administrative rules of the insurance industry, with the social realm reduced to a community of insurance. The 'solidarity' envisaged in UHI-C was not a society supporting its citizens through collective healthcare, rather solidarity was solidarity in insurance terms:

> The two-tier health system undermines SOLIDARITY within society, and encourages duplication and waste by creating two administrative systems. However, any move to abolish peoples' right to health insurance would reduce choice. The fairest solution is to ensure that everyone has health insurance. (Fine Gael, 2011: 8)
>
> The UHI system will be founded on principles of social solidarity, encompassing the fundamental tenets of financial protection, open enrolment, lifetime cover and community rating. (DoH, 2014a: 38)

Solidarity in UHI-C was defined strictly in relation to payment for health services. The 'principles of social solidarity' equated to 'equal access based on need rather than ability to pay' (*ibid.*: 5). The existence of a 'public' option for health insurance was defined as a 'social solidarity measure' (DoH, 2012: 5), implying perhaps that the private insurance companies are not. Social solidarity was also seen to exist in the devolving of the purchasing of care to insurers with controls: 'In line with the fundamental principle of social solidarity, neither insurers nor providers operating within the UHI system will be allowed to sell faster access to services covered by the UHI standard package of care' (DoH, 2014a: 38).

UHI-C was advertised as 'universal' rather than 'mandatory' health insurance, which would achieve 'social solidarity' with cost containment. The policy was carefully built on a semantic value basis of 'solidarity', 'universality' and 'fairness' to solve Ireland's 'problem' of providing health-care while containing costs. This 'values talk' (Giacomini et al., 2004) was employed as a governing device (see Dean, 1999). The term 'Universal Health Insurance' implied citizens would have access to everything, silenc-ing (for the time being at least) the prioritisation and rationing of resources which lay at the heart of its intention to reduce health system costs. The inclusion of the word 'universal' in the 'Universal Health Insurance' acted to insulate the health reform programme from widespread critique. The reaction to the policy was unlikely to be the same if it was called 'Compul-sory Health Insurance' or 'Private Health Insurance for All'.

The values of solidarity, universality, fairness and equity appeared as refrains and litanies in the UHI-C documents with little reflection on their meaning or relative importance (Giacomini et al., 2004). Solidarity 'will underpin all relevant legislation' (Government of Ireland, 2011: 32) and the system would be 'designed according to the European principle of social solidarity: access will be according to need and payment will be according to ability to pay' (Government of Ireland, 2011: 32). As McDonnell and O'Donovan (2009: 6) have demonstrated, the meaning of social solidarity in health has been confused in Ireland, with PHI represented as 'a unique cultural heritage founded on social commitments to community and inter-generational solidarity'. Fine Gael (2011: 8) identified the main problems of the current health system, stating that it 'undermines SOLIDARITY within society and encourages duplication and waste by creating two administrative systems' (emphasis original). However, it is clear that UHI-C was designed primarily to address the perceived inefficiency and politicised nature of healthcare provision in Ireland, rather than to address the lack of solidarity exposed in the unequal access to healthcare for non-PHI holders.

The social state of the Irish public health system then, albeit already fragile, would be fractured in UHI-C into conflicting communities. The insured and the uninsured, the healthy and the unhealthy, would be sepa-rated from one another, with the uninsured and the unhealthy seen as poor consumers and poor managers of their health risks.

Conclusion

This chapter has argued that UHI-C was a rationality and technology of advanced liberal governing, masquerading in claims to social solidarity. When the long-awaited policy offering universal access to healthcare was finally articulated in 2011, it was predicated on market principles and envisaged a role for the state 'at a distance' from citizens' health needs. The trade-offs identified by the DoH (2013b: 46) in the development of a single-tier health system were named as involving 'tensions between efficiency and equity or between comprehensiveness and cost control'. While UHI-C was predicated (linguistically at least) on a 'universal' health system with access for all, it contradictorily tied healthcare delivery more strongly to market processes and controls. The metaphors from economics and business practices within UHI-C came to overwhelm the ill-defined social values of solidarity, universality, fairness and equity. The subjectivity effects of the market talk contained in UHI-C transformed patients into consumers, moving the context of health policy from social obligations and dependence on one another to the contractual obligations of business transactions (Malone, 1999).

The Government claimed that UHI-C would provide 'an efficient and effective single-tier health service which promotes equitable access to high quality care on the basis of need' (DoH, 2014a: 17). My analysis here suggests that the outcome of UHI-C would be increased responsibility for citizens to manage their own healthcare needs as newly imagined citizen-consumers. Further, UHI-C as an example of advanced liberal governing would strengthen the role for private enterprise in the Irish health system. While it now appears unlikely that UHI-C will be implemented, primarily due to economic analysis showing the model is 'cost-inflationary' (Wren et al., 2015: 126), Ireland is not turning volte-face against advanced liberal models of health policy. Instead, the trajectory of health policy remains focused on the injection of competition, privatisation of provision and rationalisation of resources. These intentions are clearly visible in recent policy choices running parallel to UHI-C, including the use of market principles to 'fine' already underfunded hospitals €10,000 for each event of Emergency Department overcrowding and legislation introduced in 2014 which forces all those 35 years and older to immediately take out PHI, or face costly loading of future policies (HSE, 2015). With or without UHI-C, Ireland's healthcare system seems destined to remain a two-tier entanglement of publicly funded healthcare and state-supported PHI.

References

Amnesty International Ireland (2012) Conference report, Guaranteeing the universal in universal healthcare – delivering on the right to health in Ireland. Dublin, Amnesty International Ireland. Available from: www.amnesty.ie/sites/default/files/file/Healthcare%20Guaranteed/Conference%20Report,%20Guaranteeing%20the%20Universal%20in%20Universal%20Healthcare,%202012.pdf. Accessed 21 December 2015.

Bacchi, C. (2009) *Analysing Policy: What's the Problem Represented to Be?* Adelaide, Pearson.

Bacchi, C. (2012) Why study problematizations? Making politics visible. *Open Journal of Political Science*, 2: 1–8.

Burke, S. (2015) Government's health insurance model is a textbook case of flawed policy making. *Irish Independent*, 18 November. www.independent/opinion/comment/governments-health-insuranc-model-is-a-textbook-case-of-flawed-policy-making-34211505.html. Accessed 18 November 2015.

Clarke, J. (2004) Dissolving the public realm? The logics and limits of neo-liberalism. *Social Policy*, 33(1): 27–48.

Considine, M. and Dukelow, F. (2009) *Irish Social Policy A Critical Introduction.* Dublin, Gill and Macmillan.

Considine, M. and Dukelow, F. (2011) Ireland and the impact of the economic crisis: upholding the dominant policy paradigm. IN: Farnsworth, K. and Irving, Z. (eds) *Social Policy in Challenging Times*. Bristol, The Policy Press: pp. 181–198.

Dean, M. (1999) *Governmentality: Power and Rule in Modern Society*. London, Sage.

DoH (2012) *Future Health – A Strategic Framework for Reform of the Health Service 2012–15*. Dublin, The Stationery Office.

DoH (2013a) *Money Follows the Patient – Policy Paper on Hospital Financing*. Dublin, The Stationery Office.

DoH (2013b) *The Path to Universal Healthcare*. Dublin, The Stationery Office.

DoH (2014a) *The Path to Universal Healthcare – White Paper on Universal Health Insurance*. Dublin, The Stationery Office.

DoH (2014b) UHI explained – frequently asked questions on the proposed new model of Universal Health Insurance. http://health.gov.ie/wp-content/uploads/2014a/04/UHI-Explained-.pdf. Accessed 16 April 2014.

Doran, D. (2014) Plan for universal health cover. Letter to the Editor, *The Irish Times*, 25 February. www.irishtimes.com/debate/letters/plan-for-universal-health-cover-1.1703063. Accessed 27 February 2014.

Ferlie, E., McGivern, G. and FitzGerald, L. (2012) A new mode of organizing in health care? Governmentality and managed networks in cancer services in England. *Social Science & Medicine*, 74: 340–347.

Fine Gael (2011) *FairCare*. Dublin, Fine Gael.

Foucault, M. (1982) The subject and power. *Critical Inquiry*, 8(4): 777–795.

Fougere, G. (2001) Transforming health sectors: new logics of organizing in the New Zealand health system. *Social Science & Medicine*, 52: 1233–1242.

Giacomini, M., Hurley, J., Gold, I., Smith, P. and Abelson, J. (2004) The policy analysis of 'values talk': lessons from Canadian health reform. *Health Policy*, 67: 15–24.

Government of Ireland (2011) *Programme for Government 2011–16*. Dublin, The Stationery Office. Available from: www.taoiseach.gov.ie/eng/Work_Of_The_Department/Programme_for_Government/Programme_for_Government_2011–2016.pdf. Accessed 15 December 2015). Document with page numbers available from: www.socialjustice.ie/sites/default/files/attach/policy-issue-article/3292/2011–03–06-programmeforgovernment2011–2016.pdf. Accessed 15 December 2015.

Gross, R. and Harrison, M. (2001) Implementing managed competition in Israel. *Social Science & Medicine*, 52: 1219–1231.

Health Insurance Authority (2016) 'Community rating', www.hia.ie/regulation/community-rating-system. Accessed 23 December 2015.

HSE (2015) 'ED (Emergency Department) Congestion Escalation Directive'. Available from: www.hse.ie/eng/services/news/media/pressrel/newsarchive/archive15/nov15/congestionsscalationdirective.html. Accessed 22 December 2015.

Irish Medical Organisation (2010) *Universal Health Coverage*. Available from: www.imo.ie/policy-international-affair/research-policy/policy-archive/IMOPP-Universal_Health_Coverage.pdf. Accessed 5 May 2012.

Irish Medical Organisation (2012) *The Market Model of Health Care – Caveat Emptor*. Available from: www.imo.ie/news-media/publications/IMO-MARKET-MODEL-paper.pdf. Accessed 26 April 2012.

Joyce, P. (2001) Governmentality and risk: setting priorities in the new NHS. *Sociology of Health & Illness*, 23 (5): 594–614.

Lemke, T. (2001) 'The birth of bio-politics' – Michel Foucault's lecture at the Collège de France on neo-liberal governmentality. *Economy and Society*, 30(2): 190–207.

Lemke, T. (2002) Foucault, governmentality, and critique. *Rethinking Marxism*, 14(3): 49–64.

Light, D.W. (2001a) Comparative institutional response to economic policy managed competition and governmentality. *Social Science & Medicine*, 52: 1151–1166.

Light, D.W. (2001b) Managed competition, governmentality and institutional response in the United Kingdom. *Social Science & Medicine*, 52: 1167–1181.

Lister, R. (2010) *Understanding Theories and Concepts in Social Policy*. Bristol, The Policy Press.

Lynch, K. (2010) From a neo-liberal to an egalitarian state: imagining a different future. TASC annual lecture, Royal Irish Academy, Dublin, 17 June 2010. Available from: http://researchrepository.ucd.ie/bitstream/handle/10197/2468/Lynch,%202010%20From%20a%20neo-liberal%20to%20an%20Egalitarian%20state%20-TASC_Annual_Lecture_June_17th_2010.pdf?sequence=1. Accessed 21 December 2015.

Malone, R. (1999) Policy as product – morality and metaphor in health policy discourse. *Hastings Center Report*, 29(3): 16–22.

McDonnell, O. and O'Donovan, O. (2009) Private health insurance as a technology of solidarity? The myth of 'community' in Irish healthcare policy. *Irish Journal of Sociology*, 17(2): 6–23.

McKee, K. (2009) Post-Foucauldian governmentality: what does it offer critical social policy analysis? *Critical Social Policy*, 29(3): 465–486.

Murphy-Lawless, J. and Quin, S. (2004) Equity, efficiency and health care. IN: Fanning, B., Kennedy, P., Kiely, G. and Quin S. (eds) *Theorising Irish Social Policy*. Dublin, UCD Press: pp. 128–146.

Naderi, P.S.D. and Meier, B.D. (2010) Privatisation within the Dutch context: a comparison of the health insurance systems of the Netherlands and the United States. *Health*, 14(6): 603–618.

Nettleton, S. (2006) *The Sociology of Health and Illness* (second edition). Cambridge, Polity Press.

O'Donovan, O. and Casey, D. (1995) Converting patients into consumers: consumerism and the charter of rights for hospital patients. *Irish Journal of Sociology*, 5: 43–66.

Randall, G.E. and Williams, A.P. (2006) Exploring limits to market-based reform: managed competition and rehabilitation home care services in Ontario. *Social Science & Medicine*, 62: 1594–1604.

Rose, N. (1996) The death of the social? Refiguring the territory of government. *Economy and Society*, 25(3): 327–356.

Rose, N. (2000) Government and control. *British Journal of Criminology*, 40: 321–339.

Rose, N. (2001) The politics of life itself. *Theory, Culture & Society*, 18(6): 1–30.

Rose, N. and Miller, P. (2010) Political power beyond the state: problematics of government. *British Journal of Sociology*, 61: 271–303.

Rosenau, P.V. and Lako, C.J. (2008) An experiment with regulated competition and individual mandates for universal health care: the new Dutch health insurance system. *Journal of Health Politics, Policy and Law*, 33(6): 1031–1055.

Thomas, S., Ryan, P. and Normand, C. (2010) *Effective Foundations for the Financing and Organisation of Social Health Insurance in Ireland*. Dublin, The Adelaide Hospital Society.

Turquet, P. (2012) Health insurance system financing reforms in the Netherlands, Germany and France: Repercussions for coverage and distribution? *International Social Security Review*, 65(1): 29–51.

Varadkar, L. (2015) Coalition health plan would have pushed up costs by €650m. *The Irish Times*, 17 November. ww.irishtimes.com/nes/ireland/irishnews/coalition-health-plan-would-have-pushed-up-costs-by-650m-1.2432434. Accessed 17 November 2015.

Veitch, K. (2010) The government of health care and the politics of patient empowerment: New Labour and the NHS reform agenda in England. *Law & Policy*, 32(3): 313–331.

Wren, M.A. (2003) *Unhealthy State – Anatomy of a Sick Society*. Dublin, New Island.

Wren, M.A., Connolly, S. and Cunningham, N. (2015) *An Examination of the Potential Costs of Universal Health Insurance in Ireland*. Dublin, Economic and Social Research Institute.

Assessment of Need as a technology of government in Ireland's Disability Act 2005

Introduction

Ireland has witnessed significant developments in the domain of disability policy and legislation in the past fifteen years. In a declared commitment to furthering the participation of people with disabilities in society, the government published a National Disability Strategy in 2004, the cornerstone of which was the passing of the Disability Act 2005. The Act, which promotes a number of positive action measures designed to safeguard disabled people's access to public sector services, has proven controversial, not least in relation to Part Two, which provides that individuals with a disability be entitled to an assessment of their health and educational needs and a related service statement (known as the Assessment of Need, or AoN process). Disability organisations have argued that the Act is far from rights-based, as it fails to guarantee the resources necessary to address the service needs that may be identified from the assessment. Moreover, insofar as the Act closes down the legal route of redress for complaints made in relation to the assessment of need process, campaigners have questioned how far disabled people's rights can be protected without the potential for recourse to the courts (De Wispelaere and Walsh, 2007).

In this chapter my concern is not with whether the Act is rights-based or not per se (are disabled people's rights being achieved?), but to explore the AoN process as a governmental technology which literally brings into being a new classification of people with disabilities – and their assessed needs – as governable entities. The Disability Act 2005 marked the culmination of a significant amount of lobbying by disabled people and their organisations of the state to acknowledge disabled people's rights to be equal citizens (Commission on the Status of People with Disabilities, 1996). However, the Act must also be understood in the context of a 'programme of government' (Rose and Miller, 1992) concerned with reforming the uneven and inequitable spatialities of Ireland's residual welfare regime, which historically emerged around the presence of powerful religious and other charitable organisations. The AoN, with its emerging classificatory regime, places new responsibilities on clinical professionals within these organisations, not least through practices of standardisation in how the assessment process is completed. Moreover, the Act's requirement that tabled statistics be presented annually to the Department of Health (DoH) on assessments completed, the incidence of different types of disability, and categories of identified (met and unmet) needs, is making the work of these agencies increasingly visible and governable as a technology of performance.

In viewing the AoN as a discrete technology of government in the Irish disability policy arena, I take my lead from Foucauldian-inspired governmentality scholars such as Dean (1995: 571) who assert that social policy depends on 'particular technical conditions of existence, routines and rituals of bureaucracy, forms of expertise and intellectual technologies' as a means of constructing and rendering entities such as 'the population' and 'the economy' governable. In particular, I am interested in the constitutive power of categories, classifications and numbers to 'make up' people and spaces (Hacking, 1982, 2006; Kurunmäki and Miller, 2008; Larner and LeHeron, 2005), and the ways in which these categorisations are interpreted and made operable in various ways by those who work with them. My particular focus in this chapter is on exploring the spaces in-between the rationalities of particular policy programmes on the one hand, and the end point of many Foucauldian studies, namely the creation of self-governing subjects, on the other. Following the call of Barnett et al. (2008) for a more critical questioning of the extent to which governmental strategies more or less successfully effect their desired ends in the formation of individual subject identities, I suggest that examining how professionals and experts interpret and implement such programmes can help explain some of the 'messy actualities' (O'Malley, Weir and Clifford, 1997; Larner, 2000) of working through different classificatory techniques (see also McDonald, Marston and Buckley, 2003). Indeed, as Barnett et al. (2008: 637) note, exploring how governmental programmes work to achieve specific ends involves taking seriously the notion that 'professionals and experts are not just the passive agents of anonymous governmental rationalities; they are just as often the subjects of such interventions'.

My discussion in this chapter is based on a number of documents published by the Health Service Executive (HSE) which provide guidance to staff on how to interpret and implement the Act, but more specifically, a research report undertaken by the National Disability Authority (NDA) in 2011, which sought to evaluate how the AoN process was bedding down in different localities across the country (NDA, 2011). The research included interviews with different professionals charged with carrying out assessments as part of AoN, and provides a rich source of data with which to explore the actualities of categorising through a specific assessment tool. Drawing on this data, the chapter is divided into four parts. I begin by situating my discussion of the AoN in conceptual terms, and follow this by describing the emergence of the Disability Act 2005 and AoN process in the context of Irish disability policy. My analysis of the AoN is then structured around two key themes. First, I consider the interpretations and meanings ascribed to disability and need as categories in the AoN by those working with the assessment tool, and how it constitutes particular types of subjects. How are we to interpret the subjectivities created by an adjudication of 'disability' and 'assessed need' under the Act, and how do those carrying out AoN negotiate what an assessment of need is in these terms? What new identities are created as a result of these negotiations? Second, I explore how the AoN has been operationalised through a new bureaucratic system which has been superimposed upon existing, spatially uneven service provision for people with disabilities and which, in many cases, has forced the breaching of what Rose and Miller (1992) refer to as the professional 'enclosures' of welfare expertise (see also Kurunmäki and Miller, 2006). The Act instituted statutory Assessment Officers (AOs) (based within the HSE) to act as independent interlocutors between children being assessed and clinical professionals (usually based in disability agencies outside the HSE) who undertake the actual assessment. While AOs have no clinical training, they make the final decision on whether a child has a disability, based on assessment reports sought from relevant professionals, and have a role in ensuring that assessment reports are carried out within a particular timeframe as enacted in the legislation. I therefore seek to explore 'the tensions that exist between different actors and expertises' (Kurunmäki and Miller, 2008: 11), where clinical professionals are often forced to become calculating selves in terms of making judgements about the prioritisation of cases and appropriate caseloads in the context of AoN.

In total, then, I seek to demonstrate the multiple, and often contested, interpretations and effects of specific calculative techniques in the context of policy programmes. As entities with constitutive power, I suggest that technologies such as the AoN have the potential to create new types of subjectivities and calculable spaces which have implications both for those who are envisaged as the end recipients of specific programmes, and those who work to administer them. These spaces and subjectivities are varied, often uncertain, and frequently result from the unintended consequences of governmental rationalities. However, they demonstrate 'feedback effects' insofar as they build back into and (re)constitute new policy rationalities. For example, at the national level it is clear that the 'massifying' of individuals' disabilities and related needs – through tabled statistics based on the AoN – are building into broader concerns about the apparent rise in numbers of children with autism in the state, and also about the recent preoccupation with value for money in disability services. To that end, I suggest that an 'analytics of government' (Dean, 1999) provides a helpful way of understanding how the AoN acts not just as a way for the Irish government to deal with rights claims by people with disabilities, but also as a tactic which seeks to effect a modernising agenda in services for people with disabilities.

Deploying governmentality: programmes and technologies of government

Governmentality literature has provided a fruitful hunting ground in terms of finding conceptual tools to analyse the ways in which states problematise and govern 'the wealth, health and happiness of populations' (Rose and Miller, 1992: 174). Huxley (2008: 1635) suggests that Foucault referred to the concept of governmentality itself in two ways: 'first, as a historical analysis of the logics of government by the state, and second, as investigations of forms of governing others and the self, instantiated throughout society in institutions, organisations and regimes of self care'. As she continues, however, he did not intend it to be a totalising social theory; rather, it is best seen as a 'framework or perspective that allows certain kinds of questions to be asked about how particular aspects of taken-for-granted social relations came to be as they are' (*ibid.*: 1636).

For commentators such as Rose and Miller (1992) and Dean (1999) this perspective can best be expressed in the notion of government as a series of *problematisations* (in the eighteenth and nineteenth centuries, for example, how to deal with disease epidemics or poverty, or today, how to address issues such as unemployment or urban unrest). Taking government beyond the notion of a monolithic, centralised state, a governmental approach involves asking questions such as, Who is governed? How are those who are to be governed known about? To what ends are they to be governed? Through what tactics and techniques does governing take place? (Rose, O'Malley and Valverde, 2006). Rose and Miller's seminal (1992) paper, 'Political power beyond the state', elucidates a series of conceptual tools which facilitate exploration of these questions. Specifically, they point to programmes and technologies of government as a basis for understanding modern forms of political power and governance processes. Programmes of government link together, or translate, aspirations and goals of political projects (in the Disability Act 2005, for example, the aspiration to fulfil disabled people's right to an assessment to enable them to participate in society) into specific project or policy objectives, and modes of service provision; in other words, they 'seek to establish the legitimacy of particular ways of delivering services and organising social life' (Kurunmäki and Miller, 2006: 89). These programmes in turn are made operationable by *technologies*, which encompass the everyday processes, mechanisms and strategies through which governing takes place (*ibid.*). Technologies may include practices such as assessments, examinations, sets of standards and calculations associated with the collection of statistical and/or financial data, and have formed the basis for a variety of empirical studies which interrogate everything from the role of standards and benchmarking in higher education to classificatory practices involved in managing the unemployed (Larner and LeHeron, 2005; Caswell, Marston and Larsen, 2010; McDonald, Marston and Buckley, 2003). It is important to note, however, that technologies do not provide the translation of aspirations into ideal or anticipated outcomes. Rather, insofar as Foucault recognised the dispersed nature of power, technologies are diverse, heterogeneous and often competing: they come into being through, and are a reflection of, 'a complex assemblage of diverse forces – legal, architectural, professional, administrative, financial, judgemental – such that the decisions and actions of individuals, groups, organisations and populations come to be understood and regulated in relation to authoritative criteria' (Rose and Miller, 1992: 183).

Crucially, both programmes and technologies of government have to be understood in relation to particular forms of knowledge and epistemic communities (Rose and Miller, 1992). Knowledge plays a central role in legitimising programmes and making visible the objects of programmes, so as to render them amenable to intervention. Domains of knowledge and expertise – whether captured in the context of social science, health and medicine, or economics – define and legitimise the contours and parameters of programmes of government. Meanwhile, specific technologies often operate both as a means of working to achieve programmatic goals, but also as a way of continually knowing and (re)presenting the issue at stake in a form of a looping effect (Hacking, 2006). For example, McDonald, Marston and Buckley's (2003) study of the Job Seeker Classification Instrument (JSCI), a form of computerised classification tool used in policy programmes designed to target the unemployed in Australia, demonstrates how the instrument not only acts to administer active welfare strategies but also creates new types of knowledge about jobseekers, based around a statistical, risk-based assessment of their employability. The politics and dynamics of knowledge production, and the role(s) of expertise in acts of governing, are necessarily complex. Thus while some technologies may seek to draw on and solidify certain forms of expertise (such as the use of 'psy' discourses to assess individuals in the JSCI), others act to disrupt or alter forms of expertise. In relation to the latter, for example, advanced neoliberal welfare regimes have increasingly sought to diminish or broach the 'enclosures' of expertise centred around different professional groups (medics, nurses, social workers and others) by introducing different forms of expertise embodied in technologies focused on financial management and performance assessment (Miller, 2001; Kurunmäki and Miller, 2006, 2011).

Indeed, it is in the context of analysing changes in welfare regimes, and the playing out of neoliberal political rationalities in what Dean (1999) refers to as 'advanced liberal government', that concepts drawn from governmentality studies have been particularly helpful. For Rose and Miller (1992), advanced liberal government is associated with governing at a distance, where policy programmes and services are operationalised through distanciated networks of agencies and institutions. Technologies associated with performance assessment facilitate the indirect surveillance and regulation of those charged with translating the aspirations of welfare programmes – namely the creation of active and self-responsible citizens – into specific actions. These processes have been made visible in a range of studies which illuminate the apparent paradox embodied in contemporary welfare strategies which seek to 'govern through freedom': that is, as Dean (1999: 165) puts it, 'in order to act freely, the subject must first be shaped, guided, moulded into one capable of responsibility exercising that freedom through systems of domination'. Government welfare rhetoric as it is applied to groups such as the unemployed, people with disabilities, lone parents and so on frequently uses the clarion call of 'no rights without responsibilities', reflecting the uneasy relationship between freedom and subjection; it is a relationship which leads to a distinction between those who are able to behave responsibly and manage their own risk (what Dean (1999) terms *active citizens*), and those who are deemed to be incapable of doing so ('targeted populations') and who, as a consequence, may find themselves subject to more authoritarian modes of power.

These distinctions speak particularly to the experience of people with disabilities as a group within the population. As Tremain (2005) notes, the history of disability cannot be understood without recourse to the biopolitical strategies of states since the eighteenth century which brought disabled people into being and rendered them knowable. A huge range of governmental interventions, that include 'asylums, income support programs, quality of life assessments, special education programs', has, she argues, 'created, classified, codified, managed and controlled social anomalies through which some people have been divided from others and *objectivised* as (for instance) physically impaired, insane, handicapped, mentally ill, retarded and deaf' (Tremain, 2005: 5–6). These forms of classification remain a constant feature of advanced neoliberal welfare regimes and their treatment of people with disabilities. As many studies of disabled people's lives have shown, expertise and experts have had a dominant role in shaping disabled people as subjects of power (see, for example, Sullivan, 2005). While there has been a notable shift in the language of disability in which articulations of rights, claims to autonomy and forms of inclusion have become stated political rationalities in advanced Western nations, analyses have demonstrated how various governmental technologies presuppose a form of responsible inclusion in which disabled people remain the subjects of surveillance and regulation. Morgan (2005), for example, likens the Special Educational Needs (SEN) system for children in the UK to a kind of panopticon in which the SEN child is constantly under surveillance through forms of assessment such as the statementing process. Meanwhile, Douglas's (2010) discussion of the project of educational inclusion for autistic children demonstrates how more liberal forms of power coexist with authoritarian forms to penalise those who are unable to conform to the norms of the education system. Her study demonstrates how the project of educational inclusion as a programme of government has implications not just for children with autism but also their families and teachers, leading to the circulation of different types of knowledges, and creating new sets of relations ('school–family–community partnerships' (Douglas, 2010: 107)) and self-identities, all regulated at a distance by various technologies, including specific forms of teaching mechanisms and placement committees. These concepts have relevance in interrogating the effects of the AoN, which, as I go on to demonstrate, has instituted a new set of relations and knowledges hinged around the problematisation of disability as a form of assessed need.

Contextualising the AoN: disability policy and welfare change

The Disability Act 2005 emerged out of a number of struggles by people with disabilities and their organisations to secure equitable access to public services in Ireland. As part of a broader National Disability Strategy, the Act places obligations on public service providers to facilitate access to services, through requirements such as the provision of accessible information, adjustments to public buildings and the drawing up of 'sectoral plans' by government departments, designed to demonstrate how their services are addressing the needs of people with disabilities. However, it is the AoN process, set out in Part Two of the Act, that has defined much of the public discourse about the Act and has provoked the most controversy. Part Two specifies that individuals can apply for an assessment of their health and educational needs, and a related service statement. The outcome of the assessment, which is coordinated by designated AOs in the HSE, is a report which sets out the nature and extent of the disability (if any), the needs arising from this disability, and a statement of the appropriate services to address these needs. Where needs are found to arise, the Assessment Report triggers the production of a Service Statement (coordinated through Liaison Officers) which sets out the practicality of providing these services and the resources available to do so. In all cases, a determination of disability is based on the definition set out in the Act, as 'a substantial restriction in the capacity of the person to carry on a profession, business or occupation in the State by reason of an enduring physical, sensory, mental health or intellectual impairment' (Government of Ireland, 2005).

From the initial drafting of the Act, contestation between disability groups and the government focused around the thorny issue of rights claims

(De Wispelaere and Walsh, 2007). For the Irish government, the AoN embodies claims to rights insofar as it provides every individual with a right to a statutory assessment of their health and educational needs. However, disability organisations and activists have argued that this right is meaningless without a commitment to meeting these needs through services – a commitment which the government has failed to meet by its unwillingness to ring-fence resources that would effectively provide a right to *services*. The Act has also been criticised for closing down legal routes of complaint and redress, not just by failing to provide enforceable rights in the context of services, but also by replacing recourse to the law courts with an internal complaints system in cases where conflict emerges between individuals and service providers in the process or outcomes of the AoN (De Wispelaere and Walsh, 2007).

These disputes speak to some of the tensions that exist within the Irish disability policy arena which, prior to the Act, was punctuated by a number of high-profile legal battles in which parents of children with disabilities took actions against the state in the High Court for failure to provide services for their children. Describing Ireland's relationship with the disability sector as 'complex and ambiguous', De Wispelaere and Walsh (2007: 519) note that while historically, charitable Catholic organisations dominated disability policy and services, 'contemporary policy is framed by a neoliberal economic agenda but also by a public commitment to mainstreaming equality of opportunity, social inclusion and human rights'. This dual discourse is readily visible in the stated aims and ideals of programmes and policy documents which set out the government's modernising agenda for disability services. A recent report produced by the DoH, *Value for Money and Policy Review of Disability Services in Ireland* (DoH, 2012: xxviii), stated that implementing the vision of disability policy to support people to participate fully in society would require 'the twin goals' of 'full inclusion and self-determination through access to individualised personal social supports and services' and 'the creation of a cost-effective, responsive and accountable system, which will support the full inclusion and self-determination of people with disabilities'. From a governmentality perspective, these two imperatives may not be as contradictory as they first seem, with commentators noting how the drive to reform services around the imperative of self-determination and choice (which in many countries involves the government providing direct payments to people with disabilities to enable them to manage their own services) may act as a cost-saving measure in which state agencies and initiatives govern by inculcating disabled people to act as self-responsible, risk-managing individuals (see for example, Junne and Huber, 2014).

Although Irish disability policy may not have fully embraced service models such as individualised payments, the vocabulary of self-determination on the one hand and cost-effectiveness on the other is evident in a range of governmental practices and initiatives characteristic of advanced neoliberal welfare regimes in which (disability) services are being reformed and made accountable at a distance 'via a multitude of calculative and managerial locales' (Rose and Miller, 1992: 200). The institutions of the Irish government, which historically had a relatively residual role in terms of directing welfare provision, are increasingly engaging in regulatory behaviour by managing disability service providers through new service level agreements and sets of standards overseen by the regulatory body HIQA (Health and Information Quality Authority). Meanwhile, the focus on creating individualised and user-focused service provision is leading to the dismantling and reconfiguring of the fragmented and uneven service provision that has grown up around disparate charitable organisations. Initiatives such as *Progressing Disability Services for Children and Young People* which involve the HSE working in partnership with voluntary providers, are ambitious projects designed to equalise, and provide a single point of access to, specialist services (www.hse.ie/progressingdisabilityservices/). These projects are, however, proving controversial, not least in the way that they force the breaching of long-established organisational and professional boundaries and allegiances, and seek to bring into being new organisational hybrids and identities.

This institutional landscape is significant as it provides the context in which the actualities of the AoN process are played out. The AoN, as far as it is administered, is built around a set of often fragmented and fragile institutional arrangements which differ across the country. Initial referrals for assessments are sent to AOs based in the HSE, for example; these officers use their judgement to seek appropriate assessments from professionals in voluntary service-providing agencies, who are contracted to provide services on behalf of the health service. Based on a collation of these assessments (which sometimes may involve just one professional, in other cases, a number of different forms of professional expertise), the AO makes the final decision on whether an individual is deemed to have a disability under the Act. This process comes with particular forms of performance measurements attached: timescales specified in the Act mean that the assessments have to be completed within three months of commencement and assessments have to be completed in accordance with specific standards drawn up by HIQA. Meanwhile, Section 13 of the Act requires the HSE to report annually to the Minister regarding 'the aggregate needs identified in assessment reports prepared including an indication of the periods of time ideally required for the provision of the services, the sequence of such provision and an estimate of the cost of such provision' (Government of Ireland, 2005). This statistical work does not just make the activities of service-providing agencies and specific professional groupings increasingly visible, but also brings into being emergent categories of people with disabilities with needs for specific professional expertise.

Visibility of the AoN in the form of statistics has led to regular critique in the media about the failings of the Act, not least in relation to waiting lists for assessments (see for example, Bardon, 2015; O'Brien, 2014a), and has brought into focus shortfalls in public healthcare services for children in Ireland's two-tier health system. Insofar as commentators such as Rose and Miller (1992: 190) refer to government as a 'congenitally failing operation', much of the arrangements which surround the AoN remain partial and incomplete. The AoN process was intended to be open to all individuals (children and adults), but was only rolled out initially for 0–5 year olds from June 2007. Following a successful challenge of the HSE in the High Court by a parent whose son was refused an assessment on the basis of his age, the HSE now stipulates that anyone born after 1 June 2002 can apply for an assessment (*The Irish Times*, 2010). However, promises made in 2006 to roll out Part Two of the Act to older age groups have failed to materialise in the context of the post-2007 economic downturn which followed the boom of the Celtic Tiger years. The AoN was also meant to be complementary to a piece of legislation drafted around the same time as the Disability Act 2005, the Education for Persons with Special Educational Needs (EPSEN) Act 2004, which makes provision for 'a right to an assessment of education needs, the development of an Individual Education Plan and an independent appeals process' (NDA, 2011: 13). Once again, the provisions of the EPSEN Act were never implemented, leaving Ireland's Ombudsman and Information Commissioner, Emily O'Reilly, to state in 2012 that 'Clearly, having legislation on the statute book is not terribly useful if that legislation can be left in no-man's land indefinitely' (www.ombudsman.gov.ie/en/News/Speeches-Articles/2012/Health-Services-and-the-Law-Some-Reflections.html). As I seek to demonstrate in the rest of the chapter, these unfinished legislative ambitions have had consequences in terms of how professionals work through and understand the AoN, and have often unintended consequences in terms of programme outcomes.

Constructing subjectivities: categorising 'disability' in the AoN

As Dean (1999) and others have highlighted, identity formation is a key element of programmes of government which seek to bring into being populations as governable entities. Specific technologies embedded in the intricacies of bureaucratic systems contribute to the production of a range of different subject positions around which particular norms of behaviour are assumed. The AoN, for example, brings into focus a nexus of concerned parents, their children and various different professionals who are expected to act according to procedures set out in guidance on the implementation of the AoN. The AoN is often, however, a process laden with emotion, confusion and ambiguity, particularly for parents who on the one hand may embrace the designation of 'disability' for its conferral of value in terms of access to services (and for whom, to use Rosenberg's (2002: 252) terms, 'the diagnosis constitutes a kind of social equity'), but on the other recognise its potential to act as a stigmatising social label. Professionals working within these systems too are acutely aware of such dilemmas, and do not make decisions about the conferral of a disabled identity lightly.

What disability actually *is* under the terms of the Act is an ambiguous question. From the outset of the AoN, confusion has shaped how professionals interpret disability as a category, not least in relation to other (clinical) categories of impairment. Assessors are expected to determine whether an individual has a disability based on the definition set out in Part Two of the legislation, which is a derivation of the definition for the whole Act, and explained in the following way:

> The definition of 'disability' in Part 2 of the Disability Act is a person with a 'substantial restriction' which-
>
> (a) Is permanent or likely to be permanent, results in significant difficulty in communication, learning or mobility or in significantly disordered cognitive processes, and
> (b) Gives rise to the need for services to be provided continually to the person whether or not a child or, if the person is a child, to the need for services to be provided early in life to ameliorate the disability.

> (Government of Ireland, 2005)

The emphasis in the definition set out in the Act, when it was created, was to focus on the relationship between an individual's impairment and society; that is, to move away from purely medicalised understandings of disability which focus on limitations in physical or intellectual functioning. Guidance to assessors in the AoN, issued by the HSE, states that

> It is particularly important to note that the term 'substantial restriction' refers to a restriction in a person's capacity to participate. It does not refer to the impairment. This is important as it is the restriction in capacity to participate that must be 'permanent or likely to be permanent' according to the definition in the Act. (HSE, 2010, as cited in NDA, 2011: 93)

This apparent recognition of disability as the interplay between corporeal and societal dynamics is, however, accompanied by a more medicalised discourse which speaks of restriction, disorder and a deficit conception of disability in which difficulties can only be present in four areas: communication, learning, mobility or cognitive processes. In advising assessors that children 'should be compared with their normative peers' (*ibid*: 103), the guidance establishes assumptions about, and distinguishes between, certain normal and abnormal categories of children's behaviour and activities. The notion of need, moreover, is defined in terms of service provision, or, as Illich (1977: 24) referred to it, as 'the individual offprint of a professional pattern'; needs do not come into being in and of themselves but in a relation to a professional intervention in the arena of health and/or education.

This form of categorisation is supported by recourse to expert knowledge(s) embodied in the form of clinicians (including psychologists, occupational therapists, physiotherapists and speech therapists). Despite HIQA standards for the AoN process which stress the importance of putting the individual at the centre of the assessment process and listening to their desired outcomes (DoHC, 2007), the guidance to assessors frequently reiterates the significance of expert clinical knowledge in determining the conferral of disability, noting that the HSE-produced guidelines themselves 'are not intended to substitute for sound clinical judgement which is a matter for relevant professionals' (HSE, 2010, cited in NDA, 2011: 100). AOs too, who make the final decision about whether a child has a disability, are described as 'normally' doing so 'having received advice from clinicians' (*ibid.*). Guidance, then, establishes clinicians as experts with the knowledge to categorise and bring into being this new classification of children. Yet research conducted with such professionals about the AoN process has illustrated the complexities of negotiating this identity, particularly in the context of the politics of diagnosis that shape access to disability-related services in the state. The HSE is clear to state that the AoN 'does not make any reference to a diagnosis. Consequently, assessors are not asked to provide a diagnosis' (HSE, 2010, cited in NDA, 2011: 101). However, the majority of clinicians who are required to carry out AoN assessments work in voluntary sector bodies, many of which require a formal clinical diagnosis for children to access their services and interventions. Diagnosis has a similarly freighted status in the education system, where limited special needs resources can only be accessed if a child has been diagnosed with a specific condition.

The politics of diagnosis sits at the crux of how clinicians interpret what disability is and thus how the subject position of the 'person with a disability' is constructed under the terms of the Act. Specifically, it speaks to a context in which a legal interpretation of disability based around the identification of service needs which arise from a restricted 'capacity to participate' collides with disciplinary (medical) knowledges which seek to diagnose particular disorders and reinforce established disease categories. Research conducted by the NDA (2011) which involved interviews with professionals engaged in the AoN process, for example, highlighted that many clinicians were unsure what an assessment should look like for the purposes of the AoN; thus, while in other circumstances they may use a battery of tests to make clinical diagnoses of specific conditions, they were unsure whether a simple 'play-based assessment' (NDA, 2011: 35) or a 'pre-diagnostic services assessment' (30) would suffice. Some clinicians reported feeling 'compelled to perform full diagnostic assessments up front' insofar as they were aware that parents were looking for a diagnosis in order to access services (*ibid.*: 30). As one clinician, a speech therapist, reported,

> We understand that the idea of the Disability Act was to move away from focusing on a diagnosis and developing a system to unlock resources for a person with a disability based on their needs. However, the truth is that a child without a diagnosis gets nothing in our system ... (Cited in NDA, 2011: 50)

It is perhaps unsurprising then that assessments undertaken through the AoN process have been shown to be subject to wide variation, and particularly dependent on the different arrangement of local services.

Assessors also reported finding the language of Part Two of the Act problematic in the context of assessing young children. The NDA research noted that many clinicians expressed difficulty in stating what the extent and nature of disability was for an individual, or indeed whether a child had a disability under the terms of the Act at all. An occupational therapist explained,

> It is a dilemma to tick 'yes' or 'no' as to whether a young child has a disability. This has been a problem for our service. Now we just see a child. See where that child is at. We fill in the report saying these are the needs that presented but that standardised tests were not practical (where they are not). I suppose that gives us some cover ... (Cited in NDA, 2011: 51)

As this quote indicates, clinicians are only too aware of both their role in shaping children's subjectivities, but also, by referring to 'cover', the disciplining gaze of the HSE and the legal apparatus attached to the Act which subjects them to particular modes of surveillance (including the potential of their decisions to be challenged by parents through a complex complaints system) (see for example, Morgan, 2005).

Clinicians' confusion around appropriate assessment tools raises questions about how they make sense of, or ascribe meaning to, those children who are designated as having a disability under the AoN, as well as those who apply for assessments on their behalf (usually parents and/or teachers). A number of clinicians in the NDA research suggested that the AoN process was being used to classify those whose condition was uncertain, or who were not already accessing services for children with disabilities; or, as the research states, the AoN 'appears to have become a route to assessment for those children who do not fit into existing categories' (NDA, 2011: 45). One occupational therapist suggested that 'the children that are referred to us are those with borderline conditions or general development delay without any diagnosis of an underlying condition and those with query ASD' (cited in NDA, 2011: 43), while another psychologist stated that AoN cases were 'query autism. This would include a lot of very poor quality autism referrals' (cited in NDA, 2011: 42). The uncertainty regarding what disability *is* appears evident in the statistics that have been collated from the AoN process. Figures from the first nine months of 2011, for example, show that after the largest category of disability based on completed AoNs ('Primary Speech and Language' at 25%), the second largest classification was 'No category specified at this stage' (18%), followed by 'Autism Spectrum Disorder' (15.5%) (NDA, 2011). As Rosenberg (2002: 254) notes in the context of diagnosis and disease classification, 'once articulated, such bureaucratic categories cannot help but exert a variety of substantive effects on individuals and institutional relationships'. This is particularly the case in the context of ASD, where media reports are seeking to produce new 'truths' which explain the apparent growth in autism assessments evidenced through the AoN. These include, in one article, the notion of 'autism-lite' (Nolan, 2014) – or the broadening out of diagnostic criteria to include less severe cases of ASD – as a way of explaining the increase in diagnoses. The AoN therefore represents a technology with the productive capacity to bring into being new categories of people and identities, in a dynamic process of 'making up people' (Hacking, 2006) that begets further institutional, political and social responses.

In the context of the AoN, these subjectivities also extend beyond the individual with a disability. Clinicians' uncertainty about identifying disability and need under the terms of the Act appears to build in to a moral discourse that constructs the conduct of certain actors (most notably parents and teachers) along a continuum of responsible–irresponsible behaviour in relation to the assessment process. For example, in seeking to make sense of the definition of disability in the AoN, clinicians draw comparisons between those children who are referred directly to their services, and those who come through the AoN process. As one occupational therapist stated, 'To my mind the main difference between children on the AON list and the early intervention list is that the parents of those children who have demanded an AON are more demanding, better educated and more affluent. It certainly has nothing to do with level of need' (cited in NDA, 2011: 46–47). Another psychologist stated that 'the vast majority of school-aged AON requests are parents or schools trying to get a psychology assessment for resources for child in the school' (*ibid.*: 42). Indeed, in the NDA research, clinicians frequently constructed teachers as having made inappropriate referrals in order to try and obtain supports for children with needs that were not available through the mechanisms of the education system.

Overall, then, the AoN challenges clinicians' assumptions and knowledge about what disability is by using a definition which cuts across and sometimes diverges from clinical classifications. Despite calls for standardisation of assessment in the guidance issued to assessors, for professionals it appears as a category of exception. For them, the subject position of 'person with a disability' under the terms of the Act is a classification designed to contain those whose conditions do not fit, or 'exceed' (Evans and Colls, 2009), pre-established diagnostic categories. In this sense, the AoN reflects

Rose and Miller's (1992: 190) observation that 'Things, persons or events always appear to escape those bodies of knowledge that inform governmental programmes, refusing to respond according to the programmatic logic that seeks to govern them.' As a category, the AoN has generated particular discourses which reflect the meanings clinicians ascribe to this emergent group of people, and which for many are borne out in discussions about stratification of need between 'rivalrous' (*ibid.*) referral routes. It is a process, and classificatory regime, that gives rise to other dynamic subjectivities, including the 'demanding' parent, and the 'pushy' or 'ill-informed' teacher, many of which reflect a context of welfare restraint and change in which parents and professionals feel compelled to campaign for scarce resources and services.

Creating calculating selves: working through the AoN

As outlined earlier in the chapter, a rich seam of governmentality-inspired literature has sought to analyse the dynamics of welfare change over the past thirty years, drawing attention to the consequences of neoliberal mentalities in shifting institutional relationships and work practices in agencies charged with delivering welfare (Dean, 1999; Rose and Miller, 1992). While the dominant narrative of this literature – which suggests a shift away from Keynesian-style, interventionist welfare delivery to more marketised and managerialist arrangements – has less relevance in an Irish context where subsidiarity has historically characterised the state's approach to welfare provision (Considine and Dukelow, 2009), there is little doubt that, in the arena of disability policy at least, neoliberal principles are increasingly informing service change. These include an imperative to increasingly monitor the performance of services, and clinicians working within these services, at a distance; and an attempt to reconfigure, and often bring together, different types of experts and expertise through more complex organisational arrangements.

The AoN can be read as an intervention which increasingly requires professionals based in disability service organisations to re-evaluate and redefine their current work practices. In the first instance, the AoN has introduced a new stream of referrals in addition to those that already come direct to the service providers (via GPs, for example), with the key difference being that the AoN process demands they be completed within a specified timescale. This issue, in particular, was raised by a number of professionals in the NDA research, who described experiencing difficulty in how best to allocate their time to the AoN and other assessment duties. As a psychologist said,

> I do a lot of autism assessments. The timelines are really tight. You are making
> a determination in a very short space of time. In the back of your mind you

are thinking that this assessment could end up in court one day. But we are under pressure from managers to meet the statutory timeframes and our managers keep telling us that they are under huge pressure to meet the statutory timeframes. (Cited in NDA, 2011: 56).

Another psychologist stated, 'We frequently delay assessing or intervening with children with greater need because we are conducting AONs' (*ibid.*: 46). Many clinicians expressed a view that conducting AoNs was preventing them from actually engaging in treatment itself. The NDA research concluded, for example, that the AoN leads to 'assessment being prioritised over intervention' (*ibid.*: 20).

The AoN has therefore contributed to a discussion around appropriate workloads for different clinicians, and how this should best be managed. Attempts have been made to quantify the number of hours required by clinicians to conduct one AoN (NDA, 2011), and in an act of peer-surveillance, some clinicians involved in the research were critical of others carrying out assessments, which they believed were too extensive or time-consuming. As a psychologist stated,

> From what I have seen since I arrived here ... lots of clinicians write their reports like they are university case studies. That is not appropriate in the public service, it is a luxury that we don't have. We are all public servants, we have an obligation to all the children in our area, which means you have an obligation to do your assessments in a timely fashion and get on with your intervention. (Cited in NDA, 2011: 65)

The issue of appropriate caseloads for different disciplinary groups is something which has a profile at a national scale in terms of the HSE's reporting requirements under Section 13 of the Disability Act 2005. Since the Act's inception, the HSE has been grappling to statistically represent the relationship between the shortfall in needs that are being addressed (i.e. needs identified in AoNs but not being met by services) and resources (in this case whole-time equivalent (WTE) posts in different disciplines) required to address this needs shortfall (HSE, n.d.a, n.d.b). This is a task that has become ever-more complex with the significant rise in numbers of assessments since the Act's inception (between 2009 and 2010, for example, a 23% increase in applications for assessments received by the HSE (see HSE, n.d.a). In its most recent report to the Minister for Disability, Equality, Mental Health and Older People, the HSE argued that a key requirement for them to make this calculation is an internationally recognised appropriate average caseload for different disciplines, something which they claim they are still waiting for guidance on. Despite the absence of this data, the report collates statistics on the frequency of required services identified from assessment reports (with speech and language therapy topping the list as the most frequently required service), representing a calculative attempt to make transparent and accountable emerging service needs and resource requirements (HSE, n.d.a).

It can be argued, then, that the AoN is increasingly requiring clinicians to act as 'calculating selves'; it represents a governance tool that engenders a form of self-surveillance in which clinicians have to respond to the requirements of AOs, whose work in turn is also monitored at arm's length by the production of quarterly statistics about numbers of assessments completed and those overdue. These statistics, which provide a breakdown by geographical area, have become a regular source of contention and are widely reported in the media, bringing the performance of both AOs and those who conduct the assessments into clear view. An article published in *The Irish Times* in September 2014, for example, stated that 'Figures for the first quarter of this year show that some 1,200 children were still waiting for an assessment after six months, a 60 per cent increase over the same period in 2012. Average waiting times are now in the region of nine months' (O'Brien, 2014b; see also O'Brien, 2013). Assessments completed under the stated timescales of the Act form a key annual performance indicator for the HSE; their 2014 annual report showed that despite a target of 100% of assessments being completed on time, in 2013 only 23.2% had been completed on time, and in 2014 only 33% (HSE, 2015). AOs cited in the NDA research rationalised the production of these statistics in a number of ways, and were critical of the way in which they simplistically represent a system which appears to be problematic and inefficient. As one AO stated in the NDA research, 'We beat ourselves up about the absolute number of overdue assessments. But what does that figure tell us? I know some Local Health Office areas have made huge progress but all that gets reported on is the absolute number of overdue assessments' (cited in NDA, 2011: 56). Another AO similarly noted the need to draw attention to the dynamics underpinning the statistics:

> I could tell you the background to every single overdue or extended AoN that we have on our books at the moment. I could tell you which are the result of poorly organised, poorly managed teams, I could tell you which are late because of Child and Adolescent Mental Health service's waiting lists, which are because the child has very complex needs ... which are late because the family is so dysfunctional they don't make the appointments. To my mind, that is the information that is needed to improve the system. (*Ibid.*)

The dynamics of performance measurement which seek to make clinicians more accountable are also part of a broader shifting of institutional and professional relationships in the disability service provision arena. In much the same way that Kurunmäki and Miller (2006: 93) document the growing hybridisation of welfare delivery which requires service providers to 're-think, re-describe and re-organise their work processes so as to align them with wider political ideals', so the AoN requires staff to work with colleagues across disciplinary boundaries, and in some cases across organisations, in more hybridised arrangements. The policy shift towards multidisciplinary early intervention teams for pre-school children, for example, is becoming ever-more visible in policy rationalities expressed in initiatives such as *Progressing Disability Services for Children and Young People*. It is perhaps unsurprising, then, that the NDA research is clear to state the benefits of joint team-working structures, noting that

> Where the DoH and the HSE have configured disability services for children into geographically-integrated teams, the National Disability Authority found that the statutory assessment of need process worked better and in a more streamlined way. There was also less emphasis on using the assessment process to develop a diagnosis in order to meet the specific entry requirements of individual services. (NDA, 2011: 78)

Clinicians in the research cited differing practices and degrees of difficulty with joint working, however. For example, despite the AoN guidance which states that 'assessors whether working in a team or individually, should confer by meeting or by teleconference, using all the information received from parents, existing reports, clinical judgement and the Assessment officer's requests' (HSE, 2010, cited in NDA, 2011: 95), one psychologist reported,

> As part of query Autism assessments I usually try to do a joint session with the Occupational Therapist. That is best practice. But for AON [*sic*] the timeframes are usually so tight that the Occupational Therapist and I can't get a suitable date for a joint assessment, so we do our individual assessments. (Cited in NDA, 2011: 55)

Disciplinary and organisational 'enclosures' have also proved difficult in terms of creating more cooperative working arrangements. For example, a number of AOs referred to the reluctance of Child and Adolescent Mental Health Services to engage with AoN requests, or to do so without regard to timescales (NDA, 2011), which has again led to large differences geographically in terms of the way in which cases of children with mental health issues are dealt with.

In the context of broader governmental rationalities and organisational changes in the disability policy arena, then, the AoN is presented as a tool designed to build into, and expedite, a vision of service equity in a context of greater multidisciplinary and cooperative working. However, given the uneven geographical and historical imprint of service configuration in the state, the AoN instead highlights the challenge of standardisation in a context shaped largely by fragmentation and enclosures bounded particularly by individual service organisation identities and practices. The NDA research demonstrated that clinicians feel ambivalent about the AoN as a technology of performance, not least in the ways it is forcing them to reflect on and modify some of their work practices, including engaging with other disciplines in different ways. Meanwhile, the statistics which make assessors' expertise ever-more calculable and administrable are also, at this juncture, ambiguous in terms of their consequences: while some may view the presentation of statistics about cases completed, or about unmet needs, as a way of lobbying for more posts within their discipline, others interpret it as a form of surveillance in which their work is coming under increasing scrutiny exercised at a distance. Certainly, to date, statistics appear to have been used to 'punish' rather than 'praise' (Larner and LeHeron, 2005: 855), indicating performative effects which go beyond the stated objectives of the AoN and Disability Act as a legislative rationality.

Conclusion

In this chapter, I have sought to deploy conceptual tools drawn from governmentality literature to explore the dynamics that underpin the AoN process as set down in the Disability Act 2005. In so doing, I have demonstrated the gap that often exists between programmatic rationalities and the intricacies of specific technologies, and the way in which the visions of particular policy and legislative initiatives are far more complex and messy at the frontline of implementation than stated ideals suggest (see also McDonald, Marston and Buckley, 2003; Caswell, Marston and Larsen, 2010). As a classificatory regime and tool of categorisation, the AoN exceeds definitions laid down in HSE guidance documents and the Act itself. Professionals build their own interpretations of what and who the person with a disability is under the terms of the Act, contributing to the creation of new spaces and subjectivities. For some, the AoN reflects those cases which are 'special' – in the sense that they exceed clinical diagnostic categories – and have led to the creation of what the NDA (2011: 75) terms a 'rarefied space' within the realm of early childhood intervention. For others, the subjectivities associated with the AoN are built around a moral discourse which constructs those applying to the process as less needy individuals trying to 'queue jump' existing referral systems – with some clinicians viewing the AoN as a 'backdoor to services' (cited in NDA, 2011: 60). In the context of historical service configurations, and a politics of diagnosis, then, clinicians are engaged in a process which builds into wider welfare debates that seek to distinguish between active, responsible welfare citizens, and those who fail to play by the rules of the game (Douglas, 2010). In the case of the AoN, this is represented through a discursive stratification of need in which some are seen as more needy, and hence more deserving of priority, according to professional criteria, than others.

The construction of these subjectivities highlights the ambiguity and confusion that professionals feel about working with the AoN, particularly in a context of service reconfiguration and welfare restraint. While the stated aims of the AoN appear to acknowledge and reinforce the significance of expert knowledges in the assessment process, clinicians are finding that it is forcing them to re-examine not just how they assess disability, but also how they manage their workloads and work across disciplinary boundaries. My analysis brings into sharp relief the messiness of technologies which seek to classify individuals, and in which 'there are misclassifications, negotiations and disagreement about the categories produced' (Caswell, Marston and Larsen, 2010: 400). It also illustrates how these classifications take on a life of their own through published statistics which, by making visible assessed need, create new problematisations for the Irish government and society more broadly (not least, in this case, 'what to do' about the issue of autism). The AoN therefore bears all the hallmarks of a biopolitical strategy of advanced neoliberal government, concerned with establishing the 'problem' of disability at both the scale of the individual body *and* the population, and governing those involved in administering such strategies at a distance through a range of regulatory techniques.

Empirically, the chapter also draws attention to the importance of engaging with those people who are charged with putting policy prescriptions and programme ideals into practice, and implementing particular technologies of government. Governmentality studies have frequently been criticised for focusing too heavily on the construction of the subject as a discursive, textual formation at the expense of exploring the localised social and political contexts which explain how subjects are mobilised in practice; the central focus on discursive rationalities often suggests a neat end point in terms of constructed subject positions, but tells us less about how individuals may respond to, or indeed resist these positions (Barnett *et al.*, 2008; McKee, 2009). For McKee (2009: 273–274), 'this preference to disregard messy empirical actualities results in a fundamental inability to account for why the governable subject, constituted through discourse, fails to turn up in practice' (see also Barnett *et al.*, 2008; Larner, 2000). I therefore suggest that understanding the positioning of different actors and subjectivities in the policy and/or legislative arena (including both those charged with *implementing* policy initiatives and those who are the *end recipients* of such initiatives) has to be informed by an awareness of the situated contexts of governing, the limits to governmental projects and the capacity of subjects to actively interpret and respond to programme rationalities in multiple, and often contradictory, ways.

References

Bardon, S. (2015) More than 13,000 awaiting assessment for speech therapy. *The Irish Times*, 31 August. Available from: www.irishtimes.com/news/health/more-than-13–000-awaiting-assessment-for-speech-therapy-1.2334389. Accessed 15 September, 2015.
Barnett, C., Clarke, N., Cloke, P. and Malpass, A. (2008) The elusive subjects of neo-liberalism. *Cultural Studies*, 22(5): 624–653.

Caswell, D., Marston, G. and Larsen, J.E. (2010) Unemployed citizen or 'at risk' client? Classification systems and employment services in Denmark and Australia. *Critical Social Policy*, 30(3): 384–404.

Commission on the Status of People with Disabilities (1996) *A Strategy for Equality*. Dublin, Stationery Office.

Considine, M. and Dukelow, F. (2009) *Irish Social Policy: A Critical Introduction*. Dublin, Gill and Macmillan.

De Wispelaere, J. and Walsh, J. (2007) Disability rights in Ireland: chronicle of a missed opportunity. *Irish Political Studies*, 22(4): 517–543.

Dean, M. (1995) Governing the unemployed self in an active society. *Economy and Society* 24(4): 559–583.

Dean, M. (1999) *Governmentality: Power and Rule in Modern Society*. London, Sage.

DoH (2012) *Value for Money and Policy Review of Disability Services in Ireland*. Dublin, DoH.

DoHC (2007) *Standards for the Assessment of Need*. Available from: http://health. gov.ie/wp-content/uploads/2014/03/standards_for_need_assessment.pdf. Accessed 15 September 2015.

Douglas, P. (2010) Problematising inclusion: education and the question of autism. *Pedagogy, Culture & Society*, 18(2): 105–121.

Evans, B. and Colls, R. (2009) Measuring fatness, governing bodies: the spatialities of the Body Mass Index (BMI) in anti-obesity politics. *Antipode*, 41(5): 1051–1083.

Government of Ireland (2005) *Disability Act 2005*. Available from: www.irishstatutebook.ie/2005/en/act/pub/0014/. Accessed 15 September 2015.

Hacking, I. (1982) Biopower and the avalanche of printed numbers. *Humanities in Society*, 5(3–4): 279–295.

Hacking, I. (2006) Making up people. *London Review of Books*, 28(16): 23–26.

HSE (n.d.a) *Report to the Minister for Disability, Equality, Mental Health and Older People at the DoH as Provided for Under Section 13 of the Disability Act 2005 in Respect of Data Collected in 2010*. Available from: www.hse.ie/eng/services/Publications/Disability/discbilityact2005inrespectdata2010.pdf. Accessed 15 September 2015.

HSE (n.d.b) *Report to the Minister for Equality, Disability, and Mental Health at the DoHC as Provided for Under Section 13 of the Disability Act 2005 in Respect of Data Collected in 2008 and 2009*. Available from: www.hse.ie/eng/services/Publications/Disability/data0809.pdf. Accessed 15 September 2015.

HSE (2010) *Disability Act 2005 Guidance Note No: 29(A): 11 August 2010*. Dublin, HSE (unpublished guidance note).

HSE (2015) *Annual Report and Financial Statements 2014*. Dublin, HSE.

Huxley, M. (2008) Space and government: governmentality and geography. *Geography Compass* 2(5): 1635–1658.

Illich, I. (1977) Disabling professions. IN: Illich, I., Zola, I.K., McKnight, J., Caplan, J. and Shaiken, H. (eds) *Disabling Professions*. London, Marion Boyars.

Junne, J. and Huber, C. (2014) The risk of users' choice: exploring the case of direct payments in German social care. *Health, Risk & Society*, 16(7–8): 631–648.

Kurunmäki, L. and Miller, P. (2006) Modernising government: the calculating self, hybridisation and performance measurement. *Financial Accountability and Management*, 22(1): 87–106.

Kurunmäki, L. and Miller, P. (2008) Counting the costs: The risks of regulating and accounting for health care provision. *Health, Risk & Society*, 10(1): 9–21.

Kurunmäki, L. and Miller, P. (2011) Regulatory hybrids: partnerships, budgeting and modernising government. *Management Accounting Research*, 22: 220–241.

Larner, W. (2000) Neo-liberalism: policy, ideology, governmentality. *Studies in Political Economy*, 63: 5–25.

Larner, W. and Le Heron, R. (2005) Neo-liberalising spaces and subjectivities: reinventing New Zealand universities. *Organization*, 12(6): 843–862.

McDonald, C., Marston, G. and Buckley, A. (2003) Risk technology in Australia: the role of the Job Seeker Classification Instrument in Employment Services. *Critical Social Policy*, 23: 498–525.

McKee, K. (2009) Post-Foucauldian governmentality: what does it offer critical social policy analysis? *Critical Social Policy*, 29(3): 465–486.

Miller, P. (2001) Governing by numbers: why calculative practices matter. *Social Research*, 68(2): 379–396.

Morgan, A. (2005) Governmentality versus choice in contemporary special education. *Critical Social Policy*, 25(3): 325–348.

NDA (2011) *National Disability Authority Report on the Practice of Assessment of Need under Part 2 of the Disability Act 2005*. Dublin, NDA.

Nolan, L. (2014) 'Autism-lite' is blamed for diagnoses rise. *The Sunday Times*, 7 September. Available from: www.thesundaytimes.co.uk/sto/news/ireland/article1456057.ece. Accessed 16 September, 2015.

O'Brien, C. (2013) Major delays assessing the needs of hundreds of children with disabilities. *The Irish Times*, 8 May. Available from: www.irishtimes.com/news/social-affairs/major-delays-assessing-the-needs-of-hundreds-of-children-with-disabilities-1.1385582. Accessed 23 February 2016.

O'Brien, C. (2014a) Thousands of children with disabilities waiting years for support. *The Irish Times*, 7 February. Available from: www.irishtimes.com/news/health/thousands-of-children-with-disabilities-waiting-years-for-supports-1.1682796. Accessed 16 September 2015.

O'Brien, C. (2014b) Child speech therapy services a 'lottery'. *The Irish Times*, 22 September. Available from: www.irishtimes.com/news/social-affairs/child-speech-therapy-services-a-lottery-1.1936985. Accessed 16 September 2015.

O'Malley, P., Weir, L. and Clifford, S. (1997) Governmentality, criticism, politics. *Economy and Society*, 26(4): 501–517.

Rose, N. and Miller, P. (1992) Political power beyond the state: problematics of government. *The British Journal of Sociology*, 43(2): 173–205.

Rose, N., O'Malley, P. and Valverde, M. (2006) Governmentality. *Annual Review of Law and Social Science*, 2: 83–104.

Rosenberg, C.E. (2002) The tyranny of diagnosis. *The Millbank Quarterly*, 80: 237–260.

Sullivan, M. (2005) Subjected bodies: paraplegia, rehabilitation and the politics of movement. IN: Tremain, S. (ed.) *Foucault and the Government of Disability*. Ann Arbour, University of Michigan Press: pp. 27–44.

The Irish Times (2010) Judge rules HSE must provide assessment to autistic boy. *The Irish Times*, 19 April. Available from: www.irishtimes.com/news/crime-and-law/judge-rules-hse-must-provide-assessment-to-autistic-boy-1.653930. Accessed 23 February 2016.

Tremain, S. (2005) Foucault, governmentality and critical disability theory: an introduction. IN: Tremain, S. (ed.) *Foucault and the Government of Disability*. Ann Arbour, University of Michigan Press: pp. 1–24.

Long-term care policy for older people in Ireland: a governmental analysis

Introduction

Over the last ten years, successive governments have introduced a range of policy reforms into the long-term care sector in Ireland with the aim of offering accessible, affordable services operating to high standards and focused on responding to the specific care needs of each individual (DoHC, 2005). This chapter seeks to analyse the reform process initiated in 2005, examining the policy tools used to improve care provision and their impact on older people. The chapter also examines the impact of recent budgetary constraints on the long-term care sector, as a result of the recession in Ireland's free market economy. The chapter is guided by a governmentality perspective, critically analysing the changing power relations within the long-term care sector in Ireland in recent years. To date, little analysis has been carried out on these reforms, and none from a governmentality perspective, which is particularly useful for understanding the 'art of government' (Foucault, 1991) – namely, for problematising the normative, accepted accounts of the state and deconstructing its inconsistencies. Theories of governmentality are also useful for exploring the complex power dynamics which operate in neoliberal societies and may provide useful insights into the 'mentalities of rule' operating in Ireland's long-term care sector, exploring how older people are conceptualised within key government policy reform documents and the impact that recent reforms have had on the sector, particularly in relation to the distribution of power among different key players.

The chapter begins by briefly introducing the theoretical and analytical framework for the chapter, and then goes on to provide an overview of the evolution of care policies in Ireland. Following this, the chapter examines how older people are conceptualised and analyses the relationships between the state and other stakeholders in the design and implementation of long-term care reform policies between 2005 and 2015. The chapter concludes with a discussion of the implications of these findings, including a brief commentary about what they reveal about governmentality more generally.

Governmentality and long-term care policy

Michel Foucault's concepts and ideas on power have become influential in a variety of disciplines. One of the key characteristics of his conceptualisation of power is that, rather than an oppressive, or negative, force, it should be seen more as a pervasive, subtle force through which individuals can be influenced or manipulated to think in a certain way. This is achieved by using various 'technologies of the self', namely, the methods used by subjects to transform themselves in order to achieve a certain quality of life. Drawing on this particular conceptualisation of power, Foucault developed the concept of governmentality, or 'the art of government' (Foucault, 1991), the aim of which is 'to secure the welfare of the population, the improvement of its condition, the increase of its wealth, longevity, health et cetera' (1991: 100).

Foucault was particularly interested in understanding neoliberalism as a form of governmentality, arguing that, at its heart, neoliberalism involves a shift from a strongly welfarist, interventionist, state to one that governs at a distance, and in which the operation of free markets seek to promote individual empowerment by offering opportunities for choice (see also Larner, 2000). Neoliberal strategies of rule encourage people to see themselves as active subjects, responsible for enhancing their own well-being. Thus, Foucault believed that modern (particularly neoliberal) states had the capacity to develop 'docile citizens' by producing certain discourses of knowledge that individuals internalise, which can lead to them governing their own behaviour.

Foucault's work on governmentality has been used by many other scholars as a framework for analysing power relations in society. The intention of a governmental analytics is not to jettison the state from scholarly analysis, but to reposition how we think about power and authority in late modern societies (Marston and McDonald, 2006). Governmentality scholars have tended to use Foucault's work on power as a theoretical lens or methodology to draw attention to the 'how' of governing, by considering how we think about the nature and practice of government (McKee, 2009), to identify the specific techniques and strategies through which citizen subjectivities come to be constructed in the management of populations, and to explore how power relations subtly produce subjects within society.

In particular, Cruikshank's (1999) central concept of technologies of citizenship describes a phenomenon whereby discourses and programmes aim at improving self-esteem and empowering people to further their own ends, but always within the context of the market economy. Such strategies are often subtle and seek to maximise the subjectivities of those perceived to lack the power to act on behalf of their own interests. In other words, they are intended to help people to help themselves, and they operate according to a specific political rationality. The outcome is that democratic citizens are both the effects and the instruments of liberal governance. Subjectivity is then seen as being both enabled and constrained by the relations of power. In order to govern individuals and utilise their capacity to achieve one's own objectives, it can be necessary to reformulate commonly understood activities, concepts and ideas. For example, if the lines between health and illness become blurred and confused, we reshape what, or who, is understood as 'ill', and thus can review, and in some cases narrow, the category of those who might be in need of care and support (Rose, 2007). This type of rhetoric, persuasion and strategic use of discourse can play a critical role in exercising the will to govern.

Atkinson and Coffey (2004) have suggested that written documents are a vital way in which individuals and organisations constitute 'reality' and the forms of knowledge appropriate to it, and so analysing rhetoric, persuasion and strategic use of discourse in textual data can reveal hidden cultural norms and assumptions through which specific groups operate. In the context of this chapter, a documentary analysis was carried out to investigate the reform of long-term care services in Ireland between 2005 and 2015 in order to examine how older people are conceptualised in the recent reforms in long-term care policy as well as their impact on the sector. The main documentary sources included in the analysis were policy planning and legislative documents relating to the development and implementation of long-term care policies and statistics primarily written or commissioned by government (public) sources. Documents written or commissioned by non-governmental sources were also included to supplement the main material, and these included documents drawn up or commissioned by civil society organisations and private sector providers.

Analysis of the documents developed in two stages. The first stage involved a general reading of each document in order to develop an overview of the main policy measures in chronological order. This analysis identified stages in the development of long-term care policy over the last ten years, each of which signalled a different attitude both to older people and to care planning. As such, each phase was subsequently analysed separately. The second stage consisted of a discourse analysis of the data. The theory of discourse analysis operates on the basis that the words we choose are never neutral; rather, they are shaped by our own social, political and historical experiences (Fairclough, 2000). As such, this second stage allowed an analysis of the use of rhetoric, persuasion and strategic use of discourse utilised by policymakers in the development of long-term care policy between 2005 and 2015. It involved a closer reading of the documents in order to identify patterns and trends in the language that might reveal insights into the attitudes and beliefs of the authors, both about older people themselves and the philosophy underpinning the organisation of care services.

The analysis of the long-term care reform process was informed by theories of governmentality, viewing the reform process as a part of neoliberal discourses in advanced welfare regimes. In line with a governmentality approach, the analysis sought to explore the 'how' of governing (McKee, 2009), by analysing how the various actors involved in the long-term care sector collaborated and negotiated to develop and implement the reform programme. It sought to examine the impact of the process and its outcomes on different actors, and aimed to identify the specific techniques and strategies through which 'citizen subjectivities come to be constructed in the management of populations' (Rose, 1999: 21), namely, how 'ageing' and 'older people' are conceptualised within key documents of the reform programme, and how this shapes how older people have come to view themselves and their attitudes towards long-term care. In line with McKee's (2009) argument that the state is a pivotal actor in shaping the conceptualisation of social problems and the proposed solutions, the chapter seeks to focus on the role of the state vis-à-vis other actors in terms of its position of power within the long-term care sector.

Governmentality has already been used to great effect in the study of gerontology, where it has helped to shatter 'taken for granted' assumptions centred on ageing (Powell and Biggs, 2003). It has been argued that the emphasis on personal choice in neoliberalism has led to the ageing process itself being constructed as a choice – whereby older people are expected to make the right choice and remain active and independent in old age (the 'Third Age'), rather than slide into the Fourth Age of decline and decrepitude (Gilleard and Higgs, 2010). Drawing on this work, this chapter seeks to explore how older people are conceptualised in long-term care policy in Ireland in light of the increased privatisation of long-term care services within the state, and the extent to which it has strengthened the way in which older people are responsibilised for making the right ageing choices (Powell, 2009).

Setting the context of long-term care policy

The decision to restructure and invest in care services for older people in Ireland in 2005 marked a major shift in government policy, standing in marked contrast to decades of inadequate funding and ad hoc planning. Partly influenced by the availability of funding from the Celtic Tiger years (Ireland's economic boom), the reform process also sought to amend for serious shortcomings in the management of the sector since the 1960s. Although official government policy since this time sought to enable older people to remain living in their own homes as long as possible, in practice, successive governments failed to develop home-care and community-based services, focusing instead on providing a limited supply of residential care and relying on families to provide informal care to the majority of those in need. Incentives were introduced to encourage private providers to set up nursing homes, in part as a way of limiting government spending in the sector. Indeed, public expenditure on residential care in Ireland was significantly lower than the Organisation for Economic Co-operation and Development (OECD) average for many years (OECD, 2005).

However, due to the rising costs of care and significant shortcomings in public spending on long-term care (Office of the Ombudsman 2001; 2010), care services for older people in Ireland were highly disjointed by 2005. In particular, provision of community services throughout the country was poor, coupled with poorly targeted residential care. The focus on expanding (residential) care for older people at the lowest possible cost to the state also led to the issue of quality being largely sidelined by successive governments (Mangan, 2002; National Economic and Social Forum, 2005; Murphy *et al.*, 2006). While Ireland's care services for older people thus contained elements of a neoliberal approach, namely, a reliance on the private sector to provide services and a focus on cost containment, there was little emphasis on 'responsibilising' older people to render themselves more governable (Foucault, 1982).

The organisation of long-term care services in Ireland in the mid-2000s stood in stark contrast to the sector elsewhere in Europe. Although coverage of long-term care services for older people varied widely throughout Europe in the 1980s and 1990s, rising costs of care, population ageing and a decline in informal care networks led many Western European countries to converge on a new approach to organising long-term care, characterised by the predominance of home care over residential care, and the targeting of public services towards the most dependent (even in traditionally social-democratic countries). This was coupled with a stronger reliance on informal care for those with fewer caring needs, and the opening up of the caring 'market' to competition to drive down costs and increase choice for those in need of care. Care policies for older people in Europe now broadly conform to a neoliberal model, with a focus on privatising services in order to reduce costs for the state (Pavolini and Ranci, 2008). Moreover, population ageing is leading governments to reduce demand for long-term care by promoting 'active ageing' (European Commission, 2014), effectively constructing ageing as a choice, in which age-related disease and frailty can be avoided at will – arguably a form of collective control of older people, making them docile and economically useful subjects (Powell, 2009). As I will go on to show, the reforms introduced into the long-term care sector between 2005 and 2015 brought Ireland closer in line with the rest of Europe.

Long-term care policies in Ireland 2005–2015:
a governmental analysis

As noted earlier, events leading up to 2005 meant that the long-term care sector was ready for significant reform. This coincided with the appointment of a new Minister for Health and Children, Mary Harney, in September 2004. Ms Harney, leader of the right-wing Progressive Democrat Party, indicated her intention to develop a more strategic vision of the Irish healthcare service, seeking to rationalise services and make the health service more accountable. This section outlines the main policy reforms that took place over the proceeding ten-year period, under Mary Harney, until 2011, and succeeded by appointments in the rival party, Fine Gael, which describes itself as a 'centrist' party, but is often perceived to be more right-leaning than other parties on the Irish political spectrum.

The section examines the ten-year period in three different phases, starting with the policy-planning phase between 2005 and 2007, during which new legislation was planned, and subsequently moving on to the implementation phase between 2008 and 2012, when many of the planned policies were brought to fruition. This section describes the challenges the government faced in rolling out policies planned during an economic boom but implemented in the midst of significant recession. Finally, the impact of governing a sector under flux in the context of extremely limited financial resources is described and analysed. Throughout the section, attention is drawn to the different technologies (rhetoric, persuasion, strategic use of discourse and technologies of self and citizenship) used to produce subjects within society in the context of shifting economic conditions and political objectives.

2005–2007: policy planning

In 2005, the Fianna Fáil-Progressive Democrat Government began to plan for a major reform of long-term care services. In January 2005, the Minister for Health established a Working Group on Long-Term Care to identify the policy options for a financially sustainable system of long-term care (DoHC, 2006a). The Working Group proposed a new funding scheme for residential care based on the principle of co-payment, or cost-sharing between the state and individuals for residential care, both in private and public settings. Those deemed in need of nursing home care (through a care needs assessment) would pay no more than 80% of their assessable income towards the cost of care, plus up to 5% of the value of their assets (including their house) per annum, for a maximum of three years (15%). This approach was heavily related to the concurrent property boom in Ireland, where house prices had doubled between 2000 and 2006. Dubbed 'The Fair Deal' by the Minister for Health when it was first announced, the scheme sought to put an end to the long-standing practice of some older people receiving almost no financial support from the state to pay for private residential long-term care, while others had their care fully paid for by the state. Eventually implemented in 2009 under the Nursing Home Support Scheme (NHSS) Act, the Fair Deal was intended to be relatively cost-neutral to the state, based on the assumption that house prices in Ireland would remain stable, or continue to rise, yielding the government a significant contribution from each resident.

The Working Group also recommended the roll-out of Home Care Packages (HCPs), support packages of care tailored to meet the needs of an individual, comprising the services of nurses, home help and various therapies, including physiotherapy and occupational therapy services. The HCP scheme was established to facilitate timely discharge from acute hospitals and offer enhanced support along with existing home help and community-based care services. It was a significant departure for long-term care policy in Ireland, as the government acknowledged for the first time that it had responsibility to provide home care for older people in Ireland (Timonen and Doyle, 2008). The scheme sought to improve home-care services by providing successful applicants with a budget they could use to buy the services they required to return home, regain their independence and remain living at home.

The official rationale for the various policy reform programmes announced in 2005 was to make long-term care more 'affordable, accessible and anxiety-free' (DoHC, 2006a). In announcing the NHSS in 2006, the Minister for Health indicated that it was a way of compensating older people for their contribution to Irish society:

> I am determined to put in place comprehensive health and social care for older people, in a way that is reliable, that respects and values older people, and that is fair financially to older people, their families and taxpayers alike ... It is entirely right that we should devote substantial additional resources to services for older people. They have made a great contribution to our society and to our present-day economic and social success. In this way, we are saying that the next generations value their contribution and will respect their needs and their continuing role in our society. (DoHC, 2005)

The HCP scheme sought to be 'comprehensive, reliable and to respect and value older people and be financially fair to them, their families and taxpayers alike':

> The investment package is focused on caring for people at home, where they want to be. It is a major step in focusing new resources on home care first and foremost, while still supporting appropriate residential care. (Minister for Health and Children, cited in *ibid.*).

However, a close reading of the policy-planning documents indicated that choice, respect and compensation were not the key drivers of the reform process. Instead, the focus was in keeping the costs incurred by the state as low as possible as it planned for a projected rise in the over-65 population. Indeed, the Working Group was anxious to ensure that older people be asked to contribute towards the cost of their care: 'It is clear that a substantial burden will fall on the Exchequer … The extent of the financing burden which falls on the State will depend on the level of co-payment which is contributed by care recipients' (DoHC, 2006a: 15).

The introduction of co-payments led to the Fair Deal being described as a 'selective inheritance tax on those who have suffered stroke or dementia' (Robinson and O'Shea, 2010: 153) as older people in need of nursing home care are the only group in Irish society who are effectively being asked to contribute twice to in-patient healthcare services which had been free of charge to all citizens in the public system since 1979:

> While some illnesses are precipitated by self-neglect, many are random; any one of us may be affected … No one has adequately explained why cancer or other high-cost treatments should be paid for by the State; whereas, a person suffering a stroke or dementia that requires extended nursing care should realise some of their assets to pay for care … In the ordinary course of events, all citizens contribute to this socialised cost via the taxes they pay to the State – it might be considered unreasonable to seek additional payments from citizens in the form of assets which have been acquired using income which has already been taxed. (Robinson and O'Shea, 2010: 152)

Indeed, the focus on trying to encourage positive ageing, evident in long-term care policies elsewhere in Europe, can also been seen in references to the independence of older people in the introduction of the HCP scheme: 'The investment package … is in line with international trends and also reflects the growing independence of older people who want to stay living in their communities' (Minister for Health and Children, cited in DoHC, 2005). This suggests an alternative perception of the policy reform programme as well as the use of rhetoric and the blurring of language in order to persuade citizens to accept the new policy changes (Cruikshank, 1999; Fairclough, 2000). Rather than seeking to put in place a system that meets the needs of a highly valued group who have made a significant contribution to the state, an ulterior agenda for the care service planning was to fulfil additional needs of the state, namely, to ensure a better budgetary balance in the area of healthcare. The focus on independence and self-reliance can be seen as a technology of citizenship (Dean, 1999), seeking to send a subconscious message to older people to remain autonomous and agentic; for each older person to become 'a model individual, conducting his life according to the precepts of health, and creating a medicalized society in order to bring conditions of life and conduct in line with requirements of health' (Cousins and Hussain, 1984: 151). This arguably shows older people with caring needs as pawns in the policy process; a policy problem to be resolved rather than a group to be served. This argument is strengthened by the fact that the *quality* of care services was broadly side-lined from the reform process until an unforeseen event gave it a greater priority.

In May 2005, a documentary, *Home Truths*, was broadcast on national television containing hidden footage of the 'systematic abuse' (O'Neill, 2006: 60) of residents in a private nursing home based in North Dublin, Leas Cross. In response, the Minister for Health established a new health-care regulator, the Health Information and Quality Authority (HIQA), to regulate the residential care sector (as well as healthcare settings more widely). HIQA was tasked with developing a set of minimum quality standards to regulate the residential care sector for older people, which sought to ensure that care providers focused on the needs of each individual resident and created an atmosphere in which residents felt safe and free to express their needs.

Such an approach responds to global calls for the rights and 'personhood' of older people to be respected, and for their autonomy to be maintained (O'Dwyer, 2013). However, the Standards focused on the protection of residents' consumer (as opposed to human) rights. In the few instances where there is acknowledgement of residents living together in the Standards, the focus is largely on formalised interaction between residents and staff, rather than on social engagement. The relationship between residents and the provider is also described in impersonal terms, as that of a client–contractor. In agreeing to move into the care setting, residents enter into, and negotiate, a contract with the provider. The formality of the provider–client relationship is also emphasised in the requirement for providers to provide an accurate description of the service and its cost prior to purchasing (Criteria 1.1 and 1.3), evoking an image of residents as discerning customers. Indeed, this service-oriented model of residential care for older people has previously been described as 'hotel-style accommodation', in which the residents are seen as 'customers who are always right' (Bland, 1999: 539). Although this approach seeks to provide older residents with greater empowerment and autonomy, it fails to acknowledge the difficulties older people living in residential care have in making choices and exercising their rights without adequate facilitation, due to the high prevalence of dementia and other forms of cognitive impairments, physical disability and fear of repercussions. A consumer-driven care system has many benefits for the state and the market, turning residential care into a commodity to be traded, a phenomenon Scourfield (2007) dubs 'caretelisation'. Yet discussing social relationships in terms of 'contracts' disguises the wider, often hidden, power relationships that underpin and shape observable reality (Powell, 2009).

Overall, therefore, it appears that there were some divergences between how care-policy reform initiatives introduced in 2005–2006 were marketed by the Minister for Health and her Department, and their implications in terms of benefits to the state. The NHSS and HCP scheme and quality standards were all introduced within a discourse of choice, freedom and fairness, part of the rhetoric of neoliberalism which focuses on selling freedom – that is, the freedom for citizen-consumers to choose goods and services which help them create their identity (Rose, 1999). The new policies at first sight appeared to challenge ageism and highlight the importance of autonomy, while in practice facilitating the government's agenda of shifting responsibility and saving money (Biggs, 2001; Powell, 2009). As a result, the policy reforms appeared less about valuing the contribution made by older people to society and more about encouraging them to make the right choices – to remain active and agentic (Jones and Higgs, 2010), either by avoiding the need for care services altogether, or accepting the responsibility of identifying the care home that best suited their needs and navigating access themselves. In turn, this released the state from the burden of carrying out these functions as would generally occur under a welfare-led system (Pavolini and Ranci, 2008). This approach reflects traces of 'care management' (Powell, 2009), whereby older people's right to welfare and adequate care becomes the subjects of a restricted, consumerised care system. Thus, as is typical of neoliberal regimes, the policies seeking to devolve autonomy and responsibility from the state to older people represent a form of 'regulated freedom' in which each individual is used to secure the ends of government (Rose, 1999). In turn, 'the creation of market-mimicking choice mechanisms in public services ... will tend to reproduce social and economic inequalities' (Clarke, Newman and Westmarland, 2008) and may serve to act against those whom governmental projects identify as requiring protection.

2008–2012: roll-out and review

Determining what authorities *wanted* to happen in relation to the objectives and strategies pursued is just the start of an analytics of governmentality (Rose, 1999). There is often a difference between the design of government policy and how it is implemented in practice; such a difference can also reveal much about how power and control are exercised in society (Rose, 1999). This is particularly the case in how care policies for older people were rolled out in Ireland, with the global economic recession playing a significant role in how policies were implemented. As outlined below, this led to private care homes being forced to share some of the costs of the services which the state could no longer afford.

As noted earlier, the NHSS was intended to be relatively cost-neutral to the state, based on the assumption that the economic boom in Ireland would continue, and thereby yielding the government a significant contribution from each resident. However, with house prices in Ireland falling by more than 51% from their peak, the state faced significantly higher-than-expected bills to finance the scheme. This was potentially highly damaging to the sitting government. Older people in Ireland are strong voters and so remain important to politicians; 88% of voters aged 65 and over voted in Ireland's last general election (Centre for Ageing Research and Development in Ireland, 2011). Effectively abolishing a much-lauded long-term care scheme for older people could cause the government to lose power at the ballot box.

So, instead of ending the scheme, the government altered some of the details in order to make the overall programme financially viable. Under the 2009 NHSS Act, the National Treatment Purchase Fund (NTPF), a state company, was tasked with negotiating the price it would give each private nursing home for accepting and caring for a resident under the scheme (it should be noted that public nursing homes were not expected to negotiate with the NTPF). Private nursing homes were given little option as to what the NTPF would pay them for each resident and, where an agreement could not be reached, the home would fail to be recognised as an 'approved' nursing home, and would not be able to accept any residents under the scheme. Thus, the 2009 Act effectively made residential care for older people a monopsony, with prices determined by the buyer (the state). Furthermore, care homes were only reimbursed for 'bed and board', with no reimbursement for physiotherapy, occupational therapies, chiropody, social programmes and other specialist equipment.

In order to avoid criticism for such stringent cutbacks, the government found a scapegoat to deflect the public's ire. Press releases from the Department of Health and Children (DoHC) began to capitalise on a general negative sentiment about private nursing homes, subtly arguing that private nursing homes were overcharging for residential care and yielding high profits to the detriment of residents, and the state:

> Private nursing homes can cost about €50,000 per year. Many people ... cannot afford to pay the balance of their costs. As a result, people are sometimes forced to sell or mortgage their homes to pay for care, or must rely on contributions from their family or friends. [Under the NHSS], the State will pay all the balance, in both public and private nursing homes [and] will continue to pay for the majority of care costs overall. (www.dohc.ie/press/releases/pdfs/fair_deal_info.pdf?direct=1)

In doing so, the government was creating a 'truth' that the high costs of private care were unsustainable and that the DoHC was an altruistic actor seeking to achieve the best interests of older people. Cotoi (2011) terms this the neoliberal state's space of veridiction, where a truth is created through the use of rhetoric which serves policymakers as well as citizen-consumers. However, in practice, private-care providers had received much of their funding from the state's subvention scheme, which was not keeping up with the rising staff and building costs of providing care in private homes (O'Shea, 2003). These measures were not enough to prevent a significant overspend on the NHSS by the state. In 2010, the first full year of the scheme's operation, funding was capped, with the possibility of waiting lists emerging in the event of the limit of the scheme being reached. Indeed, the scheme was suspended for a month in May 2011 and was again suspended for older people living in their own homes in April 2013 in order to clear beds in acute hospitals. In December 2013, the waiting time for allocation to a home under the scheme was seventeen weeks.

While cost overruns underpinned the exercise of the scheme, arguably the most contentious issue about the introduction of the NHSS was the change it signified in terms of the state's responsibility to provide residential care services to older people. Research conducted by the Office of the Ombudsman (2010) found that the legislation introducing the NHSS removed the right of older people to long-term residential care. As a result, older people in need of residential care no longer have a right to care free at the point of service: 'In summary, then, each individual is liable to meet the full costs of their long-term residential care, although they can apply to the Health Service Executive (HSE) for financial support ... in accordance with the terms of the Nursing Homes Support Scheme' (Office of the Ombudsman, 2010: 84). This is a radical departure for the state. Ultimately, the costs associated with residential care have motivated the Irish government to 'dismantle' a part of the welfare state in order to save precious resources. It could be argued that the Irish state's 'governance' of the private residential care sector displayed regulatory strategies to manage the market and undercut the sector, not least as it became clear to the government that the loss of residential care supply could be replaced by cheaper home-care services. The result of this has been some private-sector nursing homes exiting the sector completely: private provision fell from 14,932 beds in 2008 to 13,375 in 2011, a reduction of 10%.

If the private residential care sector is a 'loser' in the long-term care reform process, private home-care providers are clear winners. Part of their success came about through the effective lobbying of the government by Home Care and Community Care Ireland (HCCI), a representative body of private home-care providers, of the government on the basis of financial calculations:

> This report provides evidence-based research to support the case for a phased outsourcing of home care service provision in Ireland in line with the Minister for Health and HSE calls for increased efficiencies and innovative models of care. The findings are important, not least that some €2 billion could be saved over the period to 2021, for patients, providers and the general taxpayer. The new delivery model which has been informed by emerging best practice in other jurisdictions will offer patients what they want: quality care at home, choice of provider, a more affordable service and the opportunity to stay at home for much longer. HCCI's overall view is that the Government needs to regulate and supervise the provision of home care but that does not mean the

HSE has to be involved in the actual delivery of that care. (EPS Consulting, 2013: 4)

Since the implementation of the HCP scheme, the home-care sector has increased significantly, from 10,968 individuals in receipt of services in 2011 to 13,199 in 2014, with just an 8% increase in funding (EPS Consulting, 2013; PA Consulting, 2009), representing a significant improvement in value for money. A major factor in this success was the increased use of the private sector in service provision (Timonen, Doyle and O'Dwyer, 2013). Indeed, the scheme stimulated the development of private home-care companies, which had previously only been used by those who were not entitled to any state support and could afford to pay for home-care services privately. Using private-sector organisations to supply home-care services represented considerable cost savings for the state; calculations made in 2009 by the private sector estimated the cost difference to be as much as 30% (PA Consulting, 2009). In 2012, the HSE organised a tender process for HCP delivery, the terms of which required successful organisations to offer HCPs at a set budget while adhering to minimum quality standards. Twenty-one of the twenty-four successful applicants were private, for-profit providers. As a result, the private home-care sector has almost doubled its 'market share' of the total home-care sector, from 6% in 2009 to 11% in 2013 (EPS Consulting, 2013; PA Consulting, 2009).

Increasingly, then, the idea of care as an economic, least-cost sum has become normalised within Irish society, with market actors playing an increasingly prominent role in the regulation of the choice rhetoric that benefits the state, as well as private providers. Moreover, if private home-care providers are winners in the outcomes, it is also clear that, as before, older people in need of care services can also be classed as losers in the implementation of the 2005 reforms. Although the original plan developed by the Working Group was for a stronger home-care service for older people in Ireland, with clear eligibility criteria, in practice it was rolled out as an administrative scheme. As a result, there is no automatic right to the HCP scheme, nor a right to avail of services under it. While the funding for the service has been increasing year on year, allowing expansion of the scheme (with 9,941 recipients in December 2010 to 13,199 in December 2013), there are no official figures on demand for the scheme, indicating that the control of information, as well as rhetoric, can be used as a tool to create uncertainty as to whether there is a supply shortage in the long-term care sector.

There was limited opposition to the inadequate supply of long-term care services, both residential and home-based, from older people themselves. The consistent use of persuasive and divisive language, vilifying the private residential care sector, has helped to reduce opposition to the shift in policy and service provision. In addition, older people's interest groups in Ireland are poorly resourced, and tend to focus on active older people (Doyle, 2014). Indeed, Swyngedouw (2005) suggests that financial cutbacks affecting civil society organisations during economic recessions can in themselves be a deliberate tool of governmentality to reduce resistance to a new social order that supports the creation of docile citizens. Retaining the support of the 'grey vote' in Ireland is particularly important, given that those aged 65 and over represent 17% of the electorate.

Cost overruns in care services for older people have also led to the deprioritisation of the quality of care services once again. While HIQA's standards appear to have increased the quality of residential care services (National Economic and Social Forum, 2012), the state has admitted that it does not have the resources for many of its outdated care settings to meet the minimum standards required. As a result, a duality appears to be emerging, whereby private homes are expected to meet the standards, while public (statutory) homes are exempt. Furthermore, as the state dictates the price the homes receive per resident, as well as the regulations on key aspects of the quality of the service, such as the staff ratio, care homes have little discretion in how they can maximise quality while also retaining a profit:

> Through inspections which St Monica's [residential care setting] has passed with flying colours, one arm of the State, HIQA rightly demands the highest standards of care and compliance, while now another arm of the State is demanding cuts that inevitably will result in a lowering of those standards. (Office of the Ombudsman, 2010: 96)

This arguably demonstrates that the market does not share equal power with the state in neoliberal societies, with regulation (via HIQA) acting as a technique to manage the behaviour of care homes at a distance. The prospect of an inspection attempts to responsibilise care providers as well as older people, encouraging them to strive for high quality in return for demand for their service. Thus, even in neoliberal societies, for-profit providers must also recognise and respect the ultimate market rule of value for money, or pay the ultimate price.

2012–2015: the politics of doing nothing

In February 2011, Fianna Fáil was swept from power following the worst defeat of a sitting government party since the formation of the Irish state in 1922. Seen as responsible for creating the economic recession in Ireland and failing to respond quickly and decisively enough to avoid further problems developing, it lost over fifty seats in the election. It was replaced by a Fine Gael–Labour coalition. Healthcare reform was a major plank of Fine Gael's election strategy, promising to dismantle the HSE, end efforts to privatise the health system and promote community-based services for older people (Fine Gael, 2011). However, due to the ongoing financial crisis, healthcare remained under-resourced, with spending on the sector overall reducing by 6.6% between 2008 and 2014. As outlined below, this has had the effect of compromising the policy goals of the Fine Gael–Labour government in relation to long-term care for older people. While small achievements were made in relation to home-care services, little effort was made to resolve the shortcomings in the sector, particularly the undersupply of care services. Instead, efforts have been concentrated on a type of policy rhetoric, whereby the government has sought to illustrate its commitment to the needs of older people in ways that require little concrete action.

When the Fine Gael–Labour government came to power in March 2011, the NHSS and the residential care sector more broadly were both in crisis. As outlined above, there was a large waiting list for the scheme every year and its dedicated budget had been inadequate since its inception. Approximately 2,000 individuals awaited a bed under the scheme at any one time, with an average wait of fifteen to seventeen weeks. Yet in spite of this, the budget for the scheme was cut by €35 million in 2014, with a consequent reduction of 1,700 beds funded under the scheme. A decision was taken to divert €23 million of the scheme's 2015 ring-fenced budget to be used on HCPs. In spite of the bed shortage, the Fine Gael–Labour government did not seek to increase the capacity of the residential care sector until 2015, when it announced the development of 115 short-stay 'step-down' beds to relieve the pressure on acute care settings. However, this figure appears somewhat insignificant in the context of the limited capacity of the residential care sector to keep up with growing demand, with many nursing homes operating at full capacity (AIB, 2014), and planned new homes and expansions of approximately 339 beds per annum unlikely to keep up with a forecasted demand of 1,000 beds per annum (BDO Ireland, 2014).

There has been little enthusiasm by the government for the scheme's reform. In 2012, the Department of Health (DoH) announced a review of the NHSS which has not yet been completed almost four years later. In February 2015, the Director of the HSE called the Scheme the 'Achilles Heel' of the health service, and suggested that budgetary top-ups would only reduce waiting times temporarily, as more people were coming on the waiting list due to demographic pressures (Cullen, 2015; Burke, 2015). Similarly, the Minister with responsibility for long-term care admitted that the Scheme was 'unsustainable in its present form' (cited in Cullen, 2015) in the context that the Scheme will cost €950 million in 2015 while bringing in only €75 million through resident co-payments. As she stated, 'The notion that you would pay €260–€290 for a service costing anything up to €1,200 is unsustainable' (cited in *ibid.*). However, she subsequently indicated that the budgetary shortfall will continue to come from the public purse (*ibid.*). Overall, therefore, while the scheme continues to exist in a permanent crisis mode, the response by politicians can be classified as one of inertia.

As noted above, strengthening home and community-based services was a key goal of the Fine Gael–Labour government. It showed considerable initiative in expanding home-care services by introducing a new programme in 2014 of intensive HCPs, to offer enhanced community services above the normal levels available from mainstream provision (DoH, 2014a). However, only twenty intensive HCPs were in place in December 2014, while the waiting list for the NHSS was fifteen weeks, highlighting a lack of urgency and innovation in responding to the care undersupply crisis.

Since the early 2000s, advocacy organisations for older people in Ireland had been calling on the government to develop a National Positive Ageing Strategy (NPAS) (DoH, 2013a) to replace the former national policy for older people, *The Years Ahead* (Working Party on Services for the Elderly (1988), the ageing strategy published in 1988). However, successive governments had failed to do so, largely because of the limited financial resources to develop a viable and ambitious plan. When the Fine Gael–Labour government took office in 2011, it made a commitment to complete and implement the NPAS. It established a cross-departmental working group in 2012 and, following extensive consultation with older people and their representative organisations, the NPAS was published in April 2013. However, the Strategy is a clear reflection of the weak economic environment. It does not contain any new concrete commitments to improve the system, such as increasing the availability of home- and community-based services. Instead, objectives are vague and in line with long-held objectives for care services for older people: 'Objective 2.2 Promote the development and delivery of a continuum of high quality care services and supports that are responsive to the changing needs and preferences of people as they age and at end of life' (DoH, 2013a: 33).

Furthermore, the Strategy emphasises the importance of healthy living for lowering the prevalence of many diseases often associated with later life, 'such as dementia, arthritis, diabetes, sensory impairments and congestive heart conditions, to name a few' (DoH, 2013a: 29), evoking once again the suggestion that older people have choices to make in terms of ageing well: 'While there is evidence that it is difficult to change the behaviour patterns of older people, research has also found that changes in lifestyle, even in later years can bring health benefits' (*ibid.*: 30). At the launch of the NPAS, the Minister for Older People stated that this new agency provided the blueprint for planning – for what we can and must do – individually and collectively – to make Ireland a good country in which to grow older (DoH, 2013b). While she promised an implementation plan for the strategy within six months (by December 2014) which would set out actions, timelines and performance indicators, to date (July 2015), the implementation plan has not yet been published. This may indicate that the purpose behind its development was to appear active in the area of ageing and long-term care without committing any financial resources to the sector.

However, the rhetoric on active and positive ageing indicates a continuation of the policy objective of responsibilising older people, and thus relieving the government itself of its own responsibility towards older people with caring needs.

The Fine Gael-led government also announced its commitment to develop a National Dementia Strategy by 2013. In 2013, the DoH convened a working group to oversee the development of the National Dementia Strategy which was ultimately launched in December 2014 (DoH, 2014b). However, as with the NPAS, the National Dementia Strategy clearly sets out priority actions (*inter alia* the provision of a better understanding of dementia in society; timely diagnosis and intervention, integrated services, supports and care for people with dementia and their carers), but only includes aspects which are considered to be capable of delivery within existing resources, or by reconfiguring the resources which are currently available. While the National Dementia Strategy does not have an implementation plan, the fact that over €30 million has been ring-fenced for the initiative does suggest a clearer intention for implementation compared to the NPAS. However, this could be explained by the financial contribution from a large philanthropic organisation, Atlantic Philanthropies, which donated €14.7 million for its implementation. Atlantic also noted in 2014 that, since 2012, it spend of €9.6 million on dementia in Ireland has leveraged an additional €5.8 million from the HSE. This helps to indicate how non-state actors can have a powerful role in determining the policy agenda, provided they have the financial resources to do so.

Conclusion

Although neoliberal governmentality seeks 'to secure the welfare of the population' (Foucault, 1991: 100), liberal policies typically battle to reconcile an interest in the population's well-being with a determination that the state should be frugal, and should constantly seek to curtail its activities in the interests of cost and liberty (McKinlay, Carter and Pezet, 2012). This summation is an accurate description of the formation and implementation of care policies for older people in Ireland over the last ten years. Overall, it is clear that the competing goals of successive Irish governments have been to limit spending on care services for older people, particularly following the onset of austerity, while retaining the goodwill of older voters. This may help to explain why the official rationale for the policy reform programme in 2006 was to recognise and repay older people for their contributions to society throughout their lives, while unofficially seeing the ageing population as a 'burden', with an urgent need to overhaul costly care systems. Encouraging older people to make the 'right' ageing choices allowed the government to relieve some of its own burden by shifting responsibility for care management onto older people themselves while also appealing to older people's desire to remain independent and youthful. This policy agenda mirrors that which has taken place elsewhere (Biggs, 2001; Clarke, Newman and Westmarland, 2008; Gilleard and Higgs, 2010; Powell, 2009), moving Ireland closer to the typical European organisation of long-term care services, and allowing the government to portray itself as generous and fair while in practice seeking cost savings for the state by cutting professional support for accessing care services (Pavolini and Ranci, 2008). Thus, in Ireland, as elsewhere, older people who do need support to access and use long-term care services become a silent aberration, unable to publicly highlight the challenges they face, because they have failed to meet societal expectations of the new old age (Gilleard and Higgs, 2010).

The implementation of the policy reforms in the era of austerity led to a greater focus on cost saving, with clear winners and losers in the sector. Private residential care providers, who face high costs, now have the price of care dictated by the state. Far from the introduction of the free market bringing greater choice, private providers have limited options, insofar as they either accept the new status quo or resist it by exiting the market. That the sitting government managed to bring the residential care sector under such tight control highlights the power of the use of obfuscation, rhetoric and coercion as tools of governance (McKee, 2009). The home-care sector has become the government's new champion, not only because it offers choice, independence and autonomy to older people at a lower cost to the state, but because it was able to successfully articulate its potential in a market-based economy. This highlights not only the state's indirect steering role in the market, but shows how different actors adapt to the cost-based perspective.

My analysis, particularly in highlighting the position of private providers, shows how a complex, hybrid form of governance exists in Ireland. While the state takes centre stage in the formation of the new institutional configurations, key decisions over resource allocation, use and transformation are taken by private actors who operate within the constraining or enabling regulatory framework of systems of government (Swyngedouw, 2005). In tandem, the rights of older people have been replaced with obligations. Older people in Ireland have had the automatic right to long-term care taken away, to be replaced with access to and funding for services at the discretion of the state and private-care providers. Paradoxically, this in turn raises questions about citizenship in Ireland, and in neoliberal societies; older people are seen as important only for their vote, yet get little in return. The driving down of costs, without an adequate focus on quality, or long-term sustainability, is simply a denial of the market's capacity to serve all needs (Clarke, Newman and Westmarland, 2008). As this chapter has indicated, older citizens have become mere pawns in a power struggle between the government and the market.

References

AIB (2014) *Outlook: Long Term Care report.* Dublin: AIB, Nursing Homes Ireland.

Atkinson, P. and Coffey, A. (2004) Analysing documentary realities. IN: Silverman, D. (ed.) *Qualitative Research: Theory, Method and Practice* (second edition). London, Sage: pp. 56–75.

BDO Ireland (2014) *Health's Ageing Crisis: Time for Action – A Future Strategy for Ireland's Long-term Residential Care Sector.* Dublin, Nursing Homes Ireland.

Biggs, S. (2001) Toward critical narrativity: stories of aging in contemporary social policy. *Journal of Aging Studies*, 15(4): 303–316.

Bland, R. (1999) Independence, privacy and risk: two contrasting approaches to residential care for older people. *Ageing and Society*, 19(5): 539–560.

Burke, S. (2015) The can has been kicked down the road yet again by a Government lacking courage. *Irish Independent*, 21 July.

Centre for Ageing Research and Development in Ireland (2011) *Focus on Older Voters.* Dublin, Centre for Ageing Research and Development in Ireland.

Clarke, J., Newman, J. and Westmarland, L. (2008) The antagonisms of choice: New Labour and the reform of public services. *Social Policy and Society*, 7(2): 245–253.

Cotoi, C. (2011) Neoliberalism: a Foucauldian perspective. *International Review of Social Research*, 1(2): 109–124.

Cousins, M. and Hussain, A. (1984) *Michel Foucault.* New York, St Martin's Press.

Cruikshank, B. (1999) *The Will to Empower: Democratic Citizens and Other Subjects.* Ithaca, NY: Cornell University Press.

Cullen, P. (2015) No increased payments for nursing home scheme, Minister insists. *The Irish Times*, 13 February.

Dean, M. (1999) *Governmentality: Power and Rule in Modern Society.* London, Sage.

Dean, M. (2010) *Governmentality: Power and Rule in Modern Society* (second edition). London, Sage.

DoH (2013a) *Positive Ageing Starts Now! The National Positive Ageing Strategy.* Dublin, DoH.

DoH (2013b) *Minister Kathleen Lynch Launches the National Positive Ageing Strategy.* Dublin, DoH.

DoH (2014a) Government launches Irish National Dementia Strategy. Press release, DoH, 17 December. Available from: http://health.gov.ie/blog/press-release/irish-national-dementia-strategy/.

DoH (2014b) *The Irish National Dementia Strategy.* Dublin, DoH.

DoHC (2005) €150m Budget package for new services for older people 'largest ever' –Tánaiste press release, 8 December 2005. Available from: http://health.gov.ie/blog/press-release/the-tanaiste-and-minister-for-health-mary-harney-t-d-today-set-out-the-details-of-the-wide-ranging-new-services-being-funded-with-the-e150m-package-announced-by-the-minister-for-finance-in-yesterday/. Accessed 12 July 2015.

DoHC (2006a) *Long-Term Care Report.* Dublin, DoHC.

DOHC (2006b) Minister announces Fair Deal on long term nursing home care. Press release, DOHC, 12 December. Available from: http://health.gov.ie/blog/press-release/minister-announces-fair-deal-on-long-term-nursing-home-care/.

Doyle, M. (2014) *The Politics of Old Age: Older People's Interest Organisations and Collective Action in Ireland*. Manchester, Manchester University Press.

EPS Consulting (2013) *The Business Case for the Outsourcing of Home Care Provision and a More Efficient Use of Fair Deal Funds*. Dublin, Home and Community Care Ireland.

European Commission (2014) *Adequate Social Protection for Long-term Care Needs in an Ageing Society*. Brussels, European Commission.

Fairclough, N. (2000) *New Labour, New Language?* London, Routledge.

Fine Gael (2011) *Fine Gael Manifesto*. Dublin, Fine Gael.

Foucault, M. (1982) The subject and power. *Critical Enquiry*, 8(4): 777–795.

Foucault M. (1988) Technologies of the self. IN: Martin, L., Gutman, H. and Hutton, P. (eds) *Technologies of the Self: A Seminar with Michel Foucault*. Amherst, University of Massachusetts Press: pp. 16–49.

Foucault, M. (1991) Governmentality. IN: Burchell, G., Gordon, C. and Miller, P. eds. *The Foucault Effect: Studies in Governmentality*. Hemel Hempstead, Harvester Wheatsheaf: pp. 87–104.

Foucault, M. (2008) *The Birth of Biopolitics: Lecture at the Collège de France, 1978–1979*. Basingstoke, Palgrave.

Gilleard, C. and Higgs, P. (2009) The power of silver: age and identity politics in the 21st century. *Journal of Aging and Social Policy*, 21(3): 277–295.

Gilleard, C. and Higgs, P. (2010) Ageing without agency: theorising the Fourth Age. *Ageing & Mental Health*, 14(2): 121–128.

HIQA (2009) *National Quality Standards for Residential Care Settings for Older People in Ireland*. Health Information and Quality Authority, Dublin.

Jones, I. and Higgs, P. (2010) The natural, the normal and the normative: contested terrains in ageing and old age. *Social Science & Medicine*, 71(8): 1513–1519.

Larner, W. (2000) Neo-liberalism: policy, ideology, governmentality. *Studies in Political Economy*, 63: 5–26.

Mangan, I. (2002) *Older People in Long Stay Care*. Dublin, The Human Rights Commission.

Marston, G. and McDonald, C. (2006) Introduction: reframing social policy analysis. IN: Marston, G. and McDonald, C. (eds) *Analysing Social Policy: A Governmental Approach*. Cheltenham, Edward Elgar: pp. 1–13.

McKee, K. (2009) Post-Foucauldian governmentality: what does it offer critical social policy analysis? *Critical Social Policy*, 29: 465–486.

McKinlay, A. Carter, C. and Pezet, E. (2012) Governmentality, power and organization. *Management & Organizational History*, 7(1): 3–15.

Murphy, K., O'Shea, E., Cooney, A., Shiel, A. and Hodgins, M. (2006) *Improving Quality of Life for Older People in Long-Stay Care Settings in Ireland*. NCAOP, Dublin.

National Economic and Social Forum (2005) *Care for Older People*. Report No. 32. Dublin, NESC.

National Economic and Social Forum (2012) *Implementation of the Home Care Package Scheme*. Report No. 38. Dublin, NESC.

O'Dwyer, C. (2013) Official conceptualizations of person-centred care: which person counts? *Journal of Aging Studies*, 27(3): 233–242.

OECD (2005) *Long-term Care for Older People*. Paris, OECD.

Office of the Ombudsman (2001) *Nursing Home Subventions: An Investigation by the Ombudsman of Complaints Regarding Payment of Nursing Home Subventions by Health Boards*. Dublin, Office of the Ombudsman.

Office of the Ombudsman (2010) *Who Cares? An Investigation into the Right to Nursing Home Care in Ireland*. Dublin, Office of the Ombudsman.

Older and Bolder (2008) *Older and Bolder's Closing Conference: Conference Proceedings*. Dublin, Advocacy Initiative.

O'Neill, D. (2006) *Leas Cross Review: A Review of the Deaths at Leas Cross Nursing Home 2002–2005*. Naas, HSE.

O'Shea, E. (2003) *Review of the Nursing Home Subvention Scheme*. Dublin, Stationery Office.

PA Consulting (2009) *Evaluation of Home Care Packages*. Dublin, Stationery Office.

Pavolini, E. and Ranci, C. (2008) *Restructuring* the welfare state: reforms in long-term care in Western European countries. *Journal of European Social Policy*, 18(3): 246–259.

Powell, J. (2009) Social theory, aging, and health and welfare professionals: A Foucauldian 'toolkit'. *Journal of Applied Gerontology*, 28 (6): 669–682.

Powell, J. and Biggs, S. (2003) Foucauldian gerontology: a methodology for understanding aging. *Electronic Journal of Sociology*, 7, 2.

Robinson, D. and O'Shea, D. (2010) Nursing home funding – deal or no deal? – an Irish perspective. *Age and Ageing*, 39(2): 152–153.

Rose, N. (1999) *Powers of Freedom: Reframing Political Thought*. Cambridge, Cambridge University Press.

Rose, N. (2007) *The Politics of Life Itself: Biomedicine, Power and Subjectivity in the Twenty-First Century*. Princeton, Princeton University Press.

Rose, N. and Miller, P. (1992) Political power beyond the state: problematics of government. *British Journal of Sociology*, 43(2): 172–205.

Scourfield, P. (2007) Are there reasons to be worried about the 'caretelization' of residential care? *Critical Social Policy*, 27(2): 155–180.

Seanad Public Consultation Committee (2012) *Report on The Rights of Older People*. Dublin, Oireachtas.

Swyngedouw, E. (2005) Governance Innovation and the Citizen: The Janus Face of Governance-beyond-the-State. *Urban Studies*, 42(11): 1991–2006.

Timonen, V. and Doyle, M. (2008) From the workhouse to the home. The historical origins and development of domiciliary care services for older people in Ireland. *International Journal of Sociology and Social Policy*, 28(3/4): 76–89.

Timonen, V., Doyle, M. and O'Dwyer, C. (2013) Expanded but not regulated: ambiguity in home care policy in Ireland. *Health and Social Care in the Community*, 20(3): 310–318.

Working Party on Services for the Elderly (1988) *The Years Ahead: A Policy for the Elderly*. Dublin, Stationery Office.

12   Eluska Fernández and Claire Edwards

Conclusion: governmentality, health policy and the place of critical politics

Introduction

Our starting point in gathering together this edited collection was a desire to explore the potential of governmentality-inspired ideas to develop a more nuanced and indeed critical understanding of the construction of health-based policy in Ireland. Health policy analysis in the Irish state, like much social policy research in general, has often taken its starting point from positivist approaches in social science, echoing Osborne's (1997) assertion that health policy is often conceptualised as a reaction to real, objective conditions, be that obesity, mental illness, disability or health inequalities. While critiques of Ireland's health system exist and have played a significant role in highlighting the inequitable dynamics of the health system and governmental agendas in the health arena (see for example Burke, 2009), these have had less to say about the usefulness or otherwise of specific theoretical approaches in understanding health policy, and also pay little attention to how particular health issues come to be problematised in the first place. This volume has sought to explore the potential of governmentality as a way of opening up different lines of analysis about the construction of health and health policy through specific empirical examples, while also using these examples to reflect back on the analytic potential – and indeed limits – of governmentality as a set of ideas.

In this chapter, we turn our attention to what the chapters here contribute in terms of developing theoretical debates about the use of governmentality in health policy, particularly in relation to the development of a *critical politics of health and healthcare*. In pulling together the collection, we have been only too aware of some of the critiques that have been made about governmentality-based ideas, and the way they have been deployed to understand social policy contexts. As highlighted in Chapter 1, these include an emphasis on the creation of subjectivities at the expense of exploring the precise mechanisms (social and political relations) through which these subjectivities get produced; an inability to adequately account for the role of central government and government power; a lack of attention paid to inequality as it is linked to social difference; and a limited understanding of resistance (McKee, 2009; O'Malley, Weir and Shearing, 1997; Walters, 2012). Although it is not our intention here to respond to each of these criticisms, we use them as a jumping-off point to briefly set out how this volume might respond to O'Malley, Weir and Shearing's (1997: 514) call for governmentality to be '(re)connected with critical theorizing', and in so doing, seek to develop debates about the purpose and potential of governmentality studies for health and health policy in the future.

Governmentality: whither critical politics?

In a seminal paper published almost twenty years ago, O'Malley, Weir and Shearing (1997) set out what they perceived to be some of the limits of the governmentality literature in terms of developing social and political critique, and critical politics. As they acknowledged at that time, while governmentality was armed with the potential to represent a '"progressive" post social politics' (*ibid.*: 513), studies using the approach had often failed to develop such a critical potential. Their ideas have been echoed and developed since that time in literature which cuts across a range of social science disciplines (Barnett *et al.*, 2008; Lemke, 2007; Lippert and Stenson, 2010; Walters, 2012). In the context of political science, for example, Walters (2012: 5) suggests that governmentality has displayed a deficient understanding of politics in the sense of 'official political activity' (political parties, elections and so forth), as well as the series of events or processes in which disagreements are articulated and played out between different groups in society.

For O'Malley, Weir and Shearing (1997), part of the difficulty with governmentality is the way the concept has been interpreted, or what Walters (2012: 143) refers to as 'applicationism'. Noting that governmentality was 'designed to form a mid-range explanatory level between the history of political philosophy and an empirical study of social relations' (O'Malley, Weir and Shearing, 1997: 504), they argue that studies have favoured an understanding of politics as a more abstract, theoretical 'mentality of rule', to the neglect of wider sociological concerns with politics as social relations. Thus, politics are reduced to ideal-type visions displayed in government policy pronouncements or documents, rather than the actualities of social and political relations in processes of governing (in other words, what happens in practice). This, they argue, has led to studies which are 'insensitive to social variation and social heterogeneity' (*ibid.*: 505) and has placed limits on the extent to which contestation and resistance are understood as part of the politics of governing. Indeed, as they suggest, contestation has often only been seen as a response to a governmental programme or mentality of rule, rather than as constitutive of these mentalities and practices.

In acknowledging these points of tension, we concur with O'Malley, Weir and Shearing (1997) that they should not be a basis for dismissing governmentality as an approach with little critical potential: quite the contrary. As we have sought to show in this volume, governmentality is not an approach which offers a grand social theory. Nor does it offer a vision of the future, or 'what to struggle for or against' (Walters, 2012: 150). Rather, its strength lies in its 'diagnostic' (*ibid.*: 2) capacity, as a set of conceptual tools that can be used to investigate the processes and practicalities of governing in a range of meso-level contexts. With its focus on the mentalities of rule, and the technologies and strategies through which these mentalities are made practicable, it moves away from thinking about governance in relation to specific institutions, ideologies or binary categories such as the state and citizen. Rather, in placing an emphasis on the *how* of governing, it draws attention to the ways in which the objects of policies are products of particular problematisations and categorisations (Bacchi, 2009). These problematisations are always temporally and spatially contingent; thus as Robertson (2001: 294–295) notes in the context of health, 'particular discourses on health emerge at particular historical moments and gain widespread acceptance primarily because they are more or less congruent with the prevailing social, political and economic order within which they are produced, maintained and reproduced'. Despite some commentators recognising that the way governmentality has been applied may lead to accusations of a 'cookie-cutter' approach (not least in terms of seeing neoliberalism as a 'master category' to be used to interpret a range of different governmental strategies and programmes) (Rose, O'Malley and Valverde, 2006: 97), we would suggest that one of the potential strengths of a governmentality approach is its capacity to excavate the contingent nature of governmental (health) rationalities and programmes, or in this case, the dynamics that give rise to a specifically *Irish* approach to health and health policy.

In the sections that follow, then, we point to some of the contributions of the chapters in developing the critical potential of governmentality in the arena of health and health policy. Following O'Malley, Weir and Shearing (1997) and others, we explore this critical potential under three themes. First, we consider the chapters' engagement with politics as social relations, an act which is closely related to recognising the messy actualities of governing, and the relationships between different spaces and sites of governing. Second, we consider the place of contestation and resistance in governmentality theory and consider its relevance for health policy. Finally, we ask what the volume tells us about those more 'traditional' social policy concerns of inequality and social difference, particularly in a context where poststructuralist approaches to health have often been accused of failing to recognise structural inequalities in health. We conclude the chapter by considering some future directions for governmentality-inspired health and health policy analysis.

Politics as contingent social relations

One of the key points underpinning accusations of governmentality's limited critical potential relates to the suggestion that studies often fail to capture the messy actualities of social and political relations. For O'Malley, Weir and Shearing (1997), this relates to the seeming disjuncture between governmental visions and technologies and practices. In the context of this volume, it is indeed hard to escape the discursive strategies set down in policy and other documents. However, the contributions demonstrate how these strategies always emerge out of particular contexts, and 'are themselves internally contradictory, continually changing and capable of mutation' (McKee, 2009: 474). Edwards's chapter, for example, demonstrates the tensions and contradictions created by the new category of disability in the AoN process, and the ways in which different actors – including health professionals and parents of children with disabilities – are seeking to interpret, manage and in some cases resist such categorisations. As the chapter illustrates, the AoN has created new pressures and points of tension between different governmental agencies, and the creation of new problematisations around disability which need to be responded to, and beget further governmental programmes. Similarly, O'Donovan's analysis of proposals to change the organ donation system in Ireland provides a rich empirical investigation of 'governing in action', and the complex social relations played out in the framing of the citizens' roles and responsibilities in relation to the governance of the dead body.

The empirical investigations in the volume expose the complexities of policymaking and the roles of the multiplicity of actors in the shaping of health issues and policies in Ireland. Thus, they expose how alliances are formed, expert knowledges drawn upon, policies debated and decisions made. Moreover, they draw attention to the multitude of actors at play in defining and responding to problematisations of health, whether these be government officials and departments, the media, non-governmental organisations, or specific groups of experts, such as psychiatrists (in the case of Chambers's chapter), occupational therapists and speech therapists (in Edwards's discussion of the AoN), or social scientists charged with gathering statistical data on the (health) status of Irish children (see Share and Share's analysis of obesity). In so doing, the chapters serve to further break down the idea that government is a sole practice of the state, and reflect Foucault's (1991: 102) notion of the 'ensemble' in the analytics of government; that is, the way in which individuals and communities are targeted by an extensive 'ensemble' of heterogonous authorities and personnel, including for-profit corporations, government departments, schools, teachers and 'experts' that attempt to shape our conduct and bodies. What also becomes apparent in this context is that the boundaries between agencies within this 'ensemble' are increasingly blurred, not least in thinking about distinctions between public and private or the state and citizen. Indeed, blurring the public and private has a particular place – and distinctive meaning – in the problematisations of healthcare in Ireland, as Cliona Loughnane's analysis of UHI bears witness to.

In the messy realpolitiks of policy visions and programmes, however, some of the chapters raise questions about the extent to which the state – partly evidenced in specific government departments and actors, but also in the broader system of political parties – still maintains a key role in shaping and regulating daily lives. Cliona Loughnane's analysis demonstrates how UHI emerged out of pre-election pledges from political parties, which were subsequently shelved in the context of economic austerity; Ciara O'Dwyer's chapter similarly highlights the fickleness of party political agendas in shaping long-term care for older people. While this may be so, it is still possible to avoid seeing the state as a totalising, monolithic and homogenous entity. According to Foucault, the state should be conceptualised more as a 'transactional reality' (Foucault, as cited by Lemke, 2007: 48), that is to say, 'a dynamic ensemble of relations and syntheses that at the same time produces the institutional structure of the state and the knowledge of the state' (ibid.). The state is not an object that is always already there, or 'that exists prior to political action' (ibid.: 50) but rather is constituted in and through discourses, practices and governmental actors.

In short, we would argue that many of the chapters shed light on the contingent, complex, social and political relationships which constitute processes of governing. These empirical analyses and specificities also serve as a vehicle to question the aforementioned criticism that governmentality proposes neoliberalism as a 'master category' (Rose, O'Malley and Valverde, 2006: 97) in understanding processes of governing. While the chapters here do often foreground neoliberal principles, and make reference to a minimalist role for the Irish state, especially in the context of resourcing healthcare services, it is difficult to view neoliberalism as a single coherent programme, or a unified political ideology (Larner, 2000). As researchers, this might encourage us to think about different versions of neoliberalism; the particular version of Irish neoliberalism studied here echoes many international trajectories and practices, but also reflects some of its own specificities. Thus, Órla O'Donovan's chapter, for example, illustrates how, despite attempts to steer the policy debate about organ donation to broader communal concerns, the new bodily imperative of presumed consent in the Irish context established the family of the deceased at the centre of concerns.

As O'Donovan notes, such discourses have to be understood in relation to specifically Irish commitments to familism in social policy, a commitment which arguably stems from the Irish Constitution's premising of the family as the primary unit of society.

Governmentality, contestation and resistance

Related to the dynamics of social relations, some commentators have raised the issue of how far governmentality can provide us with the tools to adequately address issues of contestation and resistance (Death, 2010; O'Malley, Weir and Shearing, 1997). Foucault's work has often been criticised for downplaying, or under-theorising resistance and contestation (Death, 2010; Sandberg, 2006). Part of this is said to relate to his understanding of power, which rather than reflecting relations of oppressor versus oppressed, or domination versus liberation, is seen to operate in a far more all-encompassing, but necessarily intricate way, which escapes ideas of structure and agency. Others suggest that given governmentality's focus again on political rationalities, resistance is only ever understood as a response to, or failure of, governmental programmes rather than as constitutive part of these programmes. Or to use O'Malley, Weir and Shearing's (1997: 510) terms, the role of contestation 'can only be a negative one of an obstacle to rule'.

While some of these criticisms may be founded, and it would be fair to say that resistance has not occupied a significant place in governmentality studies, we would concur with Rose, O'Malley and Valverde (2006) that this may be to miss the point about the potential of governmentality. In particular, Foucault – and his theorisation of power – was never concerned with large-scale exercises of revolution, the crystallisation of resistance in a single act or 'the form of a heroic meta-subject' (Rose, O'Malley and Valverde, 2006: 100); rather, contestation is to be found in numerous micro-scale practices, whether in contests over framing different health 'problems', bringing to the fore less visible, or hidden (health) knowledges, and challenging particular norms about health and healthcare.

The chapters in this volume are replete with examples of these micro-scale resistances and contestations in diverse health arenas. In the arena of mental health, for example, Derek Chambers draws attention to the contested voices – both within and outside the domain of psychiatry – which have the potential to resist dominant biomedical articulations of mental illness. Share and Share's chapter brings to the fore the contested ways in which obesity is framed by different actors. Meanwhile, Fiona Dukelow's analysis of *Stop the Spread* also acknowledges the different stances which people can adopt in responding to governmental programmes; thus as she notes, Internet discussion fora and health advocacy groups both provided sites from which resistance to the campaign was articulated, whether in expressed scepticism of the reduction of obesity to simple waist measurements, or in their offering of other types of health knowledge to understand obesity. Such instances seem to be prime examples of what Foucault (2007: 44) sought to refer to as 'counter-conducts': 'how not to be governed *like that*, by that, in the name of those principles, with such and such an objective in mind and by means of such procedures, not like that, not for that, not by them'.

Neither are these small sites of resistance separate from the processes of governing and governmental programmes, but rather are often constitutive of them. Thus O'Donovan's chapter provides a clear example of how different and often competing voices, each drawing on different types of knowledge, build into governmental visions and approaches to organ donation. Edwards's analysis of the AoN similarly highlights the ways in which those charged with implementing the procedure do not accept it as a given, but find small-scale resistive practices designed to help them circumvent some of the challenges of the assessment process.

We would suggest then that governmentality offers the potential for an exploration of contestation as 'dispersed and shifting' (Death, 2010: 239). However, we acknowledge that this may also mean looking in different places, or examining health problematisations from different perspectival starting points, in building such an analysis. Chief among these may be a focus on the mentalities and practices of the wide range of health social movements and advocacy groups which play an influential role in shaping and governing health knowledges. What, for example, are the truth claims and knowledges around which these groups build their activism? What strategies and technologies do they use? To what extent do they challenge or indeed reinforce governmental practices? All of these questions, we would suggest, are ones which governmentality has the conceptual tools to address.

Health inequalities and social difference

Another concern raised by critics has focused on where governmentality studies take us in relation to traditional concerns with issues of equality and social inequalities in social policy studies and political sociology. O'Malley, Weir and Shearing (1997), for example, argue that the focus of governmentality studies on mentalities of rule and governmental technologies has been to the detriment of asking questions about the effects or costs of these mentalities. McKee (2009) also notes the lack of attention paid by governmentality studies to how the exercise of power is linked to social inequalities. Other authors, such as Bacchi (2009), are more positive about the contribution that governmental analyses can make to critical politics and the analysis of governmental effects. In fact, Bacchi (2009) has integrated questions about the kinds of implications (or effects) that follow from particular problematisations as part of her 'what's the problem represented to be' (WPR) approach.

We would suggest that the chapters in this volume, especially in the context of exploring the nexus between political rationalities and political subjects, help reveal potential processes of exclusion that can result from neoliberal projects which presume and promote particular types of subject positions in already highly unequal societal contexts (such as the two-tier healthcare system in Ireland), and thus help point towards the '"dark side" of liberal governance' (O'Malley, Weir, and Shearing, 1997: 514). One of the key issues raised by these contributions concerns the individualising effects of neoliberal forms of governing, which, as highlighted earlier, often tend to reduce problems such as obesity, smoking, mental health and health inequalities to individual problems, and, as some have argued, individual willpower (see for example Greco, 1993). As Wilson and Prior note in Chapter 8, public health strategies in Ireland increasingly target the individual in encouraging them to engage in health-promoting behaviours. Similarly, Fiona Dukelow's chapter starkly illustrates how the management of obesity is increasingly being placed in the hands of individuals, by vesting them with a technology designed to monitor their waist circumference. Yet there is a flip side for those who are deemed unable to take responsibility, or become constructed as irrational, or uncivilised, and who are likely to find themselves on the receiving end of more disciplinary strategies. The chapters here do not suggest that technologies of force (such as penalties and fines that were introduced in order to enforce the smoking ban in Ireland) have been entirely replaced by 'technologies of the self' (i.e. pressure to do 'the right thing'); rather, as Fernández's chapter highlights, they draw attention to the way in which the boundaries between both are often blurred. This blurring can occur, for example, by incorporating strategies, which may replace the police by 'experts' in the enforcement of policies (to de-emphasise the coercive nature of enforcement), enhancing the role of the 'community' in the implementation of policies, and discursive strategies that seek to convince rather than regulate.

Strategies aimed at responsibilising are also found to carry stigmatising subtexts, which reproduce gendered and classed stereotypes that continue to place the emphasis of responsibility for health promotion upon particular groups of people. Thus Share and Share's analysis of the contested discourses around obesity, for example, draws attention to the responsibilisation of parents, and mothers in particular, for managing their children's obesity. Meanwhile, Fernández's analysis of the smoking ban demonstrates how particular groups were stigmatised in discourses – 'women as mothers, young people as irrational and young men as dangerous' (p. 111) – with little concern for the structural constraints under which different groups of people operate.

Conclusion

Arguably, some of the critiques levied against governmentality's critical potential stem from the way in which Foucault's concepts have been deployed, rather the way in which he which spoke and wrote about governmentality himself (Rose, O'Malley and Valverde, 2006). Our discussion here has, albeit briefly, sought to suggest that governmentality as an 'analytical toolbox' (*ibid.*: 100) offers significant potential to contribute to debates about critical politics in the context of health and health policymaking, not least by demonstrating that health policy is embedded within a series of complex relationships between different agencies and bodies, amongst which there are frequent tensions in the framing of health issues. The analyses offered here also raise serious questions about the unequal consequences of health-based problematisations, whether in the context of obesity, smoking or child health and well-being, as well as about the 'costs' of governmental strategies which place their trust in neoliberal strategies of privatisation and individualisation in their various guises. If nothing else, the chapters here would seem to confirm the oft-cited assertion that government is a 'congenitally failing operation' (Rose, O'Malley and Valverde, 2006: 98), in which programmes are continually being reinvented as strategies and political agendas clash, fail and emerge reconstituted in multiple different forms.

That said, we would suggest that there is a need to attend further to ways in which the critical potential of governmentality may be developed: this may include empirical approaches which move beyond the discursive world of (health) policy and programme documents; a focus on those charged with implementing and working through governmental schemes; and as mentioned earlier, a focus on the political relations of resistance and protest as articulated through the practices of health-based activism. As O'Malley (1996) and Walters (2012) suggest, there may be a need to shift perspective or angle in applying a governmentality frame, by moving away from the usual starting points of state programmes and programmers to those sites more commonly conceptualised as the 'margins' (in O'Malley's (1996) case, for example, demonstrating how resistive practices emerging from 'indigenous governance' are incorporated within, and are constitutive of, processes of liberal government).

For Walters (2012), moreover, there is a case to be made for a more politically engaged governmentality scholarship. As he and others note, governmentality has never been an approach concerned with developing a political agenda or proposals for 'what should be', despite Foucault's own role as a public intellectual, and his engagement with social movements; rather, the emphasis has been on opening up, and exploring, the complexity of (social) problems. It is, however, this tradition of critique through problematising – and particularly by problematising *historically* – that offers the potential, Walters (2012) argues, for governmentality's political contribution. As Kevin Ryan's chapter so eloquently demonstrates, governmental agendas do not appear out of nowhere, but find their echoes and continuities in different ages; nor are political discourses and logics which may appear self-evident or common sense anything other than traceable to historical, economic and political contexts. In the end, by thinking of 'history as a vast repository of techniques of governance, an immense archive storing humanity's experiences of rule and self-rule' (Walters, 2012: 149), and viewing the present with reference to the past, governmentality scholars may have the potential to question and offer up alternative ways of thinking about the problematisation of health and critical health policy trajectories.

References

Bacchi, C. (2009) *Analysing Policy: What's the Problem Represented to Be?* Adelaide, Pearson.
Barnett, C., Clarke, N., Cloke, P. and Malpass, A. (2008) The elusive subjects of neo-liberalism. *Cultural Studies*, 22(5): 624–653.
Burke, S. (2009) *Irish Apartheid: Healthcare Inequality in Ireland*. Dublin, New Island.
Death, C. (2010) Counter-conducts: a Foucauldian analytics of protest. *Social Movement Studies*, 9(3): 235–251.
Foucault, M. (1991) Governmentality. IN: Burchell, G., Gordon, C. and Miller, P. (eds) *The Foucault Effect: Studies in Governmentality*. Chicago, University of Chicago Press: pp. 87–104.
Foucault, M. (2007) What is critique? IN: Foucault, M., *The Politics of Truth*, ed. Lotringer, S., trans. Hochroth, L. and Porter, C. Los Angeles, Semiotext(e): pp. 41–81.
Greco, M. (1993) Psychosomatic subjects and the 'duty to be well': personal agency within. *Economy and Society*, 22(3): 357–372.
Larner, W. (2000) Neo-liberalism: policy, ideology, governmentality. *Studies in Political Economy*, 63(Autumn): 5–25.
Lemke, T. (2007) An indigestible meal? Foucault, governmentality and state theory. *Distinktion: Journal of Social Theory*, 8(2): 43–64.
Lippert, R. and Stenson, K. (2010) Advancing governmentality studies: lessons from social constructionism. *Theoretical Criminology*, 14(4): 473–494.
McKee, K. (2009) Post-Foucauldian governmentality: what does it offer critical social policy analysis? *Critical Social Policy*, 29(3): 465–486.
O'Malley, P. (1996) Indigenous governance. *Economy and Society*, 25(3): 310–326.
O'Malley, P., Weir, L. and Shearing, C. (1997) Governmentality, criticism, politics. *Economy and Society*, 26(4): 501–517.
Osborne, T. (1997) Of health and statecraft. IN: Petersen, A. and Bunton, R. (eds) *Foucault, Health and Medicine*. London and New York, Routledge: pp. 173–188.

Robertson, A. (2001) Biotechnology, political rationality and discourses on health risk. *Health: An Interdisciplinary Journal for the Social Study of Health, Illness and Medicine*, 5(3): 293–309.

Rose, N., O'Malley, P. and Valverde, M. (2006) Governmentality. *Annual Review of Law and Social Science*, 2: 83–104.

Sandberg, S. (2006) Fighting neo-liberalism with neo-liberal discourse: ATTAC Norway, Foucault and collective action framing. *Social Movement Studies*, 5: 3: 209–227.

Walters, W. (2012) *Governmentality: Critical Encounters*. London, Routledge.

Index

active citizen(s) 120, 195, 208
advanced neoliberal government 2,
    222
advocacy groups 11, 59, 91, 144, 145,
    153, 241, 252, 253
Agamben, Giorgio 25, 27, 28
ageing Chapter 11 *passim*
Amnesty International Ireland 133, 186
anthropological machine 29
    see also Agamben, Giorgio
anthropometry 81
anti-tobacco movement 99
ASH Ireland 101, 107
Assessment of Need Chapter 10
    passim
asylums 76, 121, 208
audit 10, 166, 168, 169, 195
austerity 4, 12, 13, 138, 148, 149,
    155, 165, 166, 168, 188, 242–243
autism 205, 209, 216, 217, 220, 222
A Vision for Change 16, Chapter 6
    passim

bioethics 137, 142, 149, 157
biological citizenship 141, 143, 155
biopedagogy 73, 75, 80
biopower 3, 5, 6, 50, 51, 74, 75, 76,
    77, 79, 80, 81, 85, 89, 91
    see also Foucault, Michel
BMI *see* Body Mass Index
body
    the cadaveric 139, 144
    the civilised 99
    collective 107, 108, 141

the dead 16, 137, 139, 14, 143,
    149–153, 156, 250
the fat 82, 83
the healthy 15, 72, 73, 82, 84, 85,
    86, 87, 89
the individual 5, 9, 13, 141, 222
    as property 141, 142
size 63, 66, 72, 73, 82–88 *passim*
the social 5, 9, 13, 32, 79
Body Mass Index 6, 15, 47, 48, 50,
    51, 62, 73, 83
Bracken, Pat 122
Bronfenbrenner, Urie 56, 60

calculating selves 10, 205, 217, 219
cancer 10, 11, 49, 73, 82, 83, 90, 99,
    101, 103, 104, 109, 138, 154,
    162, 165, 233
care management 235, 243
Carpenter, Mary 30, 31, 32
Catholic Church 12, 30
Celtic Tiger 13, 212, 239
Chief Bioethics Offer 150–154 *passim*
Chief Medical Officer 104
childhood 14–15, Chapter 2 *passim*
    conceptions of 25–27, 29, 41, 64–66
    and *Healthy Ireland* 37, 38
    as 'national asset' 30, 35, 37
    obesity Chapter 3 *passim*
Childhood Obesity Surveillance
    Initiative 54, 64
Children Act (1908) 33, 35
citizens as consumers 2, 140, 163,
    165, 168, 170, 174

class 9, 30, 32, 167, 185, 191
classification 50, 203, 204, 208, 214, 216, 217, 222
cognitive behavioural therapy 120, 128
commons 140, 143, 151, 156
community 4, 60, 101, 120, 125, 126, 128, 129, 174, 182, 196, 197, 198, 209, 254
 -based services 122, 130, 172, 230, 232, 239, 241
 development 171
 policy 66
 rating 185, 190, 197
Community Mental Health Team 129
competition *see* managed competition; Universal Health Insurance-by Competition
Constitution (Irish) 152, 252
contagion 52, 84, 104, 105, 110
counter-conducts 17, 121, 131, 149, 156, 253
criminal 30, 31, 32, 35
Critical Voices Network Ireland 122, 123
Cruikshank, Barbara 227, 233
culture 84, 96, 108, 123, 128, 192

Dean, Mitchell
 analytics of government 26, 205, 235, 250
 fields of visibility 16, 121, 124, 184
 identity formation 119, 121, 212
 regimes of practices 119, 121, 134
 technologies of citizenship 227, 231, 233
 understandings of government 1, 4, 6, 7, 121, 134, 138, 184, 191, 204, 208
delinquency 26, 30, 31, 32, 34
depression 119, 120, 133
diabetes 49, 52, 73, 82, 83, 146, 147, 155, 162, 241
diagnosis 51, 82, 129, 213–216, 220, 221, 242
Disability Act 2005 Chapter 10 *passim*
disciplinary power 55, 75, 76, 80, 86
 see also Foucault, Michel

discipline
 and bodies 9, 11, 14, 29, 77, 78, 173
discourse
 analysis 100, 228
 biomedical 73, 117, 122
 health promotion 110, 112
 public health 98, 99, 110
 truth 80, 84, 85, 91
disease
 cardiovascular 73, 82, 150, 162, 165
 categories 3, 5, 214
 chronic 168
 classification 216, 230
 conceptualisation 3, 73
 epidemics 11, 52, 84, 206
 indicators 34, 50, 73, 83, 84, 85
 infectious 105
 kidney 146, 155
 medical register 31, 54
 organ 143, 155
 risk factors 82, 83, 84, 84
docile bodies 78, 227, 231, 239

education
 and children 29, 33, 34, 132
 and obesity 55, 62, 63
 and organ donation 149
 reformatory 26, 30–32, 40, 41
 and sexual health 9
 and tobacco control 98
education system
 and disability 203, 209, 210, 212, 214, 216
 and mental health 119, 124, 135
emigration 148, 165
employability 38, 207
empowerment 162, 195, 227, 234
enterprise society 37
entrepreneur of the self 89, 140, 192
EU *see* European Union
eugenics 33, 81
EU-IMF *see* European Union-International Monetary Fund
Europe 5, 107, 109, 145, 146, 149, 152, 168, 188, 189, 198, 230, 233, 243

European Central Bank 148, 149
European Convention on Human
    Rights 152
European Union 162, 165, 167, 176
European Union Health
    Commissioner 107
European Union-International
    Monetary Fund 13
expert knowledge 3, 98, 101, 214,
    221, 250

FairCare 187
familism 152, 156, 252
fields of visibility 121, 124, 184
    see also Dean, Mitchell
financial management 10, 132, 196,
    207
Fine Gael 183, 187, 191, 198, 231
Fine Gael / Labour 137, 182, 185,
    188, 239, 240, 241, 242
Fitzgerald, Frances 36, 55, 65
Foucault, Michel
    art of government 6, 77, 97, 226,
        227
    clinical gaze 49, 73, 86
    concepts of power 3, 4–8, 14, 25,
        29, 32, 36, 37, 40, 72, 73,
        75–79, 85, 96, 97, 118, 131,
        138–140, 162, 173, 190, 191,
        195, 206, 226, 227, 250, 252,
        253, 255
    'conduct of conduct' 1, 6, 16, 78,
        85, 96, 97, 138

game of differentiation 37
game of inequality 26, 36, 37, 40, 41
genealogy 5, 27, 141
    lectures on governmentality 6, 74,
        77, 119, 206
    power/knowledge 4, 8, 50
    and subjectification 27, 78, 80, 140
gender 48, 50, 254
General Medical Service 62
General Practitioners 12, 130, 172
governing at a distance 18, 161, 164,
    169, 170, 189, 208
GPs see General Practitioners
Growing Up in Ireland 15, 39, 46, 55,
    60, 65

GUI see Growing Up in Ireland

Hacking, Ian 3, 50, 76, 80, 81, 204,
    207, 216
Harney, Mary 231
HCCI see Home Care and Community
    Care Ireland
Health Behaviours in School-Aged
    Children 39, 40, 168
health inequalities 17, 26, 35, 36, 176,
    247, 253, 254
Health Information and Quality
    Authority 12, 18, 211, 214, 234,
    239
health insurance 12, 13, 18, 98,
    182–188, 192–194, 196–198
Health Service Executive 12, 13, 59,
    122, 127, 129, 132, 148, 204,
    209, 211–218 passim, 237–239,
    240, 242
Healthy Ireland 17, 26, 36, 37, 38,
    118, 123, 125, 164, 168, 169,
    170, 175, 176, 178, 195
HIQA see Health Information and
    Quality Authority
Home Care and Community Care
    Ireland 237
homo economicus 79, 139, 140, 142,
    151
HSE see Health Service Executive

identity formation 119, 121, 212
    see also Dean, Mitchell
individualisation 161, 255
International Monetary Fund 148,
    149
internet 91, 252
Irish Cancer Society 103, 104
Irish Kidney Association 147
Irish Medical Organisation 186
Irish Taskforce on Obesity 54, 55, 56

Joint Committee on Health and
    Children 16, 137, 144, 156

kidney transplant 146, 147, 148, 154,
    155

life expectancy 76, 165–8

Lupton, Deborah 5, 6, 8, 9, 49, 63,
    64, 98, 99

managed competition 182, 186, 187,
    188, 191
marketing
  digital 86
  social 48, 63, 64, 78, 79, 85, 100,
      104, 105, 110
  techniques 80, 85, 86
markets 37, 187, 193, 227
  quasi- 192
Martin, Micheál 101–109 *passim*
McKee, Kim 7, 11, 91, 92, 222, 229,
    253
media 6, 11, 15, 46–49 *passim*, 55,
    59, 63–66, 91, 106, 109, 127,
    133, 171, 188, 212, 216, 219,
    250
medical
  care 182
  categories 8, 53, 87
  discourses 15, 16, 47, 59, 107, 110,
      118, 129, 133, 134, 150, 214
  inspection 26, 34, 35, 40
  institutions 66, 101
  interventions 6, 9, 11, 12, 52, 62,
      64, 143, 144, 146, 147, 151,
      155
  knowledge 8, 26, 30, 52, 76, 119,
      122, 214
  norms 15, 25, 30, 35, 76, 77, 78,
      130, 150, 196, 233
  professionals 8, 11, 15, 48, 49, 59,
      65, 106, 118, 122, 129, 134,
      144, 146, 154
  screening 9
  system 155
Medical Card 12, 185
mental health 1, 9, 16, Chapter 6
    passim, 168, 178, 209, 219, 220,
    252
Mental Health Act (2001) 122, 130
Miller, Peter 4, 7, 10, 13, 18, 37, 79,
    98, 183, 189, 192–196, 205–208,
    212, 219
  see also Rose, Nicholas
mixed economy of healthcare 12, 163
modernity 25, 27

moral
  decline 26
  health 31
  hospital 31
  management 32
morality and children 14, 34
motherhood 9, 105
mothers 15, 48, 52, 60, 66, 104, 105,
    111, 254

National Children's Strategy 38–39
National Disability Authority
    Chapter 10 *passim*
NDA *see* National Disability Authority
neoliberalism 6, 36–37, 74–75, 79,
    162–163
  see also advanced liberal government
neuroscience 130, 132, 133
New Right 6
  see also neoliberalism
NHSS *see* Nursing Home Support
    Scheme
normalisation 34–35, 65–66, 81
nudge-based policy 86, 89, 173, 177
nursing homes 236–237, 240
Nursing Home Support Scheme 232,
    235, 236, 237, 240, 241

obesity 1, 6, 9, 15, 146, 162, 173,
    250, 252–253, 254
  and children Chapter 3 *passim*
  'epidemic' 15, 47, 48, 51, 58, 59,
      66, 173
  prevalence of 51, 53, 54, 56–58
  and conflation with overweight 49,
      51–52, 61
  measurement of 48–49, 50–51,
      81–83
  see also Body Mass Index
  schools 55, 62–63
  see also overweight
OECD *see* Organisation for Economic
    Co-operation and Development
older people 18, 50, Chapter 11
    passim
O'Malley, Pat 3, 10, 99, 161, 204,
    248–255 *passim*
O'Malley, Tim 124
Operation Transformation 51, 66

organ
    donation 50, 251
    retention scandal 138
    scarcity 124
    transplantation 137, 152, 157
Organisation for Economic
        Co-operation and
        Development 53, 168, 230
overweight Chapter 4 *passim*, 46
    conflation with obesity 49, 51
    measurement of 51, 72, 77, 81, 83
    prevalence amongst Irish
        children 53, 54, 55, 56, 57
    see also obesity

parenting 35, 48
parents 15, 30, 35, 46, 60, 62–66
        passim, 138, 208, 210, 212, 214,
        215, 216–217, 220, 250, 254
    see also mothers
partnership 36, 56, 133, 149, 170,
        171, 177, 209, 211
pastoral power 90
    see also Foucault, Michel
paternalism 15, 162
patient(s)
    categories of 13, 185, 194
    as citizens 1, 137, 148, 172, 185
    as consumers 2, 163, 165, 166,
        191, 192, 193, 195, 196, 199,
        238
    as experts 162
    and mental health 130, 131
    moral 31
    and obesity 62, 83
    and organ transplantation 146–149,
        154, 155, 157
    rational 98
    satisfaction surveys 98, 166
patients' organisations 11, 143, 191
    see also advocacy groups
people with disabilities 10, Chapter 10
        passim
performance indicators 10, 166, 241
Phillips, Anne 139, 141, 151, 156
population(s)
    ageing 230, 242
    and biopower 55, 76–77, 80, 85, 222

as governable entities 204, 206, 207,
        212
    health of 5, 6, 14, 81, 83, 92, 161,
        166, 169, 171, 175
    management of 1, 3, 31, 204, 227,
        229
    and mental health 124, 125, 126,
        134
    and obesity 88, 89
        childhood 51
    and organ donation 146, 148
    and private health insurance 12–13,
        18, 182, 184, 185, 197
    targeted 208
poverty 37, 38, 66, 119, 148, 206
pregnancy 9, 38, 105
presumed consent 16, Chapter 7
        passim, 251
primary care 12, 126, 129, 130, 168,
        192
privatisation 2, 13, 37, 163, 184, 192,
        199, 229, 255
problematisations 11, 14, 184, 206,
        222, 249, 250, 253, 254, 255
programmes of government 121, 206,
        207, 212
psychiatry 3, 16, 117, 121–123,
        130–131, 252
psychotropic medication 122, 123
public health
    campaigns 48, 50, 83, 127
    discourses 98, 99 110
    Foucauldian approaches to 6, 8, 9
    policy 15, 17, 97, 98, 164, 177
    strategies 14, 17, 25, 55, 118,
        254
    system in Ireland 13, 30, 130, 190,
        196, 198, 212
public hygiene 26, 30, 33, 40

quality
    of healthcare services 165, 166, 167,
        170, 184, 186, 187, 190, 193,
        195, 196, 199, 230, 234, 235,
        239, 241
    of life 35, 144, 227
Quality and Fairness 17, 164, 167,
        170, 173, 176

rationalities 2, 7, 8, 16, 17, 18, 117, 121, 124, 140, 144, 148, 164, 173, 184, 189, 204, 207, 206, 222, 249, 252, 254
rationality of government 6, 7, 97, 98
recovery (in mental health) 118, 123, 129
regimes
  of practices 119, 121, 134
  of truth 119, 173
  see also Dean, Mitchell
Reilly, James 36, 65, 183
resistance 2, 14, 17, 19, 72, 82, 91, 92, 111, 131, 176, 239, 248, 249
  see also counter-conducts
responsibilisation 64, 66, 166, 254
risk
  biomedicine and 73, 82
  citizens at 1–2, 10, 48, 52, 61, 87, 99
  equalisation 174
  factors 63, 73, 83, 161, 162, 175
  governmental strategies of 9–10, 11, 15, 64, 65, 66, 77, 141, 171, 208
  management of 18, 99, 169, 170, 171, 177, 184, 191, 193, 196, 210
Rose, Nikolas 4, 6, 18, 34, 35, 74, 80, 98, 161, 183, 189, 206
  see also Miller, Peter
Rousseau, Jean Jacques 14, 25–29, 31, 32, 33, 34, 38, 41

Safefood 59, 64, 65, 84, 86, 87, 90, 91, 92
self-help 174
self-surveillance 65, 66, 219
Shaping a Healthier Future 17, 164, 165, 167, 169, 172, 176
smoking 14, 16, 38, Chapter 5 passim
  ban Chapter 5 passim
  passive 101, 103, 104, 105
social difference 248, 253, 259
sociology of health and illness 8, 11
solidarity 18, 154, 169, 171, 172, 185, 188, 193, 194, 197–199

somatic individuality 74, 75, 89
sovereign power 5, 28, 29, 75–77, 176
special educational needs 208, 212
statistics 5, 31, 65, 103, 204, 205, 212, 215, 218, 219–222 passim, 228
  see also classification
stigmatisation 61, 62, 154
Stop the Spread 15, Chapter 4 passim
STS see Stop the Spread
subjectification 75, 78, 80, 88, 89, 90, 98, 139, 140, 157
subjectivities 3–10 passim, 17, 48, 90, 91, 117, 121, 131, 139, 172, 176, 205, 212, 215, 221, 227, 229, 247
subsidiarity 4, 12, 217
suicide prevention 16, 123–124, 126–127, 135
surveillance 9, 35, 38, 39, 40, 49, 55, 66, 76, 87, 97, 168, 176, 208, 215, 221

taxation 182, 185, 186, 195
tax breaks 18, 185
taxpayer 232, 237
technologies of government 2, 3, 7, 10, 110, 139, 184, 189, 163, 206, 207–208, 222
  of citizenship 231, 233
  of domination 97
  and performance 207–208
  of power 140, 97
  of the self 7, 97, 99, 173, 175, 227, 254
  of subjectification 137, 139
Together for Health 162
two-tier health system 2, 13, 18, 182, 187, 189, 197, 199, 212, 254

UHI see Universal Health Insurance
UHI-C see Universal Health Insurance by Competition
UN Convention of the Rights of the Child 35
Universal Health Insurance 182, 183, 188, 198

Universal Health Insurance by
    Competition 182, Chapter 9
    passim

Varadkar, Leo 183
VHI *see* Voluntary Health Insurance
Vintners Federation of Ireland 106
Voluntary Health Insurance 182, 185

welfare state 6, 170, 177, 194
    dismantling of 141, 237
    and Ireland 12

wellbeing 38, 56, 120, 123, 125, 171,
    172, 175, 178
WHO *see* World Health Organization
Whole Child approach 38, 39, 41
whole system approach 36, 38
World Health Organisation 47, 60, 83,
    108, 162, 173, 178